Treatment strategy in Hodgkin's disease

Stratégie thérapeutique dans la maladie de Hodgkin

Colloques INSERM
ISSN 0768-3154

Other *Colloques* published as co-editions by John Libbey Eurotext and INSERM

133 Cardiovascular and Respiratory Physiology in the Fetus and Neonate. *Physiologie Cardiovasculaire et Respiratoire du Fœtus et du Nouveau-né.*
Scientific Committee : P. Karlberg,
A. Minkowski, W. Oh and L. Stern;
Managing Editor : M. Monset-Couchard.
ISBN : John Libbey Eurotext 0 86196 125 0
INSERM 2 85598 340 1

134 Porphyrins and Porphyrias. *Porphyrines et Porphyries.*
Edited by Y. Nordmann.
ISBN : John Libbey Eurotext 0 86196 087 4
INSERM 2 85598 281 2

137 Neo-Adjuvant Chemotherapy. *Chimiothérapie Néo-Adjuvante.*
Edited by C. Jacquillat, M. Weil and D. Khayat.
ISBN : John Libbey Eurotext 0 86196 125 0
INSERM 2 85598 340 1

139 Hormones and Cell Regulation (10th European Symposium). *Hormones et Régulation Cellulaire (10ᵉ Symposium Européen).*
Edited by J. Nunez, J.E. Dumont and R.J.B. King.
ISBN : John Libbey Eurotext 0 86196 125 0X
INSERM 2 85598 340 1

147 Modern Trends in Aging Research. *Nouvelles Perspectives de la Recherche sur le Vieillissement.*
Edited by Y. Courtois, B. Faucheux, B. Forette,
D.L. Knook and J.A. Tréton.
ISBN : John Libbey Eurotext 0 86196 126 0X
INSERM 2 85598 340 1

149 Binding Proteins of Steroid Hormones. *Protéines de liaison des Hormones Stéroïdes.*
Edited by M.G. Forest and M. Pugeat.
ISBN : John Libbey Eurotext 0 86196 125 0
INSERM 2 85598 340 1X

151 Control and Management of Parturition. *La Maîtrise de la Parturition.*
Edited by C. Sureau, P. Blot, D. Cabrol, F. Cavaillé and G. Germain.
ISBN : John Libbey Eurotext 0 86196 125 0
INSERM 2 85598 340 1

Suite page 427

TREATMENT STRATEGY IN HODGKIN'S DISEASE

STRATEGIE THERAPEUTIQUE DANS LA MALADIE DE HODGKIN

Proceedings of the Paris International Workshop and Symposium
held on June 28-30, 1989

*Compte rendu de la Réunion Internationale et du Symposium tenus à Paris
les 28-30 juin 1989*

Satellite meetings of the 17th International Congress of Radiology/Radiation Oncology
Réunions satellites du 17ème Congrès International de Radiologie/Radiothérapie

Sponsored by / *Avec le parrainage de*

Monsieur Hubert Curien, Ministre de la Recherche et de la Technologie
Monsieur Jacques Chirac, Maire de la ville de Paris
Monsieur Pierre Laffitte, Sénateur des Alpes Maritimes

Institut National de la Santé et de la Recherche Médicale (INSERM)
"Europe Against Cancer" campaign of the European Economic Community
Ligue Nationale Contre le Cancer, Comité de Paris

Edited by

R. Somers
M. Henry-Amar
J.H. Meerwaldt
P. Carde

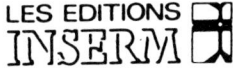

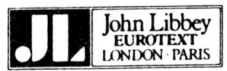

British Library Cataloguing in Publication Data
Treatment strategy in Hodgkin's disease.
1. Man. Hodgkin's disease
I. Institut national de la santé et de la recherche médicale
616.99446

ISBN 0 86196-226 5
ISSN 0768-3154

First published in 1990 by

Editions John Libbey Eurotext
6 rue Blanche, 92120 Montrouge, France. (1) 47 35 85 52
ISBN 0 86196 226 5

John Libbey & Company Ltd
13 Smiths Yard, Summerley Street, London SW18 4HR, England.
(1) 947 27 77

Institut National de la Santé et de la Recherche Médicale
101 rue de Tolbiac, 75654 Paris Cedex 13, France.
(1) 45 84 14 41
ISBN 2 85598 398 3

ISSN 0768-3154

© 1990 Colloques INSERM/John Libbey Eurotext Ltd,
All rights reserved
Unauthorised publication contravenes applicable laws

CONTENTS
SOMMAIRE

XI   Acknowledgements
Remerciements

XIII List of participants
Liste des participants

XIX INTRODUCTION
INTRODUCTION

Pr R. Flamant, Dr R. Somers, Pr M. Tubiana

PATHOLOGY AND CELL BIOLOGY OF HODGKIN'S DISEASE
HISTOPATHOLOGIE ET BIOLOGIE CELLULAIRE DE LA MALADIE DE HODGKIN

3   C. Kalle, V. Diehl, M. Jücker, H. Tesch, C. Fonatsch, M. Pfreundschuh and M. Schaadt
New developments in the pathogenesis of Hodgkin's disease
Nouvelles données dans la pathogénèse de la maladie de Hodgkin

17   **K.A. MacLennan, M.H. Bennett, J. Bosq, J. Diebold, A.M. Mandard, B. Vaughan Hudson and G. Vaughan Hudson**
The histology and immunohistology of Hodgkin's disease : its relationship to prognosis and clinical behaviour
Histologie et immuno-histologie de la maladie de Hodgkin : relations avec le pronostic et l'évolution clinique

PROCEEDINGS OF THE WORKSHOP ON TREATMENT STRATEGY IN HODGKIN'S DISEASE
COMPTE RENDU DE LA REUNION DE TRAVAIL SUR LA STRATEGIE THERAPEUTIQUE DANS LA MALADIE DE HODGKIN

29   **W. Gregory and M. Löffler**
Introduction
Introduction

♦ Early Stage Hodgkin's Disease
Maladie de Hodgkin : stades localisés

37   **J.H. Meerwaldt, M. van Glabbeke and B. Vaughan-Hudson**
Prognostic factors for stage I and II Hodgkin's disease
Facteurs pronostiques dans les stades I et II de la maladie de Hodgkin

51   **R.T. Hoppe**
Hodgkin's disease treatment strategy, stage I-II
Stratégie thérapeutique dans la maladie de Hodgkin, stades I-II

63   **J.M. Cosset, J. Thomas, and E.M. Noordijk**
The current EORTC strategy for stage I-II Hodgkin's disease
Stratégie actuelle de l'OERTC dans les stades I-II de la maladie de Hodgkin

67   **B. Hoerni**
Hodgkin's disease treatment strategy, stage I-II
Stratégie thérapeutique dans la maladie de Hodgkin, stades I-II

69   **F.B. Hagemeister and L.M. Fuller**
Treatment of patients with clinically-staged I and II Hodgkin's disease
Traitement des malades de stade clinique I-II de la maladie de Hodgkin

73 **A. Horwitch**
Approaches to treatment of early Hodgkin's disease at the Royal Marsden Hospital
Approche thérapeutique des stades localisés de la maladie de Hodgkin au Royal Marsden Hospital

77 **S. Pavlovsky**
Hodgkin's disease treatment strategy in stage I-II according to socio-economic status and therapeutic ressources
Stratégie thérapeutique dans les stades I-II de la maladie de Hodgkin en fonction des conditions socio-économiques locales et des moyens thérapeutiques disponibles

81 **L. Specht and N.I. Nissen**
Treatment strategy in Hodgkin's disease stages I-II : The Finsen Institute approach
Stratégie thérapeutique dans les stades I-II de la maladie de Hodgkin : La politique du Finsen Institute

83 **B. Vaughan Hudson**
Hodgkin's disease treatment strategy - stage I-II
Stratégie thérapeutique dans la maladie de Hodgkin - stades I-II

♦ **Advanced Stage Hodgkin's Disease**
Maladie de Hodgkin : stades disséminés

89 **M. Löffler, D.O. Dixon and R. Swindell**
Prognostic factors for stage III and IV Hodgkin's disease
Facteurs pronostiques dans les stades III et IV de la maladie de Hodgkin

105 **P. Carde, D.E. Bergsagel, N.I. Nissen and A. Hagenbeek**
The treatment of advanced Hodgkin's disease : strategy
Le traitement des stades disséminés de la maladie de Hodgkin : stratégie

119 **J.M.V. Burgers**
Management of progression/relapse in clinical stages III-IV of Hodgkin's disease : classical radio-chemotherapy?
Traitement des échecs et des rechutes dans les stades cliniques III-IV de la maladie de Hodgkin : place de l'association radio-chimiothérapie?

129 **J.O. Armitage**
The place of bone marrow transplantation in the treatment of patients with Hodgkin's disease
Place de la greffe de moelle osseuse dans le traitement des malades atteints d'une maladie de Hodgkin

LONG TERM SURVIVAL AND SIDE-EFFECTS OF TREATMENT
SURVIE A LONG TERME ET MORBIDITE THERAPEUTIQUE

139 **J. Kaldor and C. Lasset**
Second malignancies following Hodgkin's disease
Deuxièmes cancers après maladie de Hodgkin

151 **M. Henry-Amar and R. Somers**
Long term survival in early stages Hodgkin's disease: the EORTC experience
Survie à long terme dans les stades localisés de la maladie de Hodgkin : l'expérience de l'OERTC

WORKSHOP STATISTICAL REPORT
RAPPORT STATISTIQUE

169 **M. Henry-Amar, in collaboration with D.M. Aeppli, J. Anderson, S. Ashley, F. Bonichon, R.S. Cox, S.J. Dahlberg, G. DeBoer, D.O. Dixon, P.G. Gobbi, W. Gregory, D. Hasenclever, M. Löffler, V. Pompe Kirn, M.T. Santarelli, L. Specht, R. Swindell, B. Vaughan Hudson**

171 **Introduction and statistical considerations (Part I)**
Introduction et considérations statistiques (1ère partie)

177 **Pretreatment patient characteristics. Description by clinical and pathological stage (Part II)**
Caractéristiques pré-cliniques. Description en fonction du stade clinique et du stade pathologique (2ème partie)

191 **Initial treatment types. Description by clinical stage (Part III)**
Traitements initiaux. Description en fonction du stade clinique (3ème partie)

203	**Relationship between pretreatment clinical and biological parameters (Part IV)**
	Liaisons statistiques des caractéristiques cliniques et biologiques initiales entre elles (4ème partie)
217	**Prognostic study of laparotomy findings by clinical stage (Part V)**
	Analyse pronostique des résultats de la laparotomie exploratrice en fonction du stade clinique (5ème partie)
233	**Response to initial therapy. Description by clinical and pathological stage (Part VI)**
	Efficacité du traitement initial. Description en fonction du stade clinique et du stade pathologique (6ème partie)
265	**Prognostic study of relapse-free survival by clinical stage (Part VII)**
	Analyse pronostique de la durée de survie sans rechute en fonction du stade clinique (7ème partie)
311	**Prognostic study of overall survival by clinical stage (Part VIII)**
	Analyse pronostique de la survie globale en fonction du stade clinique (8ème partie)
355	**Study of second cancer risk (Part IX)**
	Risque de développement d'un deuxième cancer. Analyse pronostique (9ème partie)
381	**Long term survival and study of causes of death (Part X)**
	Survie à long terme et analyse des causes de décès (10ème partie)
419	**References**
	Bibliographie
423	**Glossary of the chemotherapy regimens used**
	Glossaire: description des chimiothérapies utilisées

AKNOWLEDGMENTS

REMERCIEMENTS

The Organizing Committee gratefully acknowledges the support of the following organisations :

Sponsors :

Institut National de la Santé et de la Recherche Médicale (INSERM)
"Europe Against Cancer" campaign of the European Economic Community
Ligue Nationale Contre le Cancer, Comité de Paris

Benefactors :

Banque Nationale de Paris
Fondation Suzanne Axel
Het Nederlands Kanker Instituut, Amsterdam
Laboratoire Beaufour
Laboratoire Bristol
Laboratoire Farmitalia-Carlo-Ebra
Laboratoire Glaxo
Laboratoire Lilly-France
Laboratoire Pierre-Fabre Oncologie
Laboratoire Rhône-Poulenc Santé
Laboratoire Roger Bellon
Laboratoire Roussel-Uclaf
Laboratoire Sandoz
Société AB Microconseil
Société AIR FRANCE
Société CGR-MeV
Société Kodack-Pathé
Société SAAS

L'organisation de ces réunions n'aurait pas été possible sans le concours de l'Institut Gustave Roussy. Nous souhaitons remercier tout particulièrement le Service Dactylographie, le Service de Reprographie, et le Service d'Iconographie, dont l'aide nous a été précieuse. Enfin, nos remerciements vont tout naturellement à Sylviane Iacobelli et Armelle Leszczynski-Kramar, qui ont assuré l'ensemble du secrétariat et de l'organisation pratique de ces journées, ainsi que Nathalie Ravinet, qui a assuré l'accueil des participants.

Organizing Committee
Comité d'organisation

P. Carde (France)
J-M. Cosset (France)
M. Hayat (France)
M. Henry-Amar, secretary (France)
J. Thomas (Belgium)
J.H. Meerwaldt (The Netherlands)
R. Somers, chairman (The Netherlands)

List and address of participants to the Workshop
Liste et adresse des participants à la réunion de travail

Aeppli D.M., Dpt of Therapeutic Radiology-Radiation Oncology, University of Minnesota Hospital and Clinic, Harvard Street at East River Road, Minneapolis, MN 55455, USA.

Anderson J., Department of Biostatistics, Harvard School of Public Health, 677 Huntington Avenue, Boston, MA 02115, USA.

Armitage J.O., Department of Internal Medicine, University of Nebraska Medical Center, 42nd and Dewey Avenue, Omaha, NE 68105-1065, USA.

Ashley S., Computer Department, The Royal Marsden Hospital, Downs road, Sutton, Surrey SM2 5PT, England.

Bergsagel D.E., Department of Medicine, The Princess Margaret Hospital, 500 Sherbourne Street, Toronto, Canada M4X 1K9.

Bloomfield C., Department of Therapeutic Radiology-Radiation Oncology, University of Minnesota Hospital and Clinic, Harvard Street at East River Road, Minneapolis, MN 55455, USA.

Bonichon F., Fondation Bergonié, 180 rue Saint-Genès, 33076 Bordeaux Cedex, France.

Bosq J., Anatomie Pathologie D, Institut Gustave-Roussy, 39-53 Rue Camille Desmoulins, 94805 Villejuif Cedex, France.

Bron D., Institut Jules Bordet, 1 Rue Héger Bordet, 1000 Brussels, Belgium.

Buerki K., University Bern, Institute of Pathology, Freiburgstraat 30, 3010 Bern, Switzerland.

Burgers J.M.V., Department of Radiotherapy, The Netherlands Cancer Institute, Antoni van Leeuwenhoek Huis, Plesmalaan 121, 1066 CX Amsterdam, The Netherlands.

Carde P., Unité Suzanne Axel, Institut Gustave-Roussy, 39-53 Rue Camille Desmoulins, 94805 Villejuif Cedex, France.

Chenal C., Département de Radiothérapie, Centre Eugène Marquis, Pontchaillou, 35033 Rennes Cedex, France.

Coleman C.N., Joint Center for Radiation Therapy, 50 Binney Street, Boston, MA 02115, USA.

Coltman C.A., Department of Clinical Medical Oncology, The University of Texas Health Sciences Center, 7703 Floyd Curl Drive, San Antonio, TX 78284-7884, USA.

Cosset J.M., Département des Radiations, Institut Gustave-Roussy, 39-53 Rue Camille Desmoulins, 94805 Villejuif Cedex, France.

Cox R.S., Department of Therapeutic Radiology-Radiation Therapy, Stanford University Medical Center, Stanford, CA 94305, USA.

Crowther D., Department of Medical Oncology, Christie Hospital and Holt Radium Institute, Wilmslow Road, Manchester M20 9BX, England.

Dahlberg S.J., SWOG Statistical Center, Fred Hutchinson Cancer Research Center, 1124 Columbia Street, Seattle, WA 98104-2092, USA.

DeBoer G., Biostatistics Department, The Princess Margaret Hospital, 500 Sherbourne Street, Toronto, Canada M4X 1K9.

Diehl V., Medizinische Universitätsklinik 1, Haus 16, Joseph-Stelzmann-Strasse 9, 5000 Köln 41, Federal Republic of Germany.

Dixon D.O., Department of Biomathematics, The University of Texas M.D. Anderson Cancer Center, 1515 Holcombe Boulevard, Houston, TX 77030, USA.

Dowling S., Department of Radiation Therapy, Yale University, 333 Cedar Street, New Haven, CT 06510-8056, USA.

Eghbali H., Fondation Bergonié, 180 rue Saint-Genès, 33076 Bordeaux Cedex, France.

Erdkamp F.L.G., Catharina Ziekenhuis, Michelangelann 2, 5602 ZA Eindhoven, The Netherlands.

Fuller L.M.,, Department of Clinical Radiotherapy, The University of Texas M.D. Anderson Cancer Center, 1515 Holcombe Boulevard, Houston, TX 77030, USA.

Gobbi P. Giorgio, Università di Pavia, Clinica Medica II, IRCCS Policlinico S. Matteo, 27100 Pavia, Italy.

Gobbi Paolo G., Università di Pavia, Clinica Medica II, IRCCS Policlinico S. Matteo, 27100 Pavia, Italy.

Gospadorowicz M., Department of Radiation Oncology, The Princess Margaret Hospital, 500 Sherbourne Street, Toronto, Canada M4X.

Gregory W., Breast Unit, Guy's Hospital, Snowfield Building, London SE1 9RT, England.

Hagemeister F.B., Department of Hematology, The University of Texas M.D. Anderson Cancer Center, 1515 Holcombe Boulevard, Houston, TX 77030, USA.

Hagenbeek A., Department of Haematology, Dr. Daniel den Hoed Cancer Center, Groene Hilledijk 301, 3075 EA Rotterdam, The Netherlands.

Hancock B.W., Royal Hallamshire Hospital, Clinical Oncology, Glossop Road, Sheffield S10 2FJ, England.

Hasenclever D., Medizinische Universtätsklinik 1, Haus 16, Joseph-Stelzmann-Strasse 9, 5000 Köln 41, Federal Republic of Germany.

Hayat M., Département de Médecine, Institut Gustave-Roussy, 39-53 Rue Camille Desmoulins, 94805 Villejuif Cedex, France.

Henry-Amar M., Département de Biostatistique et d'Epidémiologie, Institut Gustave-Roussy, 39-53 Rue Camille Desmoulins, 94805 Villejuif Cedex, France.

Hoerni B., Fondation Bergonié, 180 rue Saint-Genès, 33076 Bordeaux Cedex, France.

Hoppe R.T., Department of Therapeutic Radiology- Radiation Therapy, Stanford University Medical Center, Stanford, CA 94305, USA.

Horwich A., Academic Unit of Radiotherapy and Oncology, The Royal Marsden Hospital and Institute of Cancer Research,, Downs Road, Sutton, Surrey SM2 5PT, England.

Jouannet P., CECOS, CHU de Bicêtre, 78 rue du Général Leclerc, 94275 Le Kremlin Bicêtre Cedex, France.

Kaldor J.M., International Agency for Research on Cancer, Unit of Biostatistics Research and Informatics, 150 Cours Albert Thomas, 69372 Lyon Cedex 08, France.

Keuning J., St Joseph Ziekenhuis, Aalstrweg 259, 5600 ML Eindhoven, The Netherlands.

Kluin-Nelemans H., Department of Haematomorphology and Immunotyping, University Hospital, Bld 1, E1-Q, Rijnsburgerweg 10, 2333 AA Leiden, The Netherlands.

Lee C.K.K., Department of Therapeutic Radiology-Radiation Oncology, University of Minnesota Hospital and Clinic, Harvard Street at East River Road, Minneapolis, MN 55455, USA.

Levitt S.H., Department of Therapeutic Radiology-Radiation Oncology, University of Minnesota Hospital and Clinic, Harvard Street at East River Road, Minneapolis, MN 55455, USA.

Lister T.A., Department of Medical Oncology, St. Bartholomew's Hospital, 45-47 Little Britain, London ECA 7BE, England.

Löffler M., Medizinische Universtätsklinik 1, Haus 16, Joseph-Stelzmann-Strasse 9, 5000 Köln 41, Federal Republic of Germany.

MacLennan K.A., Department of Pathology, Royal Marsden Hospital, Fulham Road, London SW3 6JJ, England.

Mandard A.M., Anatomopathologie, Centre Régional François Baclesse, Route de Lion-sur-Mer, BP 5026, 14021 Caen Cedex, France.

Mauch P., Joint Center for Radiation Therapy, 50 Binney Street, Boston, MA 02115, USA.

Meerwaldt J.H., Department of Radiotherapy, Medisch Spectrum Twente, PO Box 50000, 7500 KA Enschede, The Netherlands.

Mellink W.A.M., Department of Radiotherapy, Dr. Daniel den Hoed Cancer Center, Groene Hilledijk 301, 3075 EA Rotterdam, The Netherlands.

Menon R.S., Department of Pathology, Dr Daniel den Hoed Cancer Center, Groene Hilledijk 301, 3075 EA Rotterdam, The Netherlands.

Michiels J.J., Academisch Ziekenhuis Dijkzigt, Dr Molenwaterplein 40, 3015 GD Rotterdam, The Netherlands.

Monconduit M., Département d'Hématologie, Centre H. Becquerel, Rue d'Amiens, 76038 Rouen Cedex, France.

Najman A., Service des Maladies du Sang, Hôpital Saint-Antoine, 184 Rue du Faubourg Saint-Antoine, 75571 Paris Cedex 12, France.

Nissen N.I., Department of Haematology, Rigshospitalet, 9 Blegdamsvej, 2100 Copenhagen Ø, Denmark.

Noordijk E.M., Department of Radiotherapy, University Hospital, Bld. 1, K1-P, PO Box 9600, 2341 CB Leiden, The Netherlands.

Obrist R., University Division of Oncology, Kantonsspittal, 4031 Basel, Switzerland.

Pavlovsky S., Pacheco de Melo 3081, (1425) Capital Federal, Buenos Aires, Argentina.

Pfreundschuh M., Medizinische Universtätsklinik 1, Haus 16, Joseph-Stelzmann-Strasse 9, 5000 Köln 41, Federal Republic of Germany.

Pompe Kirn V., Cancer Registry of Slovenia, Zaloska 2, 61000 Ljubljana, Yougoslavia.

Portlock C.S., Memorial Sloan-Kettering Cancer Center, 1275 York Avenue, New-York, NY 10021, USA.

Raemaekers J.M.M., Department of Haematology, University Hospital, PO Box 9101, 6542 TA Nijmegen, The Netherlands.

Regnier R., Institut Jules Bordet, 1 rue Héger Bordet, 1000 Brussels, Belgium.

Santarelli M.T., Pacheco de Melo 3081, (1425) Capital Federal, Buenos Aires, Argentina.

Somers R., Department of Haematology, The Netherlands Cancer Institute, Antoni Van Leeuwenhoek Ziekenhuis, Plesmanlaan 121, 1066 CS Amsterdam, The Netherlands.

Specht L., Department of Haematology, Rigshospitalet, 9 Blegdamsvej, 2100 Copenhagen Ø, Denmark.

Sutcliffe S., Department of Radiation Oncology, The Princess Margaret Hospital, 500 Sherbourne Street, Toronto, Canada M4X 1K9.

Swindell R., Department Medical Statistics, Christie Hospital and Holt Radium Institute, Wilmslow Road, Manchester M20 9BX, England.

Tanguy A., Centre Régional François Baclesse, Route de Lion-sur-Mer, BP 5026, 14021 Caen Cedex, France.

Thomas J., Department of Haematology, St Rafaël Ziekenhuis, 3000 Leuven, Belgium.

Tirelli U., Centro di Riferimento Oncologico, Via Pedemontana Occidentale, 33081 Aviano (PN), Italy.

Tubiana M., Institut Gustave-Roussy, 39-53 Rue Camille Desmoulins, 94805 Villejuif Cedex, France.

Valagussa P., Instituto Nazionale per lo Studio et la Cura dei Tumori, Via Venezian 1, 20133 Milano, Italy.

Van Bunningen B.N.F.M., The Netherlands Cancer Institute, Antoni van Leeuwenhoek Huis, Plesmanlaan 121, 1066 CX Amsterdam, The Netherlands.

Van der Schueren E., Department of Radiotherapy, St Rafaël Ziekenhuis, 3000 Leuven, Belgium.

Van Glabbeke M., EORTC Data Centre, Avenue E. Mounier 83 - B11, 1200 Brussels, Belgium.

Vaughan Hudson B., Department of Oncology, 3rd floor Jules Thorn Building, The Middlesex Hospital, Mortimer Street, London W1N 8AA, England.

Vaughan Hudson G., Department of Oncology, 3rd floor Jules Thorn Building, The Middlesex Hospital, Mortimer Street, London W1N 8AA, England.

Vovk M., Institute of Oncology, Zaloska 2, 61000 Ljubljana, Yougoslavia.

INTRODUCTION

INTRODUCTION

The E.O.R.T.C. International Workshop on Treatment Strategy in Hodgkin's Disease, organized as a satellite meeting of the first I.S.R.O. Congress (International Society for Radiation Oncology), will stand out from different points of view.

For the past 40 years, therapeutic progress in Hodgkin's disease constitutes one of the most important advances in cancer research. The way in which this progress evolved is very interesting. By successive stages and with the support of methodologically well-conducted clinical trials, the survival rate has increased from nearly zero 25 years ago to a cure rate of 80 % for early stages. These results are that much more appreciable since the patients are usually young. Ever since then, the aims of clinical research are two-fold. For favourable cases the aim is to continue to obtain good results while, at the same time, reducing sequelea to a minimum so as not to handicap the life of the cured patients. For unfavourable cases, the aim is to search for new therapies, even intensive. It is for this reason that prognostic research has been developped with such intensity in this disease and for which this symposium has provided a large opening. This is probably the first area of clinical oncology where the possibility of an individual personalized treatment based on a gravity index is offered to the patient.

The modalities for the preparation and realisation of this symposium are also original. It is quite remarkable to have been able to bring together and analyze the totality of data from the most important groups working on the subject. We should thank all of the participants and the organizers and especially Michel HENRY-AMAR.

Finally this symposium has been the occasion of pay respect to Professor Maurice TUBIANA, Honorary Director of the Institut Gustave-Roussy, who ended his hospital and university functions on October 1st 1989. Professor Maurice TUBIANA was the first president of the Lymphoma Cooperative Group of the EORTC. He initiated as early as 1963, the first large randomized trial of this group, the H1 trial. We can say today on the occasion of this symposium that he has without a doubt played an important part in the success of the cooperative work accomplished in this disease.

We do not doubt that Professor Maurice TUBIANA will preserve his numerous activities and continue to provide his extensive knowledge and his great dynamism for the benefit of medical research. He will do this as head of numerous organizations, notably as Vice-President of the EORTC. It was quite natural that he be acknowledged during the course of this meeting.

Professor Robert FLAMANT
Director of the Institut Gustave Roussy

La réunion internationale sur la Stratégie Thérapeutique dans la Maladie de Hodgkin, organisée par le Groupe Lymphome de l'O.E.R.T.C. comme manifestation satellite du 1er Congrès de l'I.S.R.O. (International Society for Radiation Oncology), fera date à plusieurs points de vue.

Les progrès thérapeutiques dans la maladie de Hodgkin constituent une des plus importantes avancées en cancérologie des 40 dernières années. La manière dont ils se sont réalisés est très intéressante. Par étapes successives et avec le support d'essais thérapeutiques méthodologiquement bien conduits, on est passé en 25 ans d'une survie quasi nulle à un taux de guérison de l'ordre de 80 % pour les formes localisées. Ces résultats sont d'autant plus appréciables que les malades sont souvent des sujets jeunes.
Dès lors, les objectifs de recherche thérapeutique sont doubles. Continuer à obtenir de bons résultats pour les cas favorables mais en réduisant au minimum les séquelles pour ne pas handicaper la vie des sujets guéris. Rechercher de nouvelles thérapeutiques, même lourdes, pour les cas moins favorables. C'est la raison pour laquelle, dans cette maladie, s'est développée avec une telle intensité une recherche pronostique élaborée, sur laquelle ce symposium donne une large ouverture. C'est probablement le premier domaine de la cancérologie clinique dans lequel on étudie maintenant la possibilité d'offrir au malade un traitement individuel personnalisé établi en fonction d'un score de gravité.

Les modalités de préparation et de déroulement de ce symposium sont également originales. Le fait d'avoir pu réunir et analyser ensemble les données des équipes les plus importantes travaillant sur le sujet est tout à fait remarquable. Il faut en remercier tous les participants et les organisateurs, notamment Michel HENRY-AMAR.

Enfin, ce symposium a été l'occasion de rendre hommage au Professeur Maurice TUBIANA, Directeur Honoraire de l'Institut Gustave-Roussy, qui a cessé ses fonctions hospitalo-universitaires le 1er octobre 1989. Le Professeur Maurice TUBIANA a été le premier président du Groupe Coopérateur Lymhomes Malins de l'O.E.R.T.C. C'est lui qui a initié dès 1963 le premier grand essai randomisé de ce groupe, l'essai H1. Il a, sans aucun doute, une très grande part dans la réussite, que l'on constate aujourd'hui à l'occasion de ce symposium, du travail coopératif effectué dans cette maladie.

Le Professeur Maurice TUBIANA va -nous n'en doutons pas- conserver de nombreuses activités et continuera à faire bénéficier la recherche médicale de ses grandes connaissances et de son grand dynamisme. Il le fera à la tête de nombreux organismes, notamment comme Vice-Président de l'O.É.R.T.C. Il était tout naturel qu'un hommage lui soit rendu au cours de cette réunion.

Professeur Robert FLAMANT
Directeur de l'Institut Gustave Roussy

In 1964 the E.O.R.T.C. Lymphoma Cooperative Group was founded, although at that time it was neither an E.O.R.T.C. Group, nor was it called the Lymphoma Cooperative Group: it's original name was the Radiotherapy-Chemotherapy Cooperative Group of the G.E.C.A. (Groupe Européen de Chimiothérapie Anticancéreuse).

The G.E.C.A. was a predecessor of the E.O.R.T.C. and the name was changed in 1968. The Group was then known as the E.O.R.T.C. Radiotherapy-Chemotherapy Group. Its aim was to study the interaction and the results of combined modality treatment in malignant tumours. Members at that time were predominantly radiotherapists as indicated by those who took the initiative to found the group: Professor Tubiana from Villejuif, the late Professor Breur from Amsterdam, and Professor v.d. Werf-Messing from Rotterdam.

In the first period attention was focused on two tumour types, the malignant lymphomas: Hodgkin's disease and non-Hodgkin's lymphoma, and bone tumours: osteosarcomas and Ewing sarcoma. In the treatment of osteosarcoma attention was given to the use of prophylactic lung irradiation (02 trial) in the prevention of lung metastases. This non-toxic treatment had a protective effect. Because of the changing pattern in the treatment of primary osteosarcoma, such as the application of reconstructive surgery and chemotherapy, the Group took the initiative to form a multidisciplinary group with orthopedic surgeons, pathologists, chemotherapists and radiotherapists, known as the European Osteosarcoma Intergroup founded in 1983.

The main interest however was the treatment of Hodgkin's disease and the non-Hodgkin's lymphomas. This resulted in five trials in stage I and II Hodgkin's disease (H1, H2, H5, H6, H7 studies), two in stage III-IV Hodgkin's disease and seven prospective studies in the non-Hodgkin's lymphomas. The questions posed in these studies show the tremendous development in this field in the last twenty-five years. In the limited stages of Hodgkin's disease treatment went from radiotherapy followed by monochemotherapy (H1 trial) in the sixties, through investigation of the role of staging laparotomy and splenectomy (H2 trial) in the early seventies, to treatment for groups of patients based on prognostic factors (H5, H6, and H7 trials) in the late seventies and the eighties. One of the aims was to define groups of patients to whom a less intensive primary treatment could be safely given without increasing the death risk from Hodgkin's disease while accepting a higher risk of relapse. On the other hand, groups could be defined for whom combined modality treatment improved the results. Lighter treatment for low risk patients is all the more important because it is clear that long-term side effects of the treatments are not negligible. In recent years the study of side effects is integrated in the protocols and the contribution of late side effects to the cause of death in long-term survivors is also receiving attention.

We were very happy to organize this first Workshop on Treatment Strategy in Hodgkin's Disease on the occasion of the 25th anniversary of the Group, but we were less happy with the second occasion, namely the retirement of Professor Maurice Tubiana. He was not only one of the founders, but he continued to activate and support the Group not only by his stimulating ideas and contributions but also by material support in the form of data management at the Institut Gustave Roussy. He played a very active role in the analysis of all Hodgkin's disease trials and in the development of the concept of the "patient adapted" treatment. He exposed his ideas in many publications and presentations. The way he approaches the disease in all its aspects can best be indicated by the term "treatment philosophy". His great erudition in other fields contributed to his attitude to Hodgkin's disease which consisted of a dual approach to develop innovation which may not only improve the results but especially may diminish the side effects to provide a better life for the patients, whithout loosing what has been achieved in recent years.

We thank Professor Tubiana for all his efforts and we would like to honour him by dedicating this Workshop and Symposium to him in the hope that this meeting may develop ideas along the lines he has set out over the last twenty-five years.

Dr. Reinier SOMERS

Le Groupe Coopérateur Lymphome de l'O.E.R.T.C. a été créé en 1964, même si à cette époque il ne s'intitulait pas encore Groupe Coopérateur Lymphome ni ne faisait partie de l'O.E.R.T.C. qui, d'ailleurs, n'existait pas. A l'origine, il avait pour nom Groupe Coopérateur Radiothérapie-Chimiothérapie du G.E.C.A. (Groupe Européen de Chimiothérapie Anticancéreuse).

Le G.E.C.A. a été le précurseur de l'O.E.R.T.C. et son nom a été modifié en 1968. A partir de ce moment, le Groupe a été connu sous le nom de Groupe Coopérateur Radiothérapie-Chimiothérapie. Son activité consistait en l'étude de l'interaction entre la radiothérapie et la chimiothérapie dans le traitement des tumeurs malignes, ainsi que l'analyse de leur efficacité. Les membres du Groupe étaient alors en majorité des radiothérapeutes à l'instar de ceux qui furent à l'initiative de sa création: le Professeur Tubiana de Villejuif, le regretté Professeur Breur d'Amsterdam, et le Professeur v.d. Werf-Messing de Rotterdam.

Au cours des premières années l'intérêt du Groupe a surtout porté sur deux types de tumeurs: les lymphomes malins, maladie de Hodgkin et lymphomes non-Hodgkiniens, et les tumeurs osseuses, ostéosarcome et sarcome d'Ewing. Dans le cas des ostéosarcomes une première étude a démontré l'intérêt de la radiothérapie pulmonaire prophylactique, traitement peu ou pas toxique, dans la survenue des métastases (essai O2). Mais du fait du changement radical des thérapeutiques de l'ostéosarcome, comme par exemple l'utilisation combinée d'une chirurgie réparatrice associée à une chimiothérapie, le Groupe prit l'initiative de créer un groupe multidisciplinaire associant chirurgiens orthopédiques, anatomopathologistes, chimiothérapeutes et radiothérapeutes. En 1983, le Groupe Européen pour l'Etude des Ostéosarcomes était créé.

Dès lors l'intérêt principal du Groupe a porté sur le traitement de la maladie de Hodgkin et des lymphomes non-Hodgkiniens. Au total le Groupe a réalisé cinq essais thérapeutiques dans les stades I-II de la maladie de Hodgkin (essais H1, H2, H5, H6, et H7), deux dans les stades III-IV de cette même maladie, et sept études prospectives sur les lymphomes non-Hodgkiniens. Chaque fois les questions posées reflétaient les problèmes du moment liés au développement extraordinaire de l'arsenal thérapeutique au cours de ces vingt-cinq dernières années. Dans les stades localisés de la maladie de Hodgkin l'évolution des thérapeutiques s'est faite en trois étapes successives: association radiothérapie + monochimiothérapie adjuvante dans les années 60 (essai H1); puis au début des années soixante-dix évaluation du rôle de la laparotomie exploratrice associée à une splénectomie (essai H2); enfin adaptation de la stratégie thérapeutique basée sur l'utilisation de facteurs de pronostic depuis la fin des années soixante-dix (essais H5, H6, et H7). L'un des buts poursuivis était d'identifier des sous-groupes de malades qu'il serait possible de traiter de manière peu agressive d'emblée sans pour autant hypothéquer les résultats en terme de survie, mais au prix éventuel d'un taux de rechute plus élevé. A l'inverse, les malades à pronostic initial péjoratif devraient être traités par association radiothérapie-chimiothérapie afin d'améliorer les résultats. Il est d'autant plus important de limiter l'intensité des thérapeutiques chez les malades au pronostic le plus favorable que les effets secondaires à long terme de ces traitements sont loins d'être négligeables. Depuis quelques années, l'évaluation des effets secondaires des traitements fait partie intégrante des protocoles et leur impact sur la survie est étudié avec beaucoup d'attention.

Nous sommes heureux d'avoir pu organiser cette première réunion internationale sur la Stratégie Thérapeutique dans la Maladie de Hodgkin à l'occasion du vingt-cinquième anniversaire du Groupe. Par contre, nous le sommes moins si l'on considère la deuxième raison pour laquelle cette réunion a eu lieu, c'est-à-dire la retraite du Professeur Maurice Tubiana. Ce dernier n'a pas été simplement l'un des fondateurs du Groupe. Il a, pendant toutes ces années, activement participé à la vie du Groupe, non seulement en proposant des idées originales mais aussi en apportant la contribution matérielle de l'Institut Gustave Roussy à la gestion des études entreprises. Il a joué un rôle fondamental dans l'analyse des résultats de tous les essais thérapeutiques entrepris sur la maladie de Hodgkin et dans le développement du concept "d'adaptation thérapeutique". La manière dont il appréhende la maladie dans son ensemble peut être considérée comme une véritable "philosophie de la thérapeutique". Son immense érudition dans d'autres domaines l'a beaucoup aidé dans son approche du traitement de la maladie de Hodgkin. Celle-ci a toujours consisté à favoriser l'innovation, dans le but non pas seulement d'améliorer les résultats mais surtout de réduire le plus possible les effets secondaires afin de préserver aux malades une vie qualitativement la plus satisfaisante possible, sans pour autant perdre le bénéfice des expériences antérieures.

Nous remercions chaleureusement le Professeur Tubiana pour tous ses efforts passés et nous souhaitions l'honorer en lui dédiant à la fois la réunion de travail et le symposium, en souhaitant que ces manifestations scientifiques participent au développement des idées qu'il a toujours défendues pendant ces ving-cinq dernières années.

Dr. Reinier SOMERS

The history of Hodgkin's disease since 1963 has been one of the most fascinating in medicine of the XXe century. Up until that date, Hodgkin's disease was inexorably fatal, to such a point that many eminent physicians, convinced that the efficacy of all treatments was limited, only considered using them parcimoniously. Suddenly, in the span of a few months, everything changed when a few pioneers, among whom we should mention Easson, Henry Kaplan and Vera Peters, demonstrated that by using increased doses of radiotherapy to larger volumes, as opposed to the use of radiotherapy as a palliative treatment, with no constant effects, it was possible to definitively cure certain patients.

This clasp of thunder was first viewed with scepticism then aroused an enormous enthusiasm. Since Hodgkin's disease could be cured, researchers on both sides of the Atlantic started to investigate on how to increase the cure rate. Henry Kaplan played an essential role in stimulating and orientating the efforts. Persuaded that only randomized clinical trials could demonstrate the validity of new therapeutic approaches, he organized the first one of them in Stanford and encouraged other groups to use the same methodology.

In France, following the Symposium in Paris on Hodgkin's disease in 1963, during which the first international classification of this disease was proposed, we were convinced, along with G. Mathé that in order to have a sufficient number of patients, those trials needed to be european, and should be realized within the framework of the E.O.R.T.C. which, along with others, we had just created. With K. Breur and B. v. d. Werf-Messing, we organized a cooperative group for this objective and in 1964, the first patients were included in the H1 trial, the aim of which was to compare radiotherapy alone to radiotherapy associated with chemotherapy. Today we are celebrating the 25th anniversary of this trial. Whereas, the objective of the group in Stanford was to evaluate the efficiency of treatment methods more and more intensive (the association of mantle and inverted Y irradiation, laparotomy and splenectomy, the combination of total lymphatic irradiation with MOPP), the E.O.R.T.C. group fixed an objective to delineate the subsets of patients in whom combinations of radiotherapy and chemotherapy are required because there is a high likelihood of relapse, and eventually death after initial treatment with radiotherapy alone. The identification of the prognostic indicators which are correlated with the relapse probability was, therefore, one of the goals of the E.O.R.T.C. trials. Eight indicators were prospectively registered : age, sex, stage, number and site of involved lymphatic areas, histological subtype, presence or absence of systemic symptoms, erythrocyte sedimentation rate; furthermore, in the group of patients who were allocated to staging laparotomy, its results were also registered. It was rapidly shown that the impact of the various prognostic factors on relapse-free survival varies with the type of treatment and, among patients treated by radiotherapy alone, with the type of radiation therapy (involved field radiotherapy, regional radiotherapy, such as mantle-field or inverted Y extended field radiotherapy or total nodal irradiation). The prognostic factors should, therefore, be envisaged in the context of the type of treatment, or of treatments, that appear optimal.

In the clinical trials initiated since 1964, the knowledge acquired from the preceeding trials were progressively introduced in order to accomodate with more precision the aggressiveness of the treatment to the severity of the disease. The validity of this strategy whose aim was to identify the subsets of patients who can be safely treated initially by radiation therapy alone was further supported when the side effects of multi-agent chemotherapy were better known *a)* the early and late toxicities which are often high and which differ according to the cytotoxic drug used, *b)* the loss of fertility which is observed in nearly all men and most women in patients treated with MOPP, and *c)* the clear increase in second neoplasia incidence.

In the first trial H1, the histological type was the prognostic factor with the best correlation with chemotherapeutic effectiveness. This factor was used to define the subgroup of patients in the second trial H2. From the third trial onwards (H5 trial), the patients were further subdivised in two subgroups according to prognostic factors and different questions were asked in each of the two subgroups. Although about 1,600 patients have been included in trials since 1964, it has recently become evident that this number is insufficient to answer, with fiability, all the questions asked:

a) The separation of the totality of the patients into two therapeutic subgroups, favourable and unfavourable, was not satisfactory. At least three subgroups seemed necessary. However, the greater the number of subgroups and variables taken into account, the more patients will be needed to be able to separate these therapeutic groups and the corresponding treatment choice, even more so since there is an interaction between prognostic factors and the initial treatment.

b) Taking survival as the only criterion in these trials is insufficient. Two other criteria are indispensable: the probability of relapse and the severity of complications caused by the treatments. Yet these criteria are not influenced by the same variables. Among young patients for instance it is easy to obtain an increased survival, but the quality of life is very important; it is conditionned by the possibility to have children and by treament sequelae especially among children by the effect of growth. On the other hand, the stress caused by a relapse among young patients is less serious than among older patients. After 40 years of age, fertility has less importance but cardiac or pulmonary toxicity become critical factors. Thus the therapeutic protocol should take age into account and at least 3 age groups should be defined: before 16 years, from 16 to 40 years, and after 40 years.

c) At least a 15 year follow-up is necessary to appreciate long term toxic effects and the frequency of second cancers. That much follow-up is only available for a few patients.

d) In the E.O.R.T.C. trials, some prognostic factors, the tumour mass in particular, were not registered prospectively. Yet it seems interesting to take it into account.

All of these considerations have led certain members of the E.O.R.T.C. group, in particular Michel HENRY-AMAR, Patrice CARDE and Jean-Marc COSSET to think that it would be useful to group together a larger number of patients so as to increase the power of the study of prognostic factors.

Other groups, in particular the British National Lymphoma Investigation (B.N.L.I.), have also conducted the study of prognostic factors on a large number of patients. Confronting the results seemed a good method for progressing. The idea for a symposium thus came about, bringing together all of the groups conducting trials in Hodgkin's disease. But in order to do this, it was necessary to meticulously prepare the collection and the handling of all of the data. This was an enormous effort which involved the cooperation of a large number of clinicians and statisticians, as well as a centralization and validation of the data. Thanks to everyone's willingness, this effort was accomplished in a remarkably short period of time. This booklet regroups the results obtained. They are considerable and the question is to know how to continue this work and prolong this effort which is susceptible, once again, to establish a model for other types of cancer.

In fact, for the other types of cancer, we can see a similar evolution in treatment. Progressive intensification in the methods of care in order to obtain an ever increasing cure rate. Then in view of the severity of sequelae, or mutilations, the data is analyzed in order to separate the population into subgroups according to optimal treatment. This effort of fitting the characteristics of a subgroup to the choice of treatment allows a deflation of treatment thus of toxic effects and a better quality of life, while, at the same time, keeping long term survival stable or even better. Two ways are possible to achieve this result: *a)* the study of prognostic factors, and *b)* biological research of the molecular mechanisms of the disease. This symposium only considers the first aspect.

For breast and thyroid cancer, spectacular results have already been obtained in this therapeutic deflation thanks to the identification of subgroup for which adjuvant treatment is not justified after surgery. As far as Hodgkin's disease is concerned, the results already obtained are very interesting and attitudes of several groups from all over the world, dedicated to the treatment of this disease, is much more similar than could have been feared. Actually, this symposium will have contributed in bringing together the different points of view. Nevertheless, efforts must be pursued since the deleterious effects of the principal treatments, radiotherapy and chemotherapy, can only be evaluated after a long follow-up. Also, the different groups of cytotoxics (MOPP, ABVD, etc.) have different advantages and disadvantages and they should be studied separately, which complicates the analysis. This first collective effort of the study of prognostic factors should be continued.

In particular the study of the induction of second cancers, one of the most important side effects, needs cohorts with large number of patients. This collection of more than 14,000 patients offers unique possibilities from this point of view. Also, the increased percentage of second cancer among patients with Hodgkin's disease after combined polychemotherapy and extended radiotherapy treatment allows prevention trials with for example $β$-carotene, retinoids, or vitamin C. The group which was formed during this symposium could serve as the infrastructure for starting up such studies. These examples show very well how interesting it is to continue this cooperation, and thanks to the commun efforts, the first fruits are already so promising.

Professor Maurice TUBIANA

L'histoire de la maladie de Hodgkin depuis 1963 a été l'une des plus fascinantes de la médecine du XXème siècle. La maladie de Hodgkin était inexorablement mortelle jusqu'à cette date, à tel point que beaucoup de médecins éminents considéraient que l'efficacité de tous les traitements étant limitée, il ne fallait les utiliser qu'avec parcimonie. Brusquement, en quelques mois, tout changea quand quelques pionniers, parmi lesquels il faut citer Easson, Henry Kaplan et Vera Peters, démontrèrent qu'alors que la radiothérapie, telle qu'elle était précédemment utilisée, n'avait qu'un effet palliatif inconstant, en utilisant des doses un peu plus élevées sur des volumes un peu plus vastes on pouvait guérir définitivement certains malades.

Ce coup de tonnerre fut d'abord accueilli avec scepticisme, puis suscita un immense élan. Puisque la maladie de Hodgkin pouvait être guérie, on recherca des deux côtés de l'Atlantique comment parvenir à augmenter le taux de guérison. Henry Kaplan joua un rôle essentiel pour stimuler et orienter les efforts. Persuadé que seuls des essais thérapeutiques comparatifs pouvaient démontrer la validité des nouvelles approches thérapeutiques, il organisa à Stanford les premiers d'entre eux et encouragea d'autres groupes à utiliser la même méthode.

En France, à la suite du symposium de Paris sur la Maladie de Hodgkin en 1963, pendant lequel fut proposée la première classification internationale de cette maladie, nous fûmes avec G. Mathé convaincus que ces essais pour réunir un nombre suffisant de malades devaient être Européens, donc s'effectuer dans le cadre de l'O.E.R.T.C. qu'avec quelques autres nous venions de créer. Avec K. Breur et B. v. d. Werf-Messing, nous organisâmes un groupe coopérateur dans ce but, et, en 1964, les premiers malades étaient inclus dans l'essai H1 dont le but était de comparer la radiothérapie seule à une association radiothérapie-chimiothérapie. Nous célébrons aujourd'hui le 25ème anniversaire de ce premier essai. Tandis que le but du groupe de Stanford fut d'évaluer l'efficacité de méthodes de soins de plus en plus lourdes (assocation d'irradiation en mantelet et en Y inversé, laparotomie et splénectomie, combinaison de l'irradiation lymphoïde totale avec le MOPP) l'objectif que s'assigna le groupe de l'O.E.R.T.C. fut d'identifier les sous-groupes de malades pour lesquels les associations radiothérapie-chimiothérapie devraient être appliquées du fait de leur haute probabilité de rechute, et éventuellement de décès, après un traitement initial par radiothérapie seule. L'identification des facteurs pronostiques liés à la probabilité de rechute était donc un des buts des essais de l'O.E.R.T.C. Parmi ces facteurs pronostiques, huit furent sytématiquement enregistrés : l'âge, le sexe, le stade clinique, le nombre et la localisation des aires ganglionnaires envahies, le type histologique, la présence ou l'absence de signes généraux, la vitesse de sédimentation. De plus, pour le groupe de malades dont le bilan incluait une laparotomie, le stade pathologique était aussi enregistré. Rapidement il apparut évident que l'influence des facteurs pronostiques sur la durée de survie sans rechute varie en fonction du type de traitement utilisé et, parmi les malades traités par radiothérapie exclusive, selon l'étendue de la radiothérapie : radiothérapie localisée, radiothérapie loco-régionale (en mantelet ou Y inversé), radiothérapie étendue (irradiation lymphoïde subtotale ou totale). Les facteurs pronostiques devaient alors être pris en compte dans le choix du ou des traitements qui paraissaient avoir une efficacité optimale.

Dans les essais thérapeutiques qui se sont succédés depuis 1964, les connaissances acquises dans les essais précédents furent progressivement introduites afin de proportionner avec de plus en plus de précision l'agressivité du traitement à la gravité de la maladie. La validité de la stratégie, dont le but était d'identifier les sous-groupes de malades qui pouvaient être traités sans risque par radiothérapie exclusive, fut d'autant plus renforcée lorsque les effets indésirables des poly-chimiothérapies furent mieux connus, à savoir : a) les toxicités précoces et tardives souvent importantes et qui varient selon les agents cytotoxiques utilisés; b) une stérilité observée chez presque tous les hommes et parmi une proportion importante de femmes traités par le MOPP; c) l'augmentation indiscutable du risque de survenue de cancers secondaires.

Dans le second essai, H2, le type histologique qui s'était révélé dans l'essai précédent être le facteur pronostique le mieux corrélé avec l'efficacité de la chimiothérapie fut utilisé pour définir le sous-groupe dans lequel celle-ci était mise en oeuvre. A partir du 3ème essai (essai H5) les malades furent divisés en deux sous-groupes en fonction des facteurs pronostiques, et des questions différentes furent posées dans chacun des 2 sous-groupes.

Cependant, bien qu'environ 1 600 malades aient été introduits dans les essais de l'O.E.R.T.C. depuis 1964, il devint récemment évident que ce nombre était insuffisant pour répondre avec fiabilité à toutes les questions posées :
a) La division de l'ensemble des malades en deux sous-groupes thérapeutiques, le favorable et le défavorable, n'était pas satisfaisante. Au moins 3 sous-groupes apparurent nécessaires. Or, plus les nombres de sous-groupes et de paramètres pris en compte augmentent et plus il faut de malades pour parvenir à la délimitation des groupes thérapeutiques et au choix du traitement, d'autant que, comme nous l'avons vu, il y a interaction entre les facteurs pronostiques et le traitement initial.
b) Prendre pour seul critère de ces essais la survie est insuffisant. Deux autres critères sont indispensables : la probabilité de rechute et la gravité des complications induites par les traitements. Or ce ne sont pas les mêmes paramètres qui influencent ces 3 critères. Chez les malades jeunes, par exemple, il est facile d'obtenir une survie élevée mais la qualité de vie est très importante, elle est conditionnée par la possibilité d'avoir des enfants et par les séquelles du traitement, notamment chez les enfants par l'effet sur la croissance staturale. Par contre, chez les jeunes, le stress causé par une rechute est moins grave que chez les sujets plus âgés. Au-delà de 40 ans, la fertilité a moins d'importance mais la toxicité cardiaque ou pulmonaire deviennent des facteurs critiques. Le protocole thérapeutique doit donc tenir compte de l'âge, et au moins 3 groupes d'âge doivent être distingués : avant 16 ans, entre 16 et 40 ans, au-delà de 40 ans.
c) Un long recul, au moins 15 ans, est nécessaire pour apprécier les effets toxiques tardifs et la fréquence des seconds cancers. Un aussi long recul n'est disponible que pour peu de malades.
d) Dans les essais de l'O.E.R.T.C., certains facteurs pronostiques, en particulier la masse tumorale, n'avaient pas été enregistrés prospectivement. Or, il apparaît intéressant d'en tenir compte.

Toutes ces considérations conduirent certains membres du groupe de l'O.E.R.T.C., en particulier Michel HENRY-AMAR, Patrice CARDE et Jean-Marc COSSET à penser qu'il serait utile de rassembler un beaucoup plus grand nombre de malades afin de rendre plus puissante l'étude des facteurs pronostiques.

D'autres groupes, en particulier le British National Lymphoma Investigation (B.N.L.I.), avaient également conduit l'étude des facteurs pronostiques sur des nombres importants de malades. Confronter les résultats représentaient une bonne méthode pour progresser. Ainsi naquit l'idée d'un symposium réunissant l'ensemble des groupes effectuant des essais de la maladie de Hodgkin. Mais, pour que celui-ci soit utile, il fallait une minitieuse préparation comportant notamment la collecte et le traitement de l'ensemble des données. C'était un gigantesque effort qui nécessitait la coopération d'un grand nombre de cliniciens et statisticiens, ainsi qu'une centralisation et une validation des données. Grâce à la bonne volonté de tous, cet effort fut accompli en un temps remarquablement bref. Cet ouvrage rassemble les résultats obtenus. Ils sont considérables, et la question se pose de savoir comment continuer cette oeuvre et prolonger cet effort qui est susceptible, une fois de plus, de constituer un modèle pour les autres types de cancer.

En effet, pour les autres types de cancer, on observe une même évolution des thérapeutiques. Alourdissement progressif des méthodes de soin afin d'obtenir un pourcentage de guérison de plus en plus élevé. Puis, devant la gravité des séquelles, ou des mutilations, un effort d'analyse est effectué pour démembrer l'entité en sous-groupes en fonction de la thérapeutique optimale. Cet effort d'adéquation entre les caractéristiques du sous-groupe et le choix du traitement permet à la fois une déflation du traitement, donc des effets toxiques, et une amélioration de la qualité de vie, tout en maintenant, voire en accroissant les pourcentages de survie à long terme. Deux voies permettent d'obtenir ces résultats : a) l'étude des facteurs pronostiques, et b) la recherche biologique des mécanismes moléculaires de la maladie. Ce symposium considère uniquement le premier aspect.

Pour le cancer du sein ou de la thyroïde, des résultats spectaculaires ont déjà été obtenus dans cette déflation thérapeutique grâce à l'identification des sous-groupes pour lesquels, après chirurgie, aucun traitement adjuvant n'est justifié. En ce qui concerne la maladie de Hodgkin, les résultats déjà obtenus sont très intéressants, et l'attitude des diverses équipes qui, dans le monde, se consacrent au traitement de cette maladie est beaucoup plus proche qu'on aurait pu le craindre. Ce symposium aura d'ailleurs contribué à rapprocher les points de vue. Cependant, l'effort doit être poursuivi car les effets délétères des principaux traitements, radiothérapie et chimiothérapie, ne peuvent être évalués qu'après de longs reculs. De plus, les différents groupes de cytotoxiques (MOPP, ABVD, etc...) ont des avantages et des inconvénients différents, et on doit les étudier séparément, ce qui rend plus complexe l'analyse. Ce premier effort collectif d'étude des facteurs pronostiques doit donc être poursuivi.

En particulier, l'étude de l'un des plus graves effets secondaires, l'induction de seconds cancers, nécessite des cohortes très importantes de malades. Ce rassemblement de plus de 14000 malades offre, de ce point de vue, des possibilités uniques. De plus, le pourcentage élevé de second cancer chez les malades atteints de maladie de Hodgkin après traitement combiné polychimiothérapie et radiothérapie étendue permet des essais de prévention par intervention avec, par exemple, b-carotène, rétinoïdes ou vitamine C. Le groupe qui s'est constitué lors de ce symposium pourrait servir d'infrastructure au lancement de telles études. Ces exemples montrent combien il serait intéressant de poursuivre cette coopération, dont, grâce aux efforts communs, les premiers fruits sont déjà si prometteurs.

Professeur Maurice TUBIANA

Reference
Bibliographie

Tubiana M., et al. (1989) : Toward comprehensive management tailored to prognostic factors of patients with clinical stages I and II in Hodgkin's disease. The EORTC Lymphoma Group controlled clinical trials : 1964-1987. *Blood* 73, 47-56.

PATHOLOGY AND CELL BIOLOGY OF HODGKIN'S DISEASE

*HISTOPATHOLOGIE ET BIOLOGIE CELLULAIRE
DE LA MALADIE DE HODGKIN*

New developments in the pathogenesis of Hodgkin's disease

C. Kalle, V. Diehl, M. Jücker, H. Tesch, C. Fonatsch, M. Pfreundschuh, M. Schaadt

Klinik I für Innere Medizin der Universität zu Köln Joseph-Stelzmann-Strasse 9, 5000 Köln 41, Federal Republic of Germany

Summary

Keeping in mind that the available data are not complete, a working hypothesis on the descent of the Hodgkin's cell can be contrived. In brief, the morphologically distinct Hodgkin and Reed-Sternberg cell has an immunophenotype characteristic of activated T or B cells (Stein et al., 1989). Dissociate from that, the genotype is immaturely lymphoid (Falk et al., 1987; Tesch et al., submitted for publication; Herbst et al., 1989). Rearrangements and expressions of the immunoglobulin super gene family are frequently incomplete or irregular (Tesch et al., submitted for publication; Herbst et al., 1989). The heterogeneity of the clinical and histological appearance of Hodgkin's disease and the multitude of different - partially controversial - cellular markers might be explained by Hodgkin's disease being a group of etio-pathophysiologically associated but not identical disease entities. The origin might be the same, probably lymphoid target cell transformed at different stages of maturation, or, alternatively, several biologically related diseases each with a different etio-pathogenesis.

Résumé

Il est possible, tout en étant conscients que les données dont nous disposons ne sont pas définitives, de bâtir une hypothèse sur l'origine de la cellule hodgkinienne. Schématiquement, cette cellule, ou cellule de Reed-Sternberg, est immunologiquement de phénotypique T ou B (Stein et al., 1989). Son génotype est lymphoide immature (Falk et al., 1987; Tesch et al., soumis pour publication; Herbst et al., 1989). Les réarrangements et les expressions des immunoglobulines sont fréquement incomplets et irréguliers (Tesch et al., soumis pour publication; Herbst et al., 1989). L'hétérogénéité clinique et histologique de la maladie de Hodgkin ainsi que le grand nombre de marqueurs cellulaires différents - et en partie controversés - pourraient trouver une explication dans une associations de plusieurs entités d'étiopathogénies différentes. Il pourrait s'agir de maladies d'origine identique, vraisemblablement une cellule cible lymphoide transformée à différents stades de maturation, ou bien de maladies biologiques d'étiopathogénies différentes.

Introduction

In contrast to the major clinical achievements in the treatment of Hodgkin's disease of the last two decades, basic research on origin and nature of Hodgkin and Reed-Sternberg cells lags behind comprehension in most other haematological malignancies. The reason for this shortcoming lies in the unique biological features of the disease. First, there is a number of heterogeneous clinical subentities to be defined rather than a monomorphous disorder. Second, the tumour cells hide, often in a one to a hundred relationships or less, in an environment of nonmalignant reactive cells from the analytical and preparatory access. Third, the obtainable cellular characteristics often do not match the conventional patterns of lineage fidelity and differentiation.

These special features, however, render the question whether the Hodgkin cell is of infectious, reactive or malignant nature all the more interesting. Not knowing the answer, it is important that no other tumour cell produces a likewise reaction of the nonmalignant specific and unspecific immune system. A comparatively low tumour cell load can cause severe clinical symptoms. Yet little knowledge is available on the true reasons for this biologic behavior.

In vitro cell lines

Within the last decade, the successful application of new techniques has shed light onto some of the pertinent questions. Cell culturing as a research tool has provided virtually unlimited amounts of tumour cell equivalents available for in-vitro research. Of the numerous attempts to culture Hodgkin tumour cells, nine tumour cell lines remain likely to be Hodgkin derived, after a necessarily strict panel of criteria had been applied (Diehl, 1985; Schaadt et al., 1989). Besides being confirmed for the histological diagnosis by two independent pathologists, the cells have to fulfill the criteria of monoclonality and aneuploidy to be considered malignant (Diehl et al., 1982). As is obvious, advanced clinical disease, the nodular sclerosing subtype and the clinical setting of an effusion are favorable for the establishment of a cell line (Table 1).

Table 1. Derivation and important characteristics of all Hodgkin's disease derived cell lines

Line	Clinical Stage	Source	Phenotype (Markers[1])	Genotype (Rearrangements)	Reference
L428	IV	PE[2]	B (CD19)	B ($Ig_{H,L}$, TCR beta)	Schaadt, 1980
L540	IV	BM	T (CD2,4)	T (TCR)	Diehl, 1982
L591	IV	PE	B (CD19,20)	B (Ig)	Diehl, 1982
Co	IV	LN	T (CD3,5,7)	T (TCR beta, gamma)	Jones, 1985
DEV	II	PE	B (CD19,20)	B ($Ig_{H,L}$)	Poppema, 1985
HD-LM2	IV	PE	T (CD2)	T (TCR)	Drexler, 1986
KM-H2	IV[3]	PE	B (CD19,21)	B (Ig_H)	Kamesaki, 1986
Ho	II	LN	T (CD3,4,7)	T (TCR beta, gamma)	Jones, 1988
Zo	II	PF	B (B-IB-Ab[4])	B ($Ig_{H,L}$)	Poppema, 1988

[1] *Important for differenciation*
[2] *PE = pleural effusion; BM = bone marrow; LN = lymph node; PF = pericardial fluid*
[3] *Histology: MC, all others NS*
[4] *B-immunoblastic NHL antibody*

Hodgkin and Reed-Sternberg Cells : In vivo and in vitro characteristics

Few haematological cell compartments have not been suspected to be the origin of Hodgkin and Reed-Sternberg cells (Table 2).

1. Phenotype

1.1. Morphology

Although morphological characteristics alone do not define the cell of origin in Hodgkin's disease, some of the histological characteristics are helpful to keep in mind when evaluating other findings.

Table 2. Historical overview of the theory formation concerning the proposed cell of origin in Hodgkin's disease

Suggestion	Group
Lymphoid Origin	
Lymphoblast	Mallory (1914)
Lymphoid subpopulation, activated	
T cell	Order (1972), Biniaminow, (1974)
B cell	Leech (1973), Garvin (1974), Boecker (1975), Poppema (1989)
Lymphoid cell (T or B)	Stein (1982?, 1984, 1985)
Immature lymphoid precursor	Falk (1987), Kamesaki (1989), Athan (1989), Herbst (1989)
Myelomonocytic Origin	
Monocytoid cell	McJunkin (1928)
Myeloblast, myeloid precursor cell,	Lewis (1941), Stein (1982),
Myelomonocytic precursor cell	Diehl (1982)
Other Origin	
Sinus endothelial cell	Reed (1902)
Megakaryocyte	Medlar (1931)
Histiocyte	Bessis (1948), Rappaport (1966), Mori (1969), Kaplan (1977), Kadin (1978), ...
Follicular dendritic cell	Curran (1978)
Dendritic ("Steinmann") cell,	
Antigen-presenting cell	Fischer (1983, 1985)
Interdigitating cell	Hansmann (1981), Kadin (1982), Hsu (1985)
Pluripotent precursor cell	Falk (1983)

In Hodgkin's disease tumours represent a majority of non malignant lymphocytes, histiocytes, plasma cells, eosinophils and others that prevail over a minority of characteristic Hodgkin and Reed-Sternberg tumour cells. The typical appearance of "large inclusion-like nucleoli, thick nuclear membranes with perinucleolar halos, and abundant eosinophilic to amphoteric cytoplasm" nevertheless is not pathognomonic (Lukes et al., 1966). It has been found as well in several reactive lymphoid and malignant diseases including infectious mononucleosis, non-Hodgkin's lymphoma, carcinomas and sarcomas (Lukes et al., 1969; Strum et al., 1971).

The distribution pattern and ratio of reactive cells and fibrosis are equally important for the diagnosis of Hodgkin's disease.

Although not offering definite conclusions, the typical yet complicated morphology of Hodgkin's disease postulates a number of characteristics a potential cell of origin has to meet. These include:
- induction of reactive cell proliferation;
- induction of collagen/fibrillar reticulum synthesis;
- initial limitation to homing in lymphatic organs.

1.2. Immunophenotype of Hodgkin Cells

Since 1980 several markers have been identified to be regularly expressed on Hodgkin and Reed-Sternberg cells, two of which were at first thought to be specific for the disease (Stein et al., 1982; Schwab et al., 1982). Hodgkin and Reed-Sternberg cells stain positive for the granulocyte staining X-Hapten (CD15) and the lectin Peanut Agglutinin (PNA), the interleukin-2 receptor (CD25), the Hodgkin's disease associated activation antigen Ki-1 (CD30), the B-cell associated antigen detected by the LN-2 antibody and the transferrin receptor (OKT9, CD71) (Hsu et al., 1984). MHC class IIa (HLA DR) antigens are constantly expressed in vivo and in vitro (Burrichter et al., 1985).

All antigens but one were initially defined only on unrelated cells. The CD30 antibodies were produced by immunizing with Hodgkin's disease derived cell line L428 (Stein et al., 1982). Except for Hodgkin and Reed-Sternberg cells, the CD30 antigen is only expressed on activated or transformed (HTLV1, EBV) T and B lymphocytes, activated and differentiated macrophages and a distinct subentity of large cell non-Hodgkin's lymphoma, the so-called "Ki-1 lymphoma" (Stein et al., 1985; Pfreundschuh et al., 1988; Andreesen et al., 1988; O'Connor et al., 1987). This reaction pattern makes CD30 antibodies a valuable diagnostic tool.

The CD30-antigen is now known to exist as a 120 kD membrane bound phosphorylated glycoprotein with a non-phosphorylated 84 kD intracellular apoprotein and a 90 kd degradation residue released into the supernatant (Hansen et al., 1989).

CD30 so far has always been associated with activated cells. Hodgkin and Reed Sternberg cells seem to comply with that rule, since the nuclear proliferation antigen Ki67 correlates well with CD30 positivity in those cells in-situ (Gerdes et al., 1987). Other data on the functional properties are not yet available.

There is, however, other data corroborating the interest in the antigen. Soluble CD30 (sCD30) antigen with a molecular weight of 90 kD as well as soluble Interleukin-2 receptor (sIl-2R) can be detected in the serum of a certain percentage of untreated Hodgkin's disease patients (Pfreundschuh et al., 1989). The clinical significance of elevated sCD30 and sIl-2R levels is currently being tested.

Attempts are being made to develop CD30 antibody conjugates for specific diagnosis and therapy of Hodgkin's disease in vivo. An immunoscintigraphy pilot study using radioiodine-labeled HRS-1 antibody was completed with promising results (Carde et al., 1989).

Data has been more diverging concerning T and B cell markers. Whereas all of the cell lines do stain positive for at least one T cell (CD 2-5, 7) or B cell (CD 19, 20, 21) antibody cluster, until recently only 11% (T) and 15% (B) of Hodgkin and Reed-Sternberg cells in biopsy specimen were considered positive for the related antigens (Drexler et al., 1988). Further optimization of antibodies and techniques in the last two years more than doubled the fraction of primary Hodgkin's cells detectable to bind lymphocyte associated antibodies. Depending on antibodies and methods, more than 60% of Hodgkin tumour cells bind either T (40%) or B cell (20%) markers (Agnarsson et al., 1989; Herbst et al., 1989; Stein et al., 1989; Casey et al., 1988; Oka et al., 1988; Falini et al., 1987). Differences between histological subtypes have been reported. Nodular sclerosing Hodgkin's disease, the most frequent histology, and mixed cellularity cells often have a T-cell associated immunophenotype. Lymphocyte predominant Hodgkin's disease has a definite B-cell phenotype with constant expression of B-cell antigens (CD20, LN1, 2, L26) and J-chain (Coles et al., 1989; Agnarsson et al., 1989; Stein et al., 1986). These findings distinguish lymphocyte predominance from the other subentities of Hodgkin's disease (Wright et al., 1989; Poppema et al., 1985).

The relevance of some markers has not yet been evaluated in detail. In 50% of mixed cellularity and lymphocyte predominant subtypes, CD45, the common leukocyte antigen (CLA) can be detected (Agnarsson et al., 1989). CD24, M2 and CFU-G(EM)M-associated antigens occur on L428 (Athan et al., 1989).

1.3. Other Markers

Rosetting of T cells with Hodgkin cells occurs both in vivo and in vitro (Stuart et al., 1977; Diehl et al., 1982). On L428 cells, both LFA3 and ICAM1 antigens are expressed (unpublished data). The presence of these ligands for T cell structures CD2 and CD11/18 might explain the adhesion mechanism responsible for T cell rosettes (Sanders et al., 1988).

Hodgkin cells are known to stimulate mixed lymphocyte reactions both in vivo and in vitro (Engelmann et al., 1980; Fischer et al., 1983). They are positive for nonspecific esterase (Diehl et al., 1982). Phagocytotic properties as well as polyclonal Ig chains in primary Hodgkin's disease may be considered artifacts (Stein 1988).

2. Genotype

2.1. Cytogenetics

Cytogenetic analysis of primary Hodgkin and Reed-Sternberg cells is hampered by the low number of obtainable mitoses and their poor chromosome banding qualities (Fonatsch et al., submitted for publication). A significant number of dividing cells with a normal karyotype represent most likely reactive lymphoid cells (Rowley et al., 1982). Depending on the histological subtype, between 75%(NS) and 42%(LP) of cases studied yielded evaluable metaphases. Short term cultures of 12 involved lymphnodes exhibited an uncommonly high number (75%) of nonclonal karyotype abnormalities (Dennis et al., 1989). In the 40 cases so far reported in complete karyotype banding studies, the percentage of abnormal karyotypes varied considerably (22% - 83%) between studies (Thangavelu et al., 1989). Although numerical and structural cytogenetic abnormalities were reported in a portion of cases studied, a specific chromosomal marker of Hodgkin's disease - like the Philadelphia chromosome in CML - could not yet be defined (Kaplan, 1980; Rowley et al., 1982; Cabanillas et al., 1988; Thangavelu et al., 1989).

Chromosome abnormalities of relapse cases or treated patients' karyotypes did not differ from examinations at the time of diagnosis (Thangavelu et al., 1989; Schouten et al., 1989). Among Hodgkin's disease associated chromosomal abnormalities, aneuploidy (100%) with hyperdiploidy (70%) is most frequent (Anastasi et al., 1987). Chromosomes 5, 2, 1, 12 and 21 are often duplicated. Rearrangements, especially translocations or deletions, were found in two thirds of cases, often involving 1p, 1q, 2q, 6q, 8q, 11q, 11p, 14q and Xq (Thangavelu et al., 1989). However, with the number of evaluable studies still low, the nonrandom involvement pattern has to be defined and correlated to clinical features in more detail. Breakpoints 11q23, 14q32, 6q, 8q24 and 11q13 have frequently been associated with B and T-cell lymphomas (Cabanillas et al., 1988).

Results with nonrandom karyotype abnormalities were also found in Hodgkin's disease derived cell lines. Interestingly, on four of the seven chromosome marker regions involved in these lines cellular oncogenes have been localized. In cell lines L428 and L540, chromosome abnormalities comprise the chromosome segments involved in Ig (L428, 14q32) and TCR (L540, 7q11-36) gene rearrangements. In-situ hybridization on L540 revealed a previously unidentified translocation of the met oncogene and TCR beta from the long arm of chromosome 7 onto the short arm of chromosome 21 (marker chromosome XIp). In this line, TCR alpha is translocated to another marker chromosome. Active nucleolus organizer regions (NOR) and active ribosomal RNA (rDNA) genes are detectable in the centromere region of both marker chromosomes IX and XI (Fonatsch et al., submitted for publication).

Peripheral blood lymphocytes from patients with Hodgkin's disease and their siblings show a much greater number of abnormal metaphases when incubated with cytostatic drugs compared to normal controls. One might well speculate about the genetic instability as an etiologic factor in Hodgkin's disease. In the future this hypothesis will have to be defined more precisely.

2.2. Gene Rearrangements

None of the phenotypic modalities of characterization allows for exact location of the Hodgkin cell within the haematopoietic differentiation system. Genetic differentiation markers add some evidence (Stein et al., 1989; Athan et al., 1989).

During differentiation of T and B lymphocytes, recombinations of immunoglobulin (Ig) or T cell receptor (TCR) genes precede the formation of functional immunoglobulin or T cell receptor molecules i.e. antigen-specific T and B cell antigen receptors (Leder et al., 1983; Hedrick et al., 1984). These rearrangements are specific for each B and T cell. The specific order of rearrangements (IgH before IgL kappa, then lambda; TCR gamma, delta before TCR beta, then alpha) allows to define the differentiation stage of such a cell clone more precisely.

In the nine available Hodgkin's disease derived cell lines results of these studies are heterogeneous concerning the differentiation into T or B lymphocytes (Table 2). Five of the lines show Ig, four have TCR re-arrangements (Falk et al., 1987; Drexler et al., 1989). Some of these lines also express Ig and/or TCR mRNA.

In primary biopsy tissue, again, the percentage of malignant cells within the tumour sample is close to the detection threshold, thus limiting the reliability of clonality studies in primary tumour material. Assembling the available data, in 4% of cases Ig, in 11% TCR rearrangements were detected.

Since B as well as T cell rearrangements occur in tested cell lines and fresh tumour material, we can not eventually determine whether the cell of origin in Hodgkin's disease is a B or T lymphocyte. Furthermore, clonal Ig or TCR rearrangements are neither specific for malignancy nor for derivation of a specific lineage. Clonal Ig rearrangements can be found in benign tissue under certain conditions like in lymphoproliferative or lymphoepithelial lesions (Cleary et al., 1984; Pelicci et al., 1983; Fishleder et al., 1987). In nonlymphocytic leukemias Ig and TCR rearrangements have also been reported (Rovigatti et al., 1984; Cheng et al., 1986). It has not eventually been determined if the rearrangements detected in primary tissue studies were derived from Hodgkin and Reed-Sternberg cells (Knowles et al., 1986). With these important doubts, the data available from in vitro and in vivo experiments favour a lymphoid origin of the Hodgkin and Reed-Sternberg cells (Stein et al., 1989; Schaadt et al., 1988; Drexler et al., 1989). Although Ig or TCR gene rearrangements have also been detected in cell lines of myeloid origin, especially the fact that all of the cell lines do have either Ig or TCR gene rearrangements (Table 1) which are often transcribed may point to an immature lymphoid origin of these cells (Hsu et al., 1989; Tesch et al., submitted for publication; Drexler et al., 1989).

2.3. Oncogenes and Oncogene Products

Proto-oncogenes are cellular genes potentially involved in tumourigenesis. Upon activation, they may affect malignant transformation. Proto-oncogenes closely associated with certain malignancies include translocated c-myc in Burkitt's lymphoma, bcr-joined c-abl in Ph+-CML and Ph+-ALL and bcl2 in follicular lymphoma (Klein, 1983; Collins et al., 1984; Fainstain et al., 1987; Cleary et al., 1984).

The analysis of proto-oncogenes in Hodgkin's disease derived cell lines revealed a heterogeneous expression pattern. Some of the proto-oncogenes (c-myc, c-myb, c-raf and N-ras) appeared in all of the four tested Hodgkin's disease derived cell lines (Jücker et al., submitted for publication). However, these proto-oncogenes are often also detected in leukemia cell lines or nonmalignant haematopoietic cells. Other genes could only be detected in some of the Hodgkin's derived cell lines. Transcripts of c-met, a proto-oncogene originally described in an osteosarcoma cell line, are expressed in Hodgkin's disease derived cell lines L428 and L540 (Dean et al., 1985). The gene is translocated into the vicinity of a transcriptionally active locus on marker chromosome XI in L540 but not in L428(see Cytogenetics section for details in Fonatsch et al., submitted for publicationc). Evidence for a rearrangement or an amplification involving c-met in these lines could not be detected. It has hitherto not been analyzed if c-met has transforming capability in hematopoietic cells.

Aberrant transcripts of the proto-oncogene c-fes occur in the L428 and Cole cell lines. A deletion or rearrangement of the gene was not detectable (Jücker et al., submitted for publication). Whether these aberrant transcripts encode a transforming protein is not clear yet.

L540 and L428 express high levels of transcripts specific for the proto-oncogene c-fms as well as the resulting protein, the CSF-1-receptor. It may be involved in autocrine stimulation of these cell lines (Paietta et al.; 1989)

The reason for the heterogeneous expression pattern of proto-oncogenes in Hodgkin's disease derived cell lines is not clear. It might represent different differentiation stages of the cells or in certain cases deregulated and probably activated proto-oncogenes (Jücker et al., submitted for publication; Paietta et al., 1989).

Oncogene expression in primary Hodgkin's cells has to date only been studied to a limited extent. Activated N-ras oncogenes have been observed in two Hodgkin cases by transfection experiments (Sklar et al., 1985). It can not be defined whether these mutations occurred in the Hodgkin and Reed-Sternberg cells. High levels of c-myc protein appeared in the nuclei of Reed-Sternberg cells as well as in surrounding lymphocytes and histiocytes (Mitani et al., 1988).

The influence of oncogenes on the tumourigenesis of Hodgkin's disease could not yet be clarified.

2.4. EBV-Infection

Epstein-Barr-Virus infection has long been suspected to exist in Hodgkin's disease. In addition to the clinical incidence of elevated anti-EBV-antibody titers and detection of EBV in Hodgkin's disease derived cell line L591 , monoclonal or oligoclonal proliferation of EBV is present in part of the biopsy specimen in Hodgkin's disease (Diehl et al., 1982; Staal et al., 1989; Weiss et al., 1987). Recently, viral DNA was detected in Hodgkin and Reed-Sternberg cells by in-situ hybridization in 19% of cases (Weiss et al., 1989). This incidence may be higher in AIDS associated Hodgkin's disease, where 4 of 7 cases displayed EBV DNA in the tumour cells (Uccini et al., 1989). Although EBV is known for its transforming capacity in B cells, its functional relevance in the pathogenesis of Hodgkin's disease remains to be elucidated (Henle et al., 1968).

EBV transformed lymphocytes may be an interesting model for the cellular transformation in Hodgkin's disease (Herbst et al., 1989). Analogous to Hodgkin cell lines, some lymphoblastoid cell lines present incomplete or no Ig rearrangements while expressing activation markers (CD25, CD30, Ki-24) (Katamine et al., 1984; Gregory et al., 1987).

3. Cytokine Production

The humoral interaction of immunocompetent cells via cytokines is a fascinating focus of interest. Judging from the intense local and systemic reactions a Hodgkin's tumour inflicts onto its host organism, the tumour cells may interfere directly or via accessory cells with the immune system through mediators. Some aspects of the typical biology of Hodgkin's disease suggest the involvement of particular cytokines (Diehl, 1985)(Table 3).

Table 3. Cytokines which could be involved in Hodgkin's disease as derived from cell line research

Biological Features in Hodgkin's disease	Possible Mediators	Molecular Weight [kD]	In-Vitro Evidence
Lymphoproliferation*, Fever, Nightsweats, Immunodeficiency	Il-1*	30-32	Immunostaining[1], Bioassay[2]
	Il-2*	15,5	Il-2R (CD25), ZO Growth
	Il-6*	26	Northern Blot
	TNF-α	17	Immunostaining, Bioassay
	TNF-β	20	Bioassay[3]
Leukocyte/Eosinophil-Infiltration, Myeloproliferation	GM-CSF	18-22	Proteinsequencing
	G-CSF	19	Bioassay[4]
	M-CSF	70-90	Northern Blot, M-CSF R[5] Autocrine Function
Fibrosis	TGF-β	16,5?	Northern Blot[6]

[1] Hsu, 1985
[2] Il1-dependent cell line
[3] cytotoxicity assay
[4] Human and murine stemm cell assay
[5] Product of c-fms proto-oncogene
[6] HD derived TGFB active at physiological pH

Diverse biological activities have been discovered in the supernatant of Hodgkin's disease derived cell lines. These include T cell rosette inhibition and costimulation of T cells, fibroblast growth induction, EBV+B cell blast proliferation and leukocyte migration inhibition (Schaadt et al., 1988; Schell-Frederick et al., 1988). It is being tested if the activities can be ascribed to any of the known cytokines, or if other factors are released.

Among evidence for several interleukins and TNF, the IL-2-receptor alpha chain (CD25) antigen is present both on most primary and cell line specimen. Hodgkin's disease derived cell line L540 expresses functional high affinity Il-2-receptors consisting of both beta and alpha chains (Tesch et al., submitted for publication).

Fibrosis is a characteristic feature of nodular sclerosing Hodgkin's disease. Cell line L428 could be demonstrated to produce a high molecular weight TGFb variety. In contrast to previously described TGFß-receptor-binding cytokines it is active at physiologic pH and does neither stand nor require acidification to be activated (Newcom et al., 1988).

Several growth factors are released by the cell lines. Both GM-CSF and G-CSF have been described (Byrne et al., 1986). An autocrine pathway involving a CSF-1 stimulation circle could be demonstrated in L540 and L428 cells using a CSF-1 assay system and mRNA probes for CSF-1 and CSF1-receptor (Paietta et al., 1989).

Until now, the existence of mediators in primary Hodgkin's material could only be demonstrated by cell surface or cytoplasmic immunostaining for Il-1 (Hsu et al., 1986). In-situ detection techniques for mRNA and proteins will help to verify cell line research results in-vivo. There is little doubt that cytokine interactions determine the pathophysiology of Hodgkin's disease (Diehl, 1985).

Conclusion

Although curable in the majority of cases, the origin of Hodgkin's disease is still a mystery to modernday research more than 150 years after the original description (Hodgkin, 1832). In this decade, however, results have been obtained that provide some more inside views concerning this puzzle (Diehl, 1989). The assumption that Hodgkin and Reed-Sternberg cells are the neoplastic cells in Hodgkin's disease is, due to the lack of other candidates, widely accepted (Diehl et al., 1982; Diehl, 1985). The availability of in-vitro cultured cells from Hodgkin's disease patients has led to a deeper understanding of the geno- and phenotypical characteristics of the Hodgkin tumour cell. The identity of in vivo and in vitro cultured counterparts and the presence of monoclonal EBV DNA in Hodgkin and Reed-Sternberg cells have demonstrated that Hodgkin and Reed-Sternberg cells are of clonal origin. Hodgkin and Reed-Sternberg cells bear the biological abnormalities that have been detected (Diehl et al., 1982; Stein et al., 1989). The generation of antibodies against epitopes of these in-vitro cells (L428, L540) has expanded knowledge on the heterogeneity of the pathological and clinical facettes of Hodgkin's disease and associated lymphomas (Ki-1-lymphomas). Remarkably, the results gained from primary material in no point openly contradict the cell line data. Most likely, these cell lines indeed stem from the tumour cell in Hodgkin's disease (Diehl et al., 1982; Diehl, 1985; Diehl et al., 1988; Schaadt et al., 1989).

Keeping in mind that the available data are not complete, a working hypothesis on the descent of the Hodgkin's cell can be contrived. In brief, the morphologically distinct Hodgkin and Reed-Sternberg cell has an immunophenotype characteristic of activated T or B cells (Stein et al., 1989). Dissociate from that, the genotype is immaturely lymphoid (Falk et al., 1987; Tesch et al., submitted for publication; Herbst et al., 1989). Rearrangements and expressions of the immunoglobulin super gene family are frequently incomplete or irregular (Tesch et al., submitted for publication; Herbst et al., 1989). The heterogeneity of the clinical and histological appearance of Hodgkin's disease and the multitude of different - partially controversial - cellular markers might be explained by Hodgkin's disease being a group of etio-pathophysiologically associated but not identical disease entities. The origin might be the same target cell transformed at different stages of maturation, or, alternatively, several biologically related diseases each with a different etio-pathogenesis.

The described set of data may well be explained by the Hodgkin's lymphoma cell being derived from an immature lymphoid stage of differentiation that is transformed prior to or during the B or T cell receptor gene rearrangement (Falk et al., 1987; Herbst et al., 1989; Kamesaki et al., 1989). The transformation process could then superimpose maturation characteristics onto the cells. Myelomonocytic features could evolve in analogy to mechanisms demonstrated by conversion of B cells into myelomonocytoid cells by oncogenes or following LPS treatment (Klinken et al., 1988; Davidson et al., 1988). An abundance of possible transformation sources is present in Hodgkin cells, including cytogenetic abnormalities and evidence for proto-oncogene and EBV involvement. The cytokine-receptor interactions of the resulting paracrine cell with the immune system are likely to produce the typical morphological and clinical manifestations of Hodgkin's disease.

References

Agnarsson, B.A. et al. (1989): The immunophenotype of Reed-Sternberg cells. A study of 50 cases of Hodgkin's disease using fixed frozen tissues. *Cancer* 63, 2083-2087.

Anastasi, J. et al. (1987): DNA aneuploidy in Hodgkin's disease. A multiparameter flow-cytometric analysis with cytologic correlation. *Am. J. Pathol.* 128, 573-582.

Athan, E. et al. (1989): Stability of multiple antigen receptor gene rearrangements and immunophenotype in Hodgkin's disease derived cell line L428 and variant subline L428KSA. *Leukemia* 3, 505-510.

Burrichter, H. et al. (1985): Hodgkin Cell Factors. In *Mediators in Oncology*. Serono Symposia Meetings. Ed. Raven Press.

Byrne, P.V. et al. (1986): Human granulocyte-macrophage colony stimulating factor purified from a Hodgkin's tumor cell line. *Biochemica Biophysica Acta* 00, 266-273

Cabanillas, F. et al. (1988): Cytogenetic features of Hodgkin's disease suggest possible origin from a lymphocyte. *Blood* 71, 1615-1617.

Carde, P. et al. (1989): Radiolabeled monoclonal antibodies against Reed-Sternberg cells for in vivo imaging of Hodgkin's disease by Immunoscintigraphy. In *New Aspects in the Diagnosis and Treatment of Hodgkin's Disease*, ed. V. Diehl, M. Pfreundschuh & M. Löffler, pp. 101-111. Rec. Results Cancer Res. Vol 117. Berlin, Heidelberg: Springer-Verlag.

Casey, T.T. et al. (1988): Immunophenotypes of Reed-Sternberg cells in plastic sections: a study of nine cases of nodular sclerosing Hodgkin's disease. *Lab. Invest.* 58, 16a.

Cheng, G.Y. et al. (1986): T cell receptor and immunoglobulin rearrangements in acute myeloblastic leukemia. *J. Exp. Med.* 163, 414-424.

Cleary, M.L et al. (1984): Immunoglobulin gene rearrangement as a diagnostic criterion of B cell lymphoma. *Proc. Nat. Ac. Sciences USA* 81, 593-597.

Cleary, M.L. et al. (1986): Cloning and structural analysis of cDNAs for bcl-2 and a hybrid bcl-2/immunoglobulin transcript resulting from the t(14;18) translocation. *Cell* 47, 19-28.

Coles, F.B. et al. (1988): Hodgkin's disease, lymphocyte-predominant type: immunoreactivity with B-cell antibodies. *Mod. Pathol.* 1, 274-278.

Collins, S.J. et al. (1984): Altered transcription of the c-abl oncogene in K-562 and other chronic myelogenous leukemia cells. *Science* 225, 72-74.

Davidson, W.F. et al. (1988): Relationships between B cell and myeloid differentiation. Studies with a B lymphocyte progenitor line, HAFTL-1. *J. Exp. Med.* 168, 389-407.

Dean, M. et al. (1985): The human met oncogene is related to the tyrosine kinase oncogenes. *Nature* 318, 385-388.

Dennis, T.R.; Stock, A.D.; Winberg, C.D.; Sheibani, K.; Rappaport, H. (1989): Cytogenetic studies of Hodgkin's disease. Analysis of involved lymph nodes from 12 patients. *Cancer Genet. Cytogenet.* 1989 37, 201-208.

Diehl, V. et al. (1982): Characteristics of Hodgkin's disease derived cell lines. *Cancer Treat. Rep.* 66, 615-632.

Diehl, V. et al. (1985): Phenotypic and genotypic analysis of Hodgkin's disease derived cell lines: histopathological and clinical implications. *Cancer Surveys* 4, 399-419.

Diehl, V. (1985): Hodgkin's disease: the Remaining Challenge. *Eur. Surg. Res.* 17, 388-398.

Diehl, V. et al. (1989). *New Aspects in the Diagnosis and Treatment of Hodgkin's Disease*. Rec. Results Cancer Res. Vol 117. Berlin, Heidelberg: Springer-Verlag.

Drexler, H.G. et al. (1988): Genotypes and immunophenotypes of Hodgkin's disease derived cell lines. *Leukemia* 2, 371-376.

Drexler, H.G. et al. (1989): Is the Hodgkin cell a T- or a B-lymphocyte? Recent evidence from geno- and immunophenotypic analysis and in vitro cell lines. *Hematol. Oncol.* 7, 95-113.

Engelmann, E.G. et al. (1980): Autologous mixed lymphocyte reaction in patients with Hodgkin's disease. *J. Clin. Investig.* 66, 149-158.

Fainstain, E. et al. (1987): A new fused transcript in Philadelphia chromosome positive acute lymphoblastic leukemia. *Nature* 330, 386-388.

Falini, B. et al. (1987): Expression of lymphoid -associated antigens on Hodgkin's and Reed-Sternberg cells of Hodgkin's disease; an immunocytochemical study on lymphnode cytospins using monoclonal antibodies. *Histopathology* 11, 1229-1242.

Falk, M.H. et al. (1987): Phenotype versus immunoglobulin and T cell receptor genotype of Hodgkin-derived cell lines: activation of immature lymphoid cells in Hodgkin's disease. *Int. J. Cancer* 40, 262-269.

Fischer, R.I. et al. (1983): Neoplastic cells from Hodgkin's disease are potent stimulators of human primary mixed lymphocyte cultures. *J. Immunol.* 130, 2666-2670.

Fishleder, A. et al. (1987): Uniform detection of immunoglobulin gene rearrangement in benign lymphoepithelial lesions. *N. Engl. J. Med.* 316, 1118-1121.

Gerdes, J. et al.: Tumor growth fraction in Hodgkin's disease. *Am. J. Pathol.* 129, 390-393.

Gregory, C.D. et al. (1987): Epstein-Barr virus-transformed human precursor B cell lines: altered growth phenotype of lines with germline or rearranged but nonexpressed heavy chain genes. *Eur. J. Immunol.* 17, 1199-1207.

Hansen, H. et al. (1989): The Hodgkin-associated Ki-1 antigen exists in an intracellular and a membrane-bound form. *Biol. Chem.* 370, 409-416.

Hedrick, S.M. et al. (1984): Isolation of cDNA clones encoding T cell specific membrane associated proteins. *Nature* 308, 149-153.

Henle, G. et al. (1968): Relation of Burkitt's tumor associated Herpes-type virus to infectious mononucleosis. *Proc. Nat. Ac. Science USA* 59, 94-101.

Herbst, H. et al: (1989): Immunoglobulin and T cell receptor gene rearrangements in Hodgkin's disease and Ki-1 positive large cell lymphoma: dissociation between phenotype and genotype. *Leukemia Res.* 13, 103-116.

Hodgkin, T. (1832): On some morbid appearances of the absorbent glands and spleen. *Med. Chir. Transactions* 17, 68-114.

Hsu, S.M. et al. (1984): Leu M1 and peanut agglutinin stain the neoplastic cells of Hodgkin's disease. *Am. J. Clin. Pathol.* 82, 29-32.

Hsu, S.M. et al. (1986): Expression of Interleukin-I in H-RS cells and neoplastuc cells from true histiocytic lymphomas. *Am. J. Pathol.* 186, 331-336.

Hsu, S. et al. (1989): Aberrant expression of T and B cell markers in myelocyte/monocyte/histiocyte derived lymphoma and leukemia cells. *Am. J. Pathol.* 134, 203-212.

Jones, D.B. et al. (1985): Phenotype analysis of an established cell line derived from a patient with Hodgkin's disease. *Hematol. Oncol.* 3, 133-145.

Kamesaki, H. et al. (1989): A new hypothesis on the cellular origin of Reed-Sternberg and Hodgkin cells based on the immunological and molecular genetic analysis of the KM-H2 Line. In *New Aspects in the Diagnosis and Treatment of Hodgkin's Disease*, ed. V. Diehl, M. Pfreundschuh & M. Löffler, pp. 83-90. Rec. Results Cancer Res. Vol 117. Berlin, Heidelberg: Springer-Verlag.

Kaplan, H.S. (1980): *Hodgkin's Disease*. Cambridge, MA: Harvard University Press.

Katamine, S. et al. (1984): Epstein-Barr virus transforms precursor B cells even before immunoglobulin gene rearrangements. *Nature* 309, 369-372.

Klein, G. (1983): Specific chromosomal translocations and the genesis of B cell derived tumors in mice and men. *Cell* 32, 311-315.

Klinken, S.P. et al. (1988): Hemopoietic lineage switch: v-raf oncogene converts En-myc transgenic B cells into macrophages. *Cell* 53, 857-867.

Knowles, D.M. et al. (1986): Immunoglobu- lin and T cell receptor ß-chain gene rearrangement analysis of Hodgkin's disease: Implications for lineage determination and differential diagnosis. *Proc. Nat. Ac. Science USA* 83, 7942-7946.

Leder, P. et al. (1983): Translocations among antibody genes in human cancer. *Science* 222, 766-771.

Lukes, R.J. et al. (1966): Report of the nomenclature committee. *Cancer Res.* 26, 1311.

Lukes, R.J. et al. (1969): Reed-Sternberg-like cells in infectious mononucleosis. *Lancet* ii, 1000-1004.

Mitani, S. et al. (1988): Expression of the c-myc oncogene product and ras family oncogene products in various human malignant lymphomas defined by immunohistochemical techniques. *Cancer* 62, 2085-2093.

Newcom, S. et al. (1988): L428 nodular sclerosing Hodgkin's cell secretes a unique transforming growth factor beta active at physiologic pH. *J. Clin. Investig.* 82, 1915-1921.

O'Connor, N.T.J. et al. (1987): Genotypic analysis of large lymphomas which express the Ki-1 antigen. *Histopathology* 11, 733-740.

Oka, K. et al. (1988): Anti-Leu-3a antibody reactivity with Reed-Sternberg cells of Hodgkin's disease. *Arch. Pathol. Lab. Med.* 112, 139-142.

Paietta, E. et al. (1989): Hodgkin's disease cells: Origin from a bipotential lymphoid/macrophage progenitor cell? *Proc. Am. Ass. Cancer Res.* 30, 430.

Pelicci, P.G. et al. (1983): Lymphoid tumors displaying rearrangements of both immunoglobulin and T cell receptor genes. *J. Exp. Med.* 162, 1015-1024.

Pfreundschuh, M. et al. (1988): Hodgkin and Reed Sternberg cell associated monoclonal antibodies HRS-1 and HRS-2 react with activated cells of lymphoid and monocytoid origin. *Anticancer Res.* 8, 217-224.

Pfreundschuh, M. et al. (1989): Soluble CD30 Antigen as a tumor marker in the sera of patients with Hodgkin's lymphoma. *Proc. 7th Int. Congr. Immunol.* 107-129.

Poppema, S. et al. (1985): Morphologic, immunologic, enzymehistochemical and chromosomal analysis of a cell line derived from Hodgkin's disease. Evidence for a B-cell origin of Sternberg-Reed cells. *Cancer* 55, 683-690.

Rovigatti, U. et al. (1984): Heavy chain immunoglobulin gene rearrangements in acute nonlymphocytic leukemia. *Blood* 63, 1023-1027.

Rowley, J.D. (1982): Chromosomes in Hodgkin's disease. *Cancer Treat. Rep.* 66, 639-643.

Sanders, M.E. et al. (1988): Molecular pathways of adhesion in spontaneous rosetting of T lymphocytes to the Hodgkin's cell line L428. *Cancer Res.* 48, 37-40.

Schaadt, M. et al. (1980): Two neoplastic cell lines with unique features derived from Hodgkin's disease. *Int. J. Cancer,* 26, 723-731.

Schaadt, M. et al. (1985): The cell of origin in Hodgkin's disease: conclusions from in vivo and in vitro studies. *Int. Rev. Exp. Pathol.* 27, 185-202.

Schaadt, M. et al. (1988): Immunologic, functional and molecular genetic properties of Hodgkin's disease derived cell lines. *Cancer Reviews* 10, 108-122.

Schaadt, M. et al. (1989): Biology of Hodgkin cell lines. In *New Aspects in the Diagnosis and Treatment of Hodgkin's Disease,* ed. V. Diehl, M. Pfreundschuh & M. Löffler, pp. 53-61. Rec. Results Cancer Res. Vol 117. Berlin, Heidelberg: Springer-Verlag.

Schell-Frederick, E. et al. (1988): Inhibition of human neutrophil migration by supernatants from Hodgkin's disease derived cell lines. *Eur. J. Clin. Investig.* 18, 290-296.

Schouten, H. et al. (1989): Chromosomal abnormalities in Hodgkin's disease. *Blood* 73, 2149-2154.

Schwab, U. et al. (1982): Production of a monoclonal antibody specific for Hodgkin and Sternberg-Reed cells on Hodgkin's lymphoma and a subset of normal lymphoid cells. *Nature* 299, 65-67.

Sklar, M.D. et al. (1985): Isolation of activated ras transforming genes from two patients with Hodgkin's disease. *Int. J. Radiat. Oncol. Biol. Phys.* 11, 49-55.

Staal, S.P. et al. (1989): A survey of Epstein-Barr Virus DNA in lymphoid tissue. Frequent detection in Hodgkin's disease. *Am. J. Clin. Pathol.* 91,1-5.

Stein, H. et al. (1982): Identification of Hodgkin and Reed-Sternberg cells as a unique cell type derived from a newly detected small-cell population. *Int. J. Cancer* 30, 445-459.

Stein, H. et al. (1985): The expression of the Hodgkin's disease associated antigen Ki-1 in reactive and neoplastic lymphoid tissue. Evidence that Reed-Sternberg cells and histiocytic malignancies are derived from activated lymphoid cells. *Blood* 66, 848-858.

Stein, H. et al. (1986): Reed-Sternberg cells and Hodgkin cells in lymphocyte predominant Hodgkin's disease of nodular subtype contain J chain. *Am. J. Clin. Pathol.* 86, 292-297.

Stein, H. (1988): Comments on Hodgkin's disease: the Reed-Sternberg cell by P. Bucsky. *Blut* 57, 143-146.

Stein, H. et al. (1989): Immunology of Hodgkin and Reed-Sternberg cells. In *New Aspects in the Diagnosis and Treatment of Hodgkin's Disease,* ed. V. Diehl, M. Pfreundschuh & M. Löffler, pp. 14-26. Rec. Results Cancer Res. Vol 117. Berlin, Heidelberg: Springer-Verlag.

Strum, S.B. et al. (1971): Interrelations of the histologic types of Hodgkin's disease. *Arch. Pathol.* 91, 127-139.

Stuart, A.E. et al. (1977): Reed Sternberg cell/lymphocyte interaction. *Lancet* ii, 768-769.

Thangavelu, M. et al. (1989): Chromosomal abnormalities in Hodgkin's disease. *Hematology/Oncology Clinics of North America* 3, 221-235.

Uccini, S. et al. (1987): High frequency of Epstein-Barr virus genome in HIV-positive patients with Hodgkin's disease. *Lancet* i, 1458.

Weiss, L. et al. (1987): Epstein-Barr viral DNA in Tissues of Hodgkin's disease. *Am. J. Pathol.* 129, 86-91.

Weiss, L. et al. (1989): Detection of Epstein-Barr viral genomes in Reed-Sternberg cells of Hodgkin's disease. *N. Engl. J. Med.* 320, 502-506.

Wright, D.H. et al. (1989): Pathology of Hodgkin's disease: anything new? In *New Aspects in the Diagnosis and Treatment of Hodgkin's Disease*, ed. V. Diehl, M. Pfreundschuh & M. Löffler, pp. 3-13. Rec. Results Cancer Res. Vol 117. Berlin, Heidelberg: Springer-Verlag.

The histology and immunohistology of Hodgkin's disease : its relationship to prognosis and clinical behaviour

K.A. MacLennan[1], M.H. Bennett[2], J. Bosq[3], J. Diebold[4], A.M. Mandard[5], B. Vaughan Hudson[6], G. Vaughan Hudson[6]

1 Royal Marsden Hospital, Fulham Road, London SW3 6JJ, England
2 Mount Vernon Hospital, Northwood, Middx HA6 2RN, England
3 Institut Gustave-Roussy, 94805 Villejuif, France
4 Hôtel-Dieu, 75181 Paris Cedex 04, France
5 Centre François Baclesse, BP 5026, 14021 Caen Cedex, France
6 Middlesex Hospital, London W1N 8AA, England

Summary

Histopathological analysis of 2819 patients, randomised into the clinical studies of the BNLI, has clearly demonstrated the clinical value of the modified Rye classification in patient management. In particular the subdivision of the numerically predominant, nodular sclerosis type, into two prognostic grades, has proved useful in selection of optimal therapy.

The distinction of Hodgkin's disease (HD) from the non-Hodgkin's lymphomas (NHL) is of major clinical importance and although the pathologist can accomplish this in the majority of cases there are a significant number that cause difficulties in resolving this differential diagnosis. These problems currently appear most prominent in "histiocyte rich" examples of HD and anaplastic large cell (Ki 1) lymphomas.

Immunocytochemistry and molecular biology have helped pathologists in establishing a diagnosis based upon more objective criteria but these techniques do not at present permit an absolute distinction between HD and the NHL's.
Good evidence now exists that there are at least two distinct forms of HD. Lymphocyte predominant nodular HD (nodular paragranuloma) appears to be a disease of the germinal centre which demonstrates a divergent clinical presentation, anatomic distribution and natural history to other histologic subtypes of HD.

Résumé

L'analyse histologique des 2819 malades inclus dans les essais thérapeutiques comparatifs du BNLI, a clairement établi que la subdivision en deux groupes de pronostic différent du sous-type sclérose nodulaire de la classification de Rye, numériquement prédominant, s'est révélée très utile pour le choix thérapique afin d'obtenir une efficacité maximum.

La distinction entre maladie de Hodgkin et lymphome non Hodgkinien est d'une importance clinique considérable. Bien que dans la plupart des cas il soit possible à l'anatomopathologiste de séparer ces deux entités, il existe un nombre non négligeable de cas pour lesquels subsistent des problèmes de diagnostic différentiel. Ces difficultés surviennent le plus souvent dans les cas de maladie de Hodgkin à prédominance lymphoïde "riche en histiocytes" et dans les lymphomes à larges cellules anaplasiques (Ki 1).

L'immunocytochimie et la biologie moléculaire ont aidé les anatomopathologistes à établir un diagnostic basé sur des critères plus objectifs mais ces techniques ne permettent pas à l'heure actuelle d'établir une distinction absolue entre maladie de Hodgkin et lymphome non Hodgkinien.

Il y a maintenant de bonnes raisons de penser qu'il existe au moins deux formes distinctes de la maladie de Hodgkin. La forme à prédominance lymphoïde de type nodulaire (paragranulome nodulaire) apparait comme une maladie se développant à partir du centre germinatif, associée à un tableau clinique, un phénotype, et une histoire naturelle différentes de celles des autres sous-types histologiques.

Introduction

Unlike the non-Hodgkin's lymphomas (NHL), the classification of Hodgkin's disease (HD) in current usage (Lukes & Butler, 1966, Lukes, Butler & Hicks, 1966; Lukes et al., 1966) has remained essentially unchanged for over 20 years and most pathologists believe they are familiar with the terminology and criteria employed. It is therefore surprising to find high levels of disagreement between pathologists in establishing the diagnosis of HD and it's classification which may range from 13 % (Chelloul et al., 1972; Miller et al., 1982) to a staggering figure of 47 % reported by Symmers (1968). The reasons for the difficulties pathologists experience in the diagnosis of HD are not difficult to understand. HD is rare and most pathologists will see only a few cases a year and this combined with the complexity of the histological picture which may be closely mimicked by a variety of neoplastic and non-neoplastic lymphoproliferative conditions will lead to errors in diagnosis.

These problems are compounded by our lack of understanding of the basic biology of HD and our ignorance of the precise identity of the Reed-Sternberg cell (R-S cell). Indeed it now appears that there may be several distinctive biological entities cohabiting under this eponymous term and the borderline between HD and the NHL's may not solely be due to our difficulties in pathological diagnosis but represent a real biological interface between the two diseases processes.

In this paper, we will present our combined experience of the diagnosis of over 3,000 cases of HD accrued in the clinical studies of the British National Lymphoma Investigation (BNLI) and Groupe Pierre et Marie Curie (GPMC). Particular emphasis will be directed to the prognostic significance of classification, the distinction of HD from the NHL's and the biological heterogeneity of different histological subtypes of HD.

The Prognostic Significance of Histological Classification in Hodgkin's Disease

Although the Lukes and Butler classification was originally intended to provide prognostic information, many now feel the recent improvements in patient management have obliterated the differences in survival between histological subtypes of Hodgkin's disease (Torti et al., 1979; Hoppe et al., 1980; Fuller et al., 1980; Culine et al., 1989) and the role of the pathologist is restricted to establishing the diagnosis and documenting the extent of spread (Dorfman & Colby, 1982).

In 1979, the BNLI analysed the survival of 1,189 patients randomised into clinical trials who had been subdivided according to the Rye classification (Figure 1). For 96 % of these patients histological subdivision provided no prognostic information and it was only the rare lymphocyte depleted variety which had a significantly reduced survival.

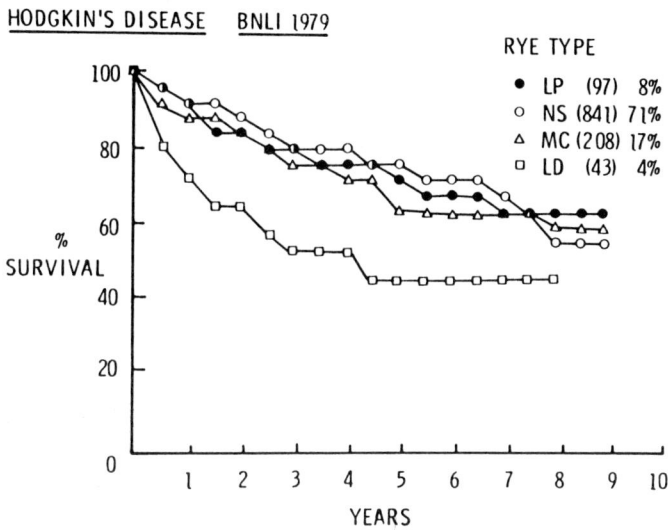

Figure 1 : *Actuarial survival of 1,189 patients classified according to the Rye classification prior to review.*

These findings prompted a critical histological review with strict application of the criteria proposed by Lukes and Butler (1966). In addition nodular sclerosis (NS) was subdivided into two prognostic grades using criteria previously described (MacLennan et al., 1985; MacLennan et al., 1989). Briefly, cases were classified as Grade 2 NS (high grade) if:
1) > 25 % of the cellular nodules showed reticular or pleomorphic, lymphocyte depleted cytology;
2) > 25 % of the cellular nodules contained numerous, anaplastic Hodgkin's cells in the absence of lymphocyte depletion;
3) > 75 % of the cellular nodules were replaced by the bland-appearing, fibro-histiocytic varient of lymphocyte depletion.

The results of this analysis clearly demonstrate the value of histopathology in predicting survival (Bennett et al., 1985; Bennett et al., 1989) (Figure 2) with the additional advantage of allowing subdivision of the numerically predominant NS group into two prognostically distinct grades (i.e. NS 1 and NS 2).

Using our published histological criteria (Bennett et al., 1985; MacLennan et al., 1985), other workers have independently demonstrated the prognostic value of this subdivision of NS (Gartner et al., 1987; Jairam et al., 1988; Ferry et al., 1989; Wijlhuizen et al., 1989).

In a series of 312 patients with clinical stage I, II and IIIa HD, collected by Groupe Pierre et Marie Curie, the prognostic value of a subdivision of NS into four histological types (Diebold, 1985) was assessed. There were no significant differences in the survival or relapse-free survival between the various histological subtypes of NS using this classification (Culine et al., 1989) even though two of the subtypes (4 S and 4 F) were similar to Grade 2 NS (high grade) as used in the BNLI study.

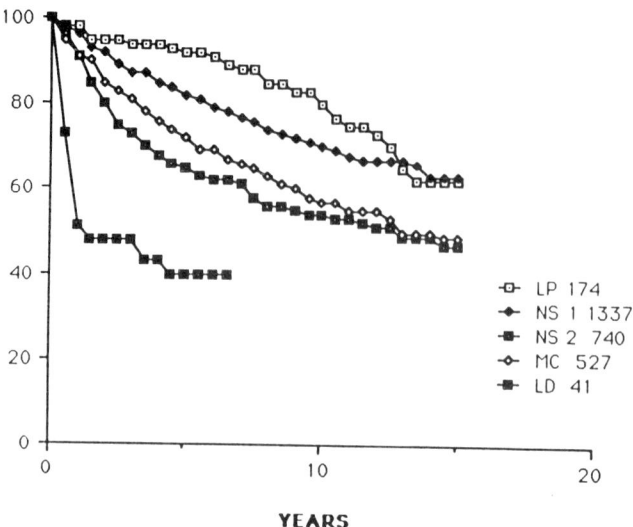

Figure 2 : *Actuarial survival of 2,819 patients classified according to the BNLI modification of the Lukes and Butler classification.*

The Recognition Of Non-Hodgkin's Lymphomas Mimicking Hodgkin's Disease

The separation of HD from the NHLs is possible, in the majority of cases, without the application of specialized techniques such as immunocytochemistry or molecular biology. However there are instances in which this distinction may prove to be extremely difficult by morphology alone; these usually occur in HD other than nodular sclerosis and particularly at the extremes of the cytological spectrum in the lymphocyte predominant (Bennett et al., 1989) and lymphocyte depleted histological subtypes (Kant et al., 1986).

In the series of cases of lymphocyte predominant (LP) HD analyzed by the BNLI (Bennett et al., 1989), it was in the diffuse variant of LP with numerous admixed epithelioid histiocytes, that difficulties in the distinction of HD from NHL occurred. Retrospective histological review, in the light of recent advances in our understanding of the pathology of peripheral T cell NHL (Suchi et al., 1987), led to the reclassification of more than a third of cases of L & H diffuse into NHL of Lennert's or peripheral T cell type. The survival of these patients reclassified as NHL was poor with 80 % dying within 3 years and it is therefore clinically important that histopathologists are able to reliably discriminate these entities. Unfortunately this may prove extremely difficult and in an excellent review of histological features of value in this differential diagnosis (Patsouris et al., 1988), Lennert states "For the near future, we will have to live with the fact that a small gray zone exists between the T-cell lymphomas of lymphoepithelioid type and HD...".

Another gray zone is present in the morphological distinction of NS with large numbers of tumours cells (Grade 2 NS) and large anaplastic cell (Ki 1) NHL's; this latter entity exhibited capsular sclerosis and intranodal collagen band formation in over half the cases studied by Agnarrson and Kadin (1988) and this combined with the cytological similarity of the malignant cells present in Ki 1 lymphoma and NS has caused difficulties in the differential diagnosis of these entities.

Because of these difficulties considerable effort has been expended in immunophenotypic studies characterising Reed-Sternberg cells and the cellular environment present in the different histologic subtypes in the hope of finding a reliable method of establishing the diagnosis of Hodgkin's disease. The results have been somewhat disappointing. On frozen sections (where the widest possible panel of reagents for immunophenotyping may be used) the combination of a very heterogeneous cellular population containing a vast predominance of reactive elements and the poor morphology associated with this technique has hampered the precise identification of labelled cells. This combined with the absence of a currently available marker with absolute specificity for the R-S cell has limited the value of frozen section immunophenotyping in establishing the diagnosis of HD in problematic cases.

A variety of recently developed monoclonal antibodies, with reactivity in routinely fixed and processed material, are currently available which have some value in the differential diagnosis of HD. The most widely studied of these are the anti-granulocyte reagent, CD 15 (Hall & D'Ardenne, 1987), antibodies to the Ki 1 antigen, CD 30, (Stein et al., 1985; Hall et al., 1988) and the leukocyte common antigen, CD 45, (Dorfman et al., 1986). Considerable heterogeneity of immunostaining patterns have been reported in HD, particularly in LPHD. Although CD 15 and CD 30 staining will highlight R-S cells in the majority of cases of HD other than LP (Chittal et al., 1988), these reagents are not specific for HD and both will stain a significant percentage of NHLs (Hall et al., 1988). In contrast to most forms of HD, the LP histological subtype is often unstained by CD 15 and CD 30 reagents and expresses CD 45 (Norton & Isaacson, 1989). Thus it would appear that immunophenotyping, whether on frozen or paraffin sections, does not provide a reliable distinction of HD from NHL in all cases. Hall et al. (1988) state "the currently available markers that have reactivity in conventionnaly fixed and processed material... do not provide a clear-cut method for distinguishing Hodgkin's from non-Hodgkin's lymphoma".

The application of molecular biological techniques to the study of HD have produced conflicting results. The study of tumour tissue from patients with HD has revealed immunoglobulin gene rearrangement in a percentage of cases (Weiss et al., 1986; Brinker et al., 1987) as was demonstrated in a case of Hodgkin's cell leukaemia (Linch et al., 1985). Rearrangement of T cell receptor genes has been less commonly observed (Greisser et al., 1986). Other workers have been unable to demonstrate a clonal rearrangement of immunoglobulin or T cell receptor genes (O'Connor et al., 1987; Raghavachar et al., 1988; Linden et al., 1988). The literature is thus somewhat confusing and further studies are required before the value of gene rearrangement studies in the diagnosis of HD can be assessed.

The Biological Heterogeneity of Hodgkin's Disease

Careful morphological studies of lymphocyte predominant nodular HD suggested to some workers that this form of the disease may be different from other histological subtypes (whose earliest site of nodal involvement is in the paracortex (Lukes, 1971)) and may originate in germinal centres (Poppema et al., 1979a). Ultrastructural and immunohistochemical studies confirmed these findings by demonstrating the presence of dendritic reticulum cells (Poppema et al., 1979b) and by showing the nodules contained a predominance of polyclonal B-cells (Abdulaziz et al., 1984; Tiemens et al., 1986; Pinkus & Said, 1988). Further strong evidence of the B-cell nature of LP nodular is provided by the demonstration of J chain (Poppema, 1980; Stain et al., 1986) and B-cell markers on the L & H, Reed-Sternberg cell varients found in this type of HD (Hansmann et al., 1986; Hall et al., 1988; Pinkus & Said, 1988). In addition L & H cells commonly express the leukocyte common antigen (CD 45) (Hall et al., 1988), epithelial membrane antigen (EMA) (Jack et al., 1986) and a sialyated form of the CD 15 antigen which is not detectable without prior neuraminidase digestion (Hsu et al., 1986). The Ki 1 antigen (CD 30) is also less commonly expressed by the L & H cell (8 % of cases of LP nodular in the study of Chittal et al. (1988).

These findings are in sharp contrast to those observed in other histological subtypes of HD and NS in particular, where the majority of the lymphoid cell population presents is of a peripheral T cell type with a helper cell predominance (CD 4 + ve) (Borowitz et al., 1982).

There are also profound differences in the phenotype of the R-S cells present in NS the majority of which are CD 15 + ve, CD 30 + ve and fail to express CD 45, EMA and B cell antigens (Dorfman et al., 1986; Hall et al., 1988).

These clear phenotypic differences between LP nodular and NS are mirrored by differences in the patient populations affected, the anatomic distribution and the response to therapy of these two forms of HD.

The sex distribution of LP nodular shows an overwhelming male predominance (M:F; 4.2:1) compared to NS which has a sex ratio of M:F; 1.5:1. There are also differences in the age distribution with LP nodular showing a peak age incidence in the 4th decade; a decade later than that of NS.

The anatomic distribution of disease also differs between the two subtypes with LP nodular most commonly presenting with localised disease exhibiting a peculiar predilection for involvement of suprahyoid cervical and inguinal lymph nodes. NS on the other hand shows a pronounced mediastinal orientation with 52% of cases demonstrating radiological evidence of mediastinal involvement (65% of cases of Grade 2 NS) compared to only 7% of cases of LP.

LP nodular appears to be a highly radiosensitive neoplasm; in a series of 767 patients with clinical stage I and IIa upper half Hodgkin's disease, treated initially with radiotherapy, patients with LP did not experience any relapses within the irradiated area. This contrasts sharply with a much higher relapse rate observed in patients with NS within the irradiated area (6.9% for Grade 1 NS and 13.8% for Grade 2 NS) (Vaughan Hudson et al., 1987).

Patients with LP nodular have been demonstrated to have an increased risk of developing second neoplasms, particularly high grade NHL (Miettinen et al., 1983; Trudel et al., 1987) compared to other forms of HD and transitional states with increased numbers of large cells have been observed (Sundeen et al., 1988; Banks et al., 1989; Grossman et al., 1989). It would thus appear that the biological partition of this subtype of HD from some examples of NHL's (eg the T cell rich B cell lymphomas (Ramsey et al., 1988)) may not be as precise as we believe.

Conclusion

This brief review has attempted to highlight some of the areas of controversy that currently exist in the study of Hodgkin's disease. In particular we have demonstrated heterogeneity within this disease process and it now appears highly probable that there are at least two (and possibly more) distinct biologic entities which are currently termed HD.

The distinction of HD from the NHL is clinically important but in a small percentage of cases proves to be extremely difficult for the pathologist to perform reliably.

Unfortunately immunocytochemistry and molecular biology have so far proved of limited value and it is in these problematic cases that careful clinico-pathological liaison is so essential to ensure optimal patient management.

In BNLI studies, histopathological classification is a valuable indicator of response to treatment and ultimate prognosis and although some workers have supported these findings others have been unable to confirm them (Culine et al., 1988; Masih et al., 1989). Further studies of large numbers of patients receiving intensive therapy may be required to resolve this issue.

References

Abdulaziz, Z., et al. (1984): An immunohistological study of the cellular constituents of Hodgkin's disease using a monoclonal antibody panel. *Histopathology* 8, 1-25.

Agnarrson, B.A. & Kadin M.E. (1988): Ki-1 positive large cell lymphoma: A morphological study of 19 cases. *Am. J. Surg. Pathol.* 12, 264-274.

Banks, P.M., et al. (1989): Nodular lymphocyte predominance Hodgkin's disease (NLPHD) and its transition to large cell lymphoma (LCL): Immunophenotypic and genetic probe analysis. *Lab. Invest.* 60, 5A (28).

Bennett, M.H., et al. (1985): Analysis of histological subtypes of Hodgkin's disease in relation to prognosis and survival. In *The cytobiology of leukaemias and lymphomas*, ed. D. Quaglino & F.G.J. Hayhoe. Vol. 20, pp. 15-32. New-York: Raven Press (Serono Symposia Publications).

Bennett, M.H., et al. (1989): The clinical and prognostic relevance of histophatological classification in Hodgkin's disease. *Progress in surgical pathology*, Vol. 10 (in press).

Borowitz, M.J., et al. (1982): Immunohistochemical analysis of the distribution of lymphocyte subpopulations in Hodgkin's disease. *Cancer Treat. Rep.* 66, 667-674.

Brinker, M.G.L., et al. (1987): Clonal immunoglobulin rearrangements in tissues involved by Hodgkin's disease. *Blood* 70, 186-191.

Chelloul, N., et al. (1972): HL-A antigens and Hodgkin's disease. Report on the histological analysis. In *Histocompatibility Testing*, ed. J. Dausset & J. Colombani, pp. 769-771. Copenhagen: Munksgaard.

Chittal, S.M., et al. (1988): Monoclonal antibodies in the diagnosis of Hodgkin's disease: The search for a rational panel. *Am. J. Surg. Pathol.* 12, 9-21.

Culine, S., et al. (1989): Relationship of histological subtypes to prognosis in early stage Hodgkin's disease: A review of 312 cases enrolled in a controlled clinical trial. *J. Cancer Clin. Oncol.* 25, 551-556.

Diebold, J. (1985): Maladie de Hodgkin. Données morphologiques récentes. In *Maladie de Hodgkin*, ed. G. Hoerni-Simon & T. Gisselbrecht. Progrès en hématologie. Vol. 7, pp. 19-43. Paris: Doin.

Dorfman, R.F. & Colby, T.V. (1982): The pathologists role in the management of patients with Hodgkin's disease. *Cancer Treat. Rep.* 66, 675-680.

Dorfman, R.F., et al. (1986): An evaluation of the utility of anti-granulocyte and antileukocyte monoclonal antibodies in the diagnosis of Hodgkin's disease. *Am. J. Pathol.* 123, 508-519.

Ferry, J.A., et al. (1989): The prognostic importance of subclassification of Hodgkin's disease, nodular sclerosis type. *Lab. Invest.* 60, 28A (162).

Fuller, L.M., et al. (1980): Evaluation of the significance of prognostic factors in stage III Hodgkin's disease treated with MOPP and radiotherapy. *Cancer.* 45, 1352-1364.

Gartner, H.V., et al. (1987): Nodular sclerosing Hodgkin's disease: Prognostic relevance of morphological parameters. *Proceedings of the First International Symposium on Hodgkin's Lymphoma.* Cologne. 27A.

Grossman, D.M., et al. (1989): Simultaneous lymphocyte predominant Hodgkin's disease (LPHD) and large cell lymphoma (LCL). *Lab. Invest.* 60, 36A (212).

Hall, P.A. & D'Ardenne, A.J. (1987): Value of CD 15 immunostaining in diagnosing immunohistochemistry. II. Hodgkin's disease and large cell anaplastic (Ki 1) lymphoma. *Histopathology* 13, 161-169.

Hansmann, M.L., et al. (1986): Paragranuloma in a variant of Hodgkin's disease with a predominance of B-cells. *Virchow Arch. (Pathol. Anat.)* 409, 171-181.

Hoppe, R.T., et al. (1980): Prognostic factors in pathological stage IIIa Hodgkin's disease. *Cancer* 46, 1240-1246.

Kant, J.A., et al. (1986): A critical reappraisal of the pathologic and linical heterogeneity of lymphocyte depledted Hodgkin's disease. *J. Clin. Oncol.* 4, 284-294.

Hsu, S.M., et al. (1986): L & H variants of Reed-Sternberg cells express sialyated Leu M1 antigen. *Am. J. Pathol.* 122, 199-203.

Jack, A.S., et al. (1986): Use of Leu M1 and antiepithelial membrane antigen monoconal antibodies for diagnosing Hodgkin's disease. *J. Clin. Pathol.* 39, 267-270.

Jairam, R., et al. (1988): Histological subclassification of the nodular sclerotic subtype of Hodgkin's disease. *Neth. J. Med.* 33, 160-167.

Jones, S.E., et al. (1977): Histopathologic review of lymphoma cases from the Southwest Oncology Group. *Cancer* 39, 1071-1076.

Linch, D.C., et al. (1985): Hodgkin's cell leukaemia of B-cell origin. *Lancet* i, 78-80.

Linden, M.D., et al. (1988): Absence of B-cell or T-cell clonal expansion in nodular, lymphocyte predominant Hodgkin's disease. *Hum. Pathol.* 19, 591-594.

Lukes, R.J. & Butler, J.J. (1966): The pathology and nomenclature of Hodgkin's disease. *Cancer Res.* 26, 1063-1081.

Lukes, R.J. et al. (1966): Natural history of Hodgkin's disease as related to its pathologic picture. *Cancer* 34, 317-344.

Lukes, R.J., et al. (1966): Report of the nomenclature committee. *Cancer Res.* 26, 1311.

MacLennan, K.A., et al. (1985): Prognostic significance of cytologic subdivision in nodular sclerosis Hodgkin's disease: An analysis of 1156 patients. In *Malignant Lymphomas and Hodgkin's disease: Experimental and therapeutic advances*, ed. F. Cavalli, G. Bonadonna & M. Rozencweig, pp. 187-200. Boston, Dordrecht, Lancaster: Martinus Nijhoff Publishing.

MacLennan, K.A., et al. (1989): The relationship of histopathology to survival and relapse: A study of 1659 patients. *Cancer* (in press).

Masih, A.S., et al. (1989): Histologic grade in nodular sclerosing Hodgkin's disease does not predict outcome. *Lab. Invest.* 60, 59A (347).

Miller, T.P., et al. (1982): Mistaken clinical and pathological diagnoses of Hodgkin's disease: A Southwest Oncology Group Study. *Cancer Treat. Rep.* 66, 645-651.

Norton, A.J. & Isaacson, P.G. (1989): Lymphoma phenotyping in formalin-fixed and paraffin wax-embedded tissue: II. Profiles of reactivity in the various tumour types. *Histopathology* 14, 557-579.

O'Connor, N.J.T., et al. (1987): Cell lineage in Hodgkin's disease. *Lancet* i, 158.

Patsouris, E., et al. (1988): Histological and immunohistological findings in lymphoepithelioid cell lymphoma (Lennert's lymphoma). *Am. J. Surg. Pathol.* 12, 341-350.

Pinkus, G.S. & Said, J.W. (1988): Hodgkin's disease, lymphocyte predominance type, nodular - further evidence for a B cell derivation. *Am. J. Pathol.* 133, 211-217.

Poppema, S., et al. (1979a): Hodgkin's disease with lymphocytic predominance, nodular type (nodular paragranuloma) and progressively transformed germinal centres. A cytohistological study. *Histopathology* 3, 295-308.

Poppema, S., et al. (1979b): Nodular paragranuloma and progressively transformed germinal centres: Ultrastructural and immunohistologic findings. *Virchows Arch. (B Cell Path.)* 31, 211-225.

Raghavachar, A., et al. (1988): Immunoglobulin and T-cell receptor gene rearrangements in Hodgkin's disease. *Cancer Res.* 48, 3591-3594.

Ramsey, A.D. et al. (1988): T-cell rich B-cell lymphoma. *Am. J. Surg. Pathol.* 12, 433-443.

Strum, S.B. & Rappaport, H. (1970): Observations of cells resembling Reed-Sternberg cells in conditions other than Hodgkin's disease. *Cancer* 26, 176-190.

Suchi, T., et al. (1987): Histopathology and immunohistochemistry of peripheral T cell lymphomas: a proposal for their classification. *J. Clin. Pathol.* 40, 995-1015.

Sundeen, J.T., et al. (1988): Lymphocyte predominant Hodgkin's disease with coexistent "large cell lymphoma": Histological progression or composite malignancy? *Am. J. Sur. Pathol.* 12, 599-606.

Symmers, W. st. C. (1968): Survey of the eventual diagnosis in 600 cases referred for a second histologic opinion after an initial biopsy diagnosis of Hodgkin's disease. *J. Clin. Pathol.* 21, 650-653.

Tiemens, W., et al. (1986): Nodular lymphocyte predominance type of Hodgkin's disease is a germinal centre lymphoma. *Lab. Invest.* 54, 457-461.

Torti, F.M., et al. (1979): The changing significance of histology in Hodgkin's disease. *Proc. Am. Assoc. Cancer Res. and ASCO* 20, 401 (C-454).

Vaughan Hudson, B., et al. (1987): A retrospective evaluation of radiotherapy as a curative agent in localised Hodgkin's disease. *Brit. J. Cancer* 56, 872.

Weiss, L.M., et al. (1986): Immunoglobulin gene rearrangements in Hodgkin's disease. *Hum. Pathol.* 17, 1009-1014.

Wijlhuizen, T.J., et al. (1989): Grades of nodular sclerosis (NS I - NS II) in Hodgkin's disease: Are they of independent prognostic value ? *Cancer* 63, 1150-1153.

**PROCEEDINGS OF THE WORKSHOP ON TREATMENT STRATEGY
IN HODGKIN'S DISEASE**

*COMPTE RENDU DE LA REUNION INTERNATIONALE SUR LA STRATEGIE
THERAPEUTIQUE DANS LA MALADIE DE HODGKIN*

Introduction

W. Gregory[1], M. Löffler[2]

1 *Breast Unit, Guy's Hospital, Snowfield Building, London SE1 9RT, England*
2 *Biometric Division, Medical University Clinic, 5000 Köln 41, Federal Republic of Germany*

Summary

Although a great many analyses have already been performed on this data, there are still many questions remaining. For instance, it has yet to be discovered whether biological parameters can replace the significance of "B" symptoms. Alternatives to the proportional hazards model involving fewer or different assumptions may be appropriate. Some of the possible treatment differences can be (cautiously) investigated in a multivariate fashion.

However, some answers have been produced, including a set of "standard" prognostic factors, with appropriate relative risks and survival rates. New trial results can be measured and evaluated against these standards, and the results provide a means of possibly selecting treatment more appropriately in some categories. The second malignancy data is fascinating, and has implications for treatment. The workshop has induced new collaborations, and encouraged the exchange of ideas.

As an extension of the reporting methods suggested, it should be possible to produce simple computer programs that could use all this prognostic information to estimate the survival and disease-free survival of groups of patients treated by the particular broad treatment strategies suggested. This could provide a further comparative baseline for future studies. These programs would use each patient's prognostic information to predict his or her likely survival, and an amalgamation of these predictions could produce expected survival curves, with confidence limits.

In conclusion, the workshop has produced some initial useful results, but promises considerably more for the future.

Résumé

Bien qu'un certain nombre d'analyses aient déjà été réalisées à partir des données recueillies, plusieurs questions restent en suspens. Par exemple, peut-on substituer aux signes généraux les paramètres biologiques, et si oui, lesquels? D'autres modèles que le modèle de Cox, nécessitant moins d'hypothèses ou des hypothèses différentes, pourraient être utilisés. Enfin, l'efficacité de certaines stratégies thérapeutiques pourraient être (avec prudence) comparées au moyen d'analyses multivariées.

Cependant, la valeur pronostique de certains paramètres "classiques" a pu être confirmée, et des risques relatifs et des taux de survie leur être associés. Les résultats des prochains essais thérapeutiques pourront être analysés en tenant comptant de ces paramètres, ces derniers permettant une meilleure approche du choix thérapeutique pour certaines catégories de malades. Les données concernant les secondes tumeurs malignes sont extrèmement intéressantes et influeront sur les choix des traitements. Cette réunion de consensus a d'autre part favorisé l'échange d'idées et fourni un point de départ à de nouvelles collaborations.

L'exposé de nouvelles méthodes d'analyse pourrait avoir comme conséquence directe l'élaboration de programmes informatiques permettant de prendre en considération les caratéristiques pronostiques des malades afin d'estimer la survie de groupes de profil défini en fonction d'une stratégie thérapeutique particulière. Ceci aurait comme intérêt de fournir une base de dicussion pour des études futures. Ces programmes devraient être capables d'utiliser toute l'information disponible afin de prédire, pour un malade donné, sa probabilité de survie. Une sommation des ces probabilités permettrait d'estimer des courbes de survie théoriques avec intervalles de confiance.

On peut dire, en conclusion, que les informations obtenues à l'occasion de cette réunion sont déja très utiles, et qu'elles le seront certainement encore beaucoup plus dans l'avenir.

Background

This report summarises an examination of prognostic factors in Hodgkin's Disease (HD), and their relationship to treatment, and to possible treatment strategies.

Data was obtained from 20 centres, on 14,315 cases of HD, using a common data collection form, designed to include all major prognostic factors and treatment details.

The aim was to discover factors which might predict for achievement of complete remission (CR), duration of CR, and survival. A study of the incidence of second malignancies was also undertaken. It was hoped that evaluation of prognostic factors across such a wide spectrum of patients and specialist treatment groups might facilitate:

1) Better design of future studies, including:
- recommended stratifications;
- recommended reporting procedures, leading to more comparability between results from different centres.

2) Suggestions for new staging criteria in HD:
- possible incorporation of "biological" parameters, such as ESR and albumin into staging classifications;
- clear evaluation of the relevance of additional disease within each stage, e.g. number of lymph nodes involved, extra localised disease, mediastinal involvement.

3) Understanding the treatment implications of prognostic factors:
- could "good" risk and "poor" risk groups be identified;
- could particular strategies, e.g. intensification or reduction of treatment, use of extra supportive measures, e.g. GCSF, or possibly BMT be recommended for particular groups.

Subsidiary questions included the possible prediction of groups where laparotomy would have a high chance of being positive, and the possibility of using biological parameters to replace the prognostic information provided by "B" symptoms.

Methodological issues

Before describing the results of the workshop, it is important to state and discuss the methods used, giving the rationale and philosophy behind them, as well as the assumptions, possible drawbacks, and alternatives.

1. Selection of patients for the analysis

The primary aims of this analysis were to make a definitive evaluation of the important prognostic factors in Hodgkin's Disease. It was felt important to obtain data on as many patients as possible, since many of the equivocal questions were relevant in relatively small subgroups, e.g. does the number of lymph node areas matter in each of the stage IIA, IIB, IIIA?

Since we also wished to examine the occurrence of second malignancies, larger patient numbers were even more important. Whether the patients came from randomised studies or not was relatively immaterial for this latter question.

Thus data were requested on all patients included in defined studies, treated with some known protocol, but not necessarily in randomised trials. Since it was also desired to involve as many centres as possible, this approach seemed particularly appropriate.

An alternative approach would have been to seek to answer specific treatment questions by requesting data from trials addressing such questions in a randomised fashion, and performing an overview analysis.

The overview approach hypothesises that, where a true difference between treatments is sufficiently small that individual trials have not given a clear cut answer to a question, any overall trend of the trials in one direction will provide this definitive answer. This study was not set up to answer such direct treatment questions, largely because this would have severely limited the patients to be included, and thus interfered with the prognostic factor analyses.

The lack of patient numbers entered into randomised trials over the last 20 years results from single institutions rarely having sufficient numbers to embark on such trials. However, many well studied and well documented sequential (essentially phase III) trials have been undertaken in this period, with larger multi-centre studies only becoming more prevalent in the last few years. The duration of follow-up in many of these more recent studies is insufficient to answer questions in a disease where events occur over such long timespans.

2. Selection of data to be collected

It is unrealistic to collect all data that may possibly affect prognosis for a disease. The possible benefits do not merit the extra effort involved, and much of the data is likely to be unavailable. In this study we restricted ourselves to variables that had previously been reported to be of prognostic importance. Patients were classified according to treatment prescribed although it proved necessary to amalgamate treatments into several broad categories, e.g. MOPP-like, alternating. No attempt was made to take account of the actual doses of treatment received.

3. Analytical methods

To examine prognostic factor effects on failure times (e.g. survival, relapse-free survival), multivariate methods involving hazard functions were employed. (Multivariate methods were necessary to distinguish the *independent* contributions of the different prognostic factors). The "hazard" gives the probability of an event within an infinitesimal interval for a population at risk at some time t. This quantifies the intensity of events to be expected at time t. If the hazard function has large values, the survival curve will fall steeply. If the hazard function is zero, the curve will have a "plateau" (Figure 1).

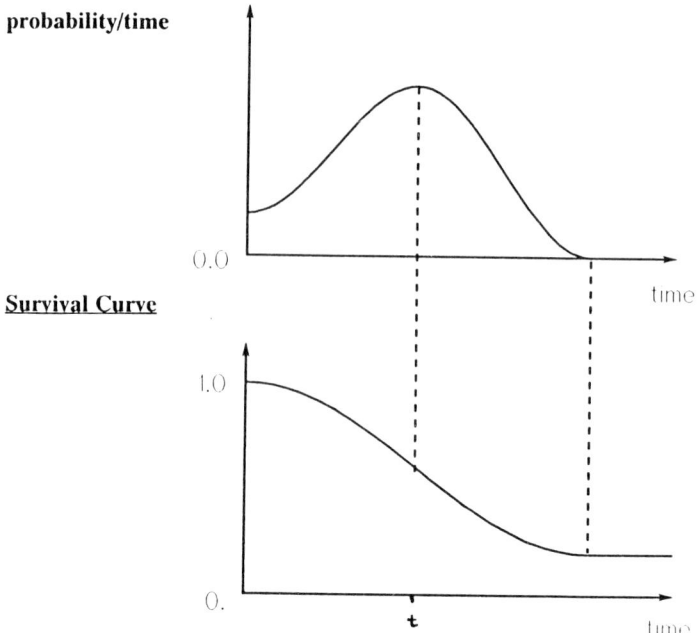

Figure 1. *Hazard function and survival curve. Hazard function h(t): Probability of an event (e.g. death) within an infinitesimal interval (t, t+ Δt) for the population at risk at time t.*

The multivariate method used for failure times was the proportional hazards model (PHM) described by Cox. The basic assumption of this model is that the presence or absence of specific factors does not change the shape of the hazard function, but transforms it in a multiplicative way (Figure 2).

For example, the curves on the left-hand side of Figure 2 have the same general humped shape, but are increased or decreased over the entire time period by a constant factor (2 or 1/2 in the figure). The same holds true for the monotonically declining curves on the right-hand side of figure 2. They differ by the same factors. In contrast, the analysis should be stratified if there is good reason to believe that the *shape* of the hazard functions is different for the different strata, as for the two strata shown in figure 2. However, although the shapes of the hazard functions are different in the two strata it is assumed that the effects of the factors are the same in both. In the analyses therefore, stratification was introduced whenever there was good reason to believe a priori that the baseline hazard functions had a different shape in different strata. This was likely to be the case for treatment types (RT, CT, RT+CT), treatment periods (1960s, 1970s, 1980s) and laparotomy (performed or not).

To analyse rates (for example of remission) logistic regression methods were used.

4. Prognostic factors

These can be defined as disease characteristics present before treatment, which appear to affect prognosis. It is necessary to make some assumptions about the way in which prognosis is affected in order to perform any analyses. Having chosen to use the PHM for the analysis of failure times (see above), the analysis was conducted with the following assumptions:

a) The prognostic factors were assumed to be independent of treatment, i.e. to be effective in the same manner for all treatments;
b) They were assumed to be likewise effective in all strata;
c) They were assumed to be effective over the whole time period.

These assumptions are in potential conflict with the clinical experience that specifically designed "risk adapted" treatments can abrogate unfavourable prognostic factors (for example, combined modality treatment is effective against large mediastinal tumours). As data were pooled from various differently designed risk adapted treatment strategies, hopes of detecting many new prognostic factors were inevitably moderate. One could reasonably expect to identify only the dominant general prognostic factors given the above assumptions and the heterogeneity of the data.

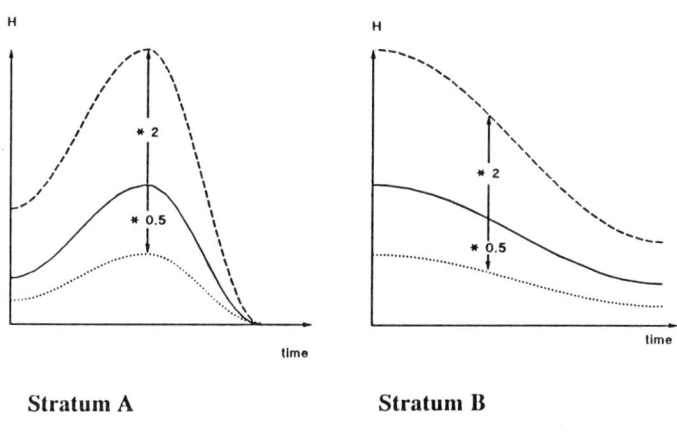

Stratum A   Stratum B

<u>Stratification</u>:   The same pattern of factor effects is expected but the shape of the hazard function differs in different strata

Figure 2. *Proportional hazards model. Assumption: Presence or absence of specific factors does not change the basic shape of the hazard function but transforms (multiplies) it proportionally.*

5. Treatment and its relation to prognostic factors

A third area for analysis involved the possible interaction of treatment with prognostic factors, and thus some treatment questions needed to be addressed.

Historically, the Ann Arbor I-IV staging criteria in Hodgkin's Disease has been primarily concerned with the extent and distribution of disease. Treatment modifications have involved giving more intensive, and/or more systemic treatment as the stage worsens. Thus, improvements in the last 25 years have been most marked in the poor prognosis groups. This has resulted in a lessening of the relevance of the prognostic factors. The primary treatment/prognostic factor interactions addressable in this study thus centre on bulk and degree of dissemination. For example, the introduction of chemotherapy for bulky stage II disease has to some extent negated the relevance of bulk as a prognostic factor in this group.

However, bulk and degree of dissemination should not be confused. Combination chemotherapy (CCT) for disseminated disease will not necessarily, on its own, eliminate local areas of bulk. For example, although the question needs to be addressed more rigorously, adjusting for all the relevant prognostic factors, it appears that CCT alone is inadequate treatment for a number of stages (e.g. for stage IIIB patients the 10 year survival rates are 47% (+/- 2%) for CCT and 55% (+/- 2%) for radiotherapy + CCT), despite many patients still being treated with this single modality. While CCT appears necessary to eradicate systemic disease, radiotherapy may be required in addition to eliminate bulky disease.

Thus, some treatment questions can be addressed and may produce clear answers. Since all the known prognostic factors have been gathered, and can be adjusted for in a multivariate fashion, if large treatment differences are still observed, they are very unlikely to be a result of unknown prognostic factors. Such findings should not be dismissed merely on the grounds that these were not randomised trials. Obviously a similar result from a randomised trial would carry even greater conviction, but relevant data will be more sparse. Both methods are thus useful, and can indeed be complementary.

A further approach to analysis of treatment questions would be to use the randomised trials within the collected data to perform an overview analysis. If the remaining data were consistent with the results of this overview analysis, they could be used to confirm findings that did not otherwise reach statistical significance. This could be extended to include further testing of any other past or on-going overviews. This option is clearly still possible, and should be explored.

Treatment questions have been difficult to address, but some hypotheses have been raised and clear results may still be forthcoming. There is clearly much work still to be done. The questions raised have been interesting, and not always obvious to the participants, as demonstrated by the answers to the survey undertaken at the Paris meeting in June 1989. (For example many oncologists appear to believe that CCT alone is adequate treatment for many patients with stages II and III disease).

The results will now be presented separately for stages I and II, and then for stages III and IV.

Early Stage Hodgkin's Disease

Maladie de Hodgkin : stades localisés

Prognostic factors for stage I and II Hodgkin's disease

J.H. Meerwaldt[1], M. Van Glabbeke[2], B. Vaughan Hudson[3]

1 Dr Daniel den Hoed Cancer Center, 3075 EA Rotterdam, The Netherlands
2 EORTC Data Centre, 1000 Brussels, Belgium
3 British National Lymphoma Investigation, University College and Middlesex School of Medicine, London W1N 8AA, England

Summary

The overall survival of 9,090 clinical stage I-II patients was 60%-71% at 15 years (70%, 71%, and 60% for clinical stage IA, clinical stage IIA, and clinical stage IB-IIB patients respectively). Initial treatment achieved complete remission in 94%-98% of patients, of whom 25% -31 % later relapsed or died without Hodgkin's disease. The overall survivals of patients who relapsed or who failed to achieve complete remission were of the order of 50% and 30% respectively, indicating only partial success from further salvage therapy.

Patients receiving initial radiotherapy had a higher complete remission rate than those receiving initial chemotherapy alone, and patients receiving combined modality treatments a higher relapse-free survival than those receiving radiotherapy or chemotherapy alone (though apparently not a higher overall survival) : however these findings should be interpreted with considerable caution, since treatment groups had been previously selected by prognostic factors in many cases.

The difference in relapse-free survival and overall survival between the prognostic subgroups studied was relatively small in most cases, with the exception of the different age groups, between which there were large differences in overall survival in patients over the age of 30 years at presentation. This was possibly due to a combination of prior use of prognostic factors for treatment group selection, to more extensive use of combination chemotherapy in recent years, and to the appreciate fraction of the total deaths recorded as being due to causes other than Hodgkin's disease and for which these factors would not have had prognostic value.

The decrease in survival with increasing age was due in large mesure to death associated with Hodgkin's disease [Statistical Report, Figure X-11]. An appreciable number of deaths from causes operative in the general population would also be expected to have occurred, mainly in the older age groups. However the cumulative incidence of death recorded as due to causes other than Hodgkin's disease rose progressively throughout the 20 year period, and after around 15 years was greater than that from HD related death [Statistical Report, Figure X-14]. An appreciable number of deaths occurred from second cancers, and for a number of them the frequency observed was significantly greater than that expected in the general population. These included acute leukaemias and non-Hodgkin's lymphomas, though their cumulative incidences were less than 2% at 15 years, whereas that for solid tumours was 6% and still increasing [Statistical Report, Figure IX-3]. As well as age, the use of extended radiotherapy and combined modality treatments including MOPP-like regimes were strongly associated with increased risk of solid tumour.

Résumé

Globalement, le taux de survie à 15 ans des 9090 stades cliniques I-II était compris entre 60% et 71% (70% pour les stades IA, 71% pour les stades IIA, et 60% pour les stades IB-IIB). Une rémission complète a été obtenue dans 94% à 98% des cas, parmi lesquels 25% à 31% ont rechuté ou sont morts d'autre cause que de maladie de Hodgkin. Le taux de survie des malades ayant rechuté ou de ceux non mis en rémission complète par le traitement initial était respectivement de l'ordre de 50% et de 30%, ce qui laisse à penser que les traitements de rattrapage n'ont été que partiellement efficaces.

Le taux de rémission complète était supérieur parmi les malades ayant été traités par radiothérapie par rapport à ceux ayant été initialement traités par chimiothérapie. De même, les malades initialement traités par une association radio-chimiothérapie ont présenté un taux de rémission complète plus élevé que celui obtenu pour ceux traités par radiothérapie seule ou chimiothérapie seule. Globalement les taux de survie ne différaient pas d'un groupe de malades à l'autre. Toutefois ces résultats doivent être interprétés avec précaution, un grand nombre de malades ayant été traités après que l'on eut pris en compte certains facteurs de pronostic.

La différence entre les divers groupes pronostiques, que l'on prenne comme critère le taux de survie sans récidive ou le taux de survie globale, était en général faible, sauf pour ce qui concerne l'âge. Les différences les plus grandes concernaient les taux de survie des malades âgés de plus de 30 ans au moment du diagnostic de la maladie. Ces différences peuvent être liées soit à l'utilisation de facteurs pronostiques dans la sélection des groupes thérapeutiques, soit à l'utilisation plus fréquente de chimiothérapie dans les années les plus récentes, soit enfin au nombre non négligeable de décès non liés à la maladie et pour lesquels ces paramètres peuvent ne pas avoir de valeur pronostique.

La diminution du taux de survie en fonction de l'âge était en grande partie associée à une plus grande fréquence des décès liés à la maladie [Rapport Statistique, Figure X-11]. On pourrait d'autre part supposer que les malades en rémission complète aient la même probabilité de décès que n'importe quel inidividu de même âge et même sexe issu de la population générale, en particulier parmi les malades les plus âgés. Cependant, le taux cumulatif de décès dus à d'autres causes que la maladie elle-même augmentait progressivement en fonction du temps, dépassant même dés la quinzième année le taux de décès directement lié à la maladie de Hodgkin [Rapport Statistique, Figure X-14]. Un nombre non négligeable de décès étaient secondaires à des deuxièmes cancers, et pour certains d'entre eux, la rapport du nombre observé au nombre attendu était significativement supérieur à 1. C'était le cas pour les leucémies aiguës et les lymphomes non Hodgkiniens, bien que le taux d'incidence cumulatif de ces cancers ne dépassait pas 2% à 15 ans, alors que celui des tumeurs solides était de l'ordre de 6% en constante augmentation [Rapport Statistique, Figure IX-3]. De même que l'âge, les traitements antérieurs par radiothérapie étendue ou association radio-chimiothérapie incluant le MOPP ou ses dérivés étaient largement associés à un risque augmenté de deuxième cancer.

Historical

The advent of combination chemotherapy in the 1960's made it possible to cure patients with generalised disease, and it became important to differentiate between localised and generalised disease, which was accomplished by clinical staging. For localised disease (Stages I and II), radiotherapy (RT) alone had been shown to be effective, and was preferred to chemotherapy (CT), since the latter resulted in the sterilisation of a large proportion of patients, was believed to cause secondary leukaemia in a significant number of them, and could be held in reserve as 'salvage treatment' if RT failed, since it was believed to be as effective when given at the time of relapse as when given initially. For most generalised disease CT was preferred, since it treated any occult disease which was not evident clinically, and also treated disease present in areas difficult to treat with RT due to the presence of vital organs which would be damaged and which therefore reduced dosage to suboptimal levels. It was tacitly assumed that CT was equally as effective as RT in treating clinically overt disease.

The high frequency of relapse below the diaphragm in patients clinically staged (CS) I-II suggested that a significant proportion of these patients had occult disease below the diaphragm at presentation (in paraaortic and hilar nodes, spleen, liver, etc.), and had in fact stage III-IV disease, and a routine policy of "pathological" staging, involving diagnostic laparotomy + splenectomy was instituted by many centres. Relapses in CS I-II patients also frequently occurred in non-supradiaphragmatic sites. The radiation field was therefore progressively extended by some groups, through mantle and extended mantle to subtotal nodal irradiation, in an attempt to prevent relapses. More recently many groups have added CT to initial RT, as combined modality therapy (CMT), in order to treat occult disease initially, instead of waiting until relapse. Many use prognostic factors such as stage, laparotomy, systemic symptoms, ESR, etc. to identify "low" and "high" risk groups, and giving more aggressive therapy in the form of wide field RT or CMT to the "high" risk groups.

EORTC workshop

The collection by the EORTC of over 14,000 patients entered into trials and studies in many different parts of the world and followed up for as long as 20 years has enabled a global view of many aspects of Hodgkin's disease (HD) to be taken for the first time. It has been possible to quantitate many values in a definitive manner from so many patients with such long follow up, particularly relatively rarely occuring events, such as second malignancies, intercurrent deaths, and late relapses.

Some important limitations should be mentioned. The relative paucity of data provided by the collaborating groups for haematological parameters has limited the assessment of their prognostic value. A further limitation may have been the omission of a request for the lymphocyte count and eosinophil count, both of which have been reported to be of prognostic value (MacLennan et al., 1981; Wagstaff et al., 1988; Specht et al., 1988; Vaughan Hudson et al., 1987). A further limitation is that prognostic factors have already been used by the collaborating groups in order to select particular treatments appropriate to prognosis. This may have reduced or nullified the effects of some prognostic factors. For example, stage II might have been considered a poor prognostic factor, and stage II patients accordingly given more aggressive treatment, and their survival thereby increased to that of stage I patients. The two stages would now have the same survival, and it would not be evident that stage had been a prognostic factor without the knowledge that the two stages had been treated differently. Since the data set does not include such information the results of treatment are difficult to interpret. A further, conceptual problem is that most of the analyses were made separately upon subgroups already identified by the classic prognostic factors, i.e. stage, symptoms, and laparotomy findings. Further analysis without such subdivisions may establish whether the "newer" factors are capable of giving similar, or more comprehensive prognostic information.

Results

Patients characteristics (Table 1)

The characteristics at presentation of patients with CS II disease differed considerably from those with CS I disease. Their mean age was lower, a higher proportion were female, a high proportion had involvement of the mediastinum, a greater proportion exhibited systemic symptoms, and a higher proportion were classified as belonging to the nodular sclerotic (NS) histopathological subtype. (As with CS III-IV patients the proportion of CS I-II patients diagnosed as belonging to this subtype has increased over the last 20 years).

Table 1. Patient characterisics

		CS I	CS II
Total patients		2,986	6,105
Age (mean)		37 yrs	31 yrs
Sex ratio		2.1	1.1
Presentation	above diaphragm	96 %	93 %
Mediastinum	involved	11 %	70 %
	"bulky" involvement	32 %	34 %
Histopathological subtypes			
	Nodular sclerosis	47 %	73 %
	Myxed cellularity	34 %	19 %
	Lymphocyte predominant	15 %	5 %
	Lymphocyte depleted	1 %	2 %
	Unclassified	2 %	2 %
Systemic symptoms	present	9 %	28 %

Laparotomy (Table 2)

Approximately half of the CS I-II patients were investigated by laparotomy. In approximately three quarters of the CS I-IIA patients investigated, and two thirds of the CS IB-IIB patients, laparotomy findings were negative.

The percentage of patients undergoing laparotomy decreased from 57% in 1970-1979 to 39% in 1980+ for CS I patients, and from 63% to 40% for CS II patients.

Initial treatment (Table 3)

Relatively few CS I-II patients received initial CT alone. Over a quarter of CS I and over a third of CS II patients received initial RT+CT. Approximately two thirds of CS I patients and half of the CS II patients received initial RT alone. The radiotherapy field was confined to the involved area(s) in less than a quarter of patients receiving initial RT.

The proportion of CS I-II patients receiving initial RT+CT without laparotomy approximately doubled between 1970-79 and 1980+, rising to 23% for CS I and 31% for CS II.

Table 2. Laparotomy.

	CS I	CS II	
Laparotomised	40 %	50 %	
	CS IA	CS IIA	CS IB-IIB
Laparotomy positive	25 %	28 %	33 %
	CS I	CS II	
Laparotomy staging			
PS I	73 %		
PS II		69 %	
PS III	25 %	29 %	
PS IV	2 %	2 %	
	CS IA	CS IIA	CS IB-IIB
Prognostic factors for positive laparotomy	Sex ***(a)	Med. ***	Sex ***
	Hist.***	LNA ***	Med. ***
	Age **	Hist.***	EL ***
		Sex **	
Poor prognosis	50+ years; Mixed cellularity/Lymphocyte depletion; Male; Mediastinal involvement; Extra localisation		

Biological parameters had no influence when included in model.

(a) p value: ** $p < 0.01$; *** $p < 0.001$
Hist. = histological type; Med. = mediastinalm involvement; LNA = number of lymph node areas involved; EL = extra localisation E+.

Table 3. Initial treatment

	CS I	CS II
Radiotherapy alone	66.0 %	51.3 %
Chemotherapy alone	5.6 %	10.1 %
Radiotherapy + chemotherapy	28.4 %	38.6 %
Radiotherapy fields		
Involved fields	26.1 %	16.3 %
Mantle / inverted Y	40.9 %	40.7 %
(Sub)total nodal	31.1 %	41.9 %
Chemotherapy		
Single- or bi-agent	12.0 %	5.7 %
Combination	87.8 %	94.3 %
Combination chemotherapy		
MOPP or MOPP-like	88.4 %	84.0 %
Adriamycin containing	7.7 %	8.4 %
Alternated	3.0 %	6.8 %

Response to initial treatment (Table 4)

The overall response to initial treatment was very high, with 98% of CS I and 94% of CS II patients achieving complete remission (CR). The response was lower in CS I and considerably lower in CS II after initial CT alone than after initial RT, whether the latter was used alone or in combination with CT.

The main prognostic factors were age 50+ and B-symptoms, together with ESR and serum albumin, in non-laparotomised patients; in laparotomised patients they were B-symptoms overall, and ESR and infradiaphragmatic presentation in patients without B-symptoms.

Table 4. Response to initial treatment

	CS I	CS II
% complete response overall	98 %	94 %

% complete response in relation to type of initial treatment	CS I			CS II		
	No Lap	PS I	PS III-IV	No Lap	PS II	PS III-IV
RT +/- single- or bi- agent CT	99 %	99 %	94 %	94 %	97 %	96 %
Combination CT	84 %		87 %	63 %	48 %	76 %
RT + combination CT	97 %	98 %	96 %	93 %	97 %	94 %

Relapse-free survival (Table 5)

The relapse-free survival (RFS) from the initial treatment of CSI-II was 73%-80% at 5 years and 69%-75% at 10 years. The RFS in patients who received initial RT+CT was consistently higher than in those who received initial RT alone, with those receiving initial CT alone occupying an intermediate position (except for CS IA, in which the RFS from CT alone was lower than that from RT alone).

Relapses continued to occur in CS I-II patients for 15-16 years from the start of initial treatment, with 12% occurring later than 5 years (Table 6).

Prognostic factors for RFS are shown in Table 7. Haematological parameters were associated with RFS, as were age and sex, together with histology, topography and number of lymph node sites involved.

Table 5. Relapse-free survival

	CS IA	CS IIA	CS IB-IIB
% RFS at 5 years overall	80 %	74 %	73 %

% RFS et 5 years in relation to type of initial treatment	CS IA		CS IIA		CS IB-IIB	
	No LAP	LAPs (All PS patients)	No LAP	LAPs (All PS patients)	No LAP	LAPs (All PS patients)
RT +/- single- or bi-agent CT	71 %	84 %	64 %	71 %	49 %	66 %
Combination CT	59 %		69 %	78 %	72 %	81 %
RT + Combination CT	92 %	90 %	88 %	88 %	84 %	87 %

Table 6. Relapse

	CS I A	CS II A	CS IB-IIB
Number of patients who relapsed	564/2707 (21%)	1134/4406 (26 %)	460/1974 (23%)
Delay from start of initial treatment			
1st year	109	300	146
2nd year	175	315	131
3rd year	79	198	86
4th year	54	125	38
5th year	47	70	18
6th year	39	41	11
7th year	19	35	13
8th year	17	16	6
9th year	6	9	3
10th year	4	6	1
11th+ year	15	19	7
Median (months)	23	21	18
Range (years)	0-16	0-16	0-15

Table 7. Relapse-free survival - Prognostic factors

	CS I A		CS II A		CS IB-IIB	
Age	***(a)	Histology (4)	**	Sex	**
Topography	***			LNA 5+	**
Sex	**				
Poorer prognosis	40+ years; supradiaphragmatic disease; male gender; mixed cellularity/lymphocyte depletion				
Biological parameters	ESR was major prognosis indicator in IA, IIA Hb significant factor in IA, IB-IIB Albumin (decreased) predictive in IB-IIB				

(a) ** $p < 0.01$; *** $p < 0.001$
LNA : number of lymph node areas involved; ESR : erythrocyte sedimentation rate (first hour); Hb : haemoglobin;

Overall survival (Table 8)

The survival of CS I-II patients who failed to achieve sustained complete remission from initial treatment was poor, being approximately 30% and 50% at 10 years for patients failing to achieve CR and patients later relapsing respectively, indicating that salvage therapy was relatively unsuccessful [*Statistical Report, Figure VIII-7*]. The survival of those patients who achieved CR and remained relapse free was approximately 90%, approximately 10% dying from causes other than HD.

Table 8. Overall survival

	CS IA	CS IIA	CS IB-IIB
No initial complete remission			
5-year survival rate	52 %	45 %	39 %
10-year survival rate		34 %	28 %
Complete remission - relapse			
5-year survival rate	75 %	77 %	64 %
10-year survival rate	56 %	58 %	47 %
Complete remission - no relapse			
5-year survival rate	95 %	96 %	94 %
10-year survival rate	87 %	92 %	89 %

Prognostic factors related to CS I-II survival are shown in Table 9. Deaths recorded as being due to causes other than HD were related to age and sex. Deaths recorded as being due to HD were also related to age, and sex, but were related to histology in addition (and in stages IB-IIB to the number lymph node areas involved).

Table 9. Overall survival - Prognostic factors

CS IA		CS IIA		CS IB-IIB	
A. Death from Hodgkin's disease					
Age 60+	***(a)	Age 60+	***	Age 60+	***
Hist. LD	***	Age 50-59	***	Hist. LD	***
Hist. MC	***	Hist. LD	**	Sex	***
Sex	**	Hist. MC	**	LNA 5+	**
Age 40-49	**				
Age 50-59	**				
Hist. NS	*				
B. Death from causes other than Hodgkin's disease					
Age 60+	***	Age 60+	***	Age 60+	***
Age 50-59	***	Age 50-59	***	Age 50-59	***
Age 40-49	***	Age 40-49	**	Age 40-49	***
Age 30-39	***	Sex	**	Age 30-39	**
Sex	***	Age 30-39	**		

(a) ** $p < 0.01$; *** $p < 0.001$;
Hist. : histological subtypes (NS : nodular sclerosis; MC : mixed cellularity; LD : lymphocyte depletion); LNA : number of lymph node areas involved
Sex : female gender favourable; MC/LD : unfavourable

Causes of death - all stages (Table 10)

Approximately one third of deaths for which the cause was specified were recorded as being due to causes other than HD (treatment-related deaths, deaths from second cancer, and intercurrent deaths).

Table 10. Causes of death (All stages)

Total patients	14225	
Total deaths	4139	
Deaths with cause unspecified	3634	
Hodgkin's disease related	2404	(66 %)
Treatment realted	237	(7 %)
Second cancer	404	(11 %)
Intercurrent disease	589	(16 %)

Second cancers - all stages (Table 11)

The relative risk (RR) of second cancer was significantly higher than that expected from general population incidence rates for non-Hodgkin's lymphoma (NHL), acute leukaemia (AL), and for many solid tumours (ST) [*Statistical Report, Table IX-2*]. An increase in RR for solid tumours was observed in most of the sites potentially submitted to radiation therapy, both in males and females.

The overall cumulative incidence rates of second cancers is shown in Table 11 [*Statistical Report, Figures IX-3* and *IX-4*]. Over half of the cancers were solid tumours, and the rise in the cumulative incidence of the latter was progressive thoughout the 20 year period. The rises for NHL and AL were much more modest, and the last case of AL was at 16 years.

Second cancers are discussed in detail in part X of the *Statistical Report*.

Table 11. Second cancers (All stages)

Total number of second cancers	653	
Solid Tumours	393	(60 %)
Acute Leukaemias	154	(24 %)
Non-Hodgkin's lymphomas	106	(16 %)

Cumulative incidence of second cancers

	10-year	15-year	20-year
All second cancers	6.4 %	11.2 %	18.6 %
Solid tumours	3.7 %	7.5 %	13.6 %
Acute leukaemias	1.8 %	2.2 %	2.4 %
Non-Hodgkin's lymphomas	1.0 %	1.8 %	3.2 %

Causes of death in HD

Measurements of the success of treatment for HD commonly include death as an end point (RFS, disease-free survival (DFS), and overall survival (OS) since whilst treatment cures patients of their HD it also results in the short and long term death of some patients (from marrow depression, cardiovascular disease, etc.). However HD patients form a subset of the general population, which is subject to death from causes other than HD. Deaths from these causes would be expected to have little effect on the 20 year survival of HD patients aged less than 30 at presentation, since relatively few people in the general population die before the age of 50, but to have a considerable effect on the 20 year survival of older HD patients. (For example, the 20 year survival of HD patients aged 70-79 at presentation will be only a few percent even if all have been cured of their HD, since any who are still alive will be in their nineties). Survival in the general population is also markedly influenced by gender, with females surviving appreciably longer than males.

Age, and to a lesser extent sex would therefore be expected a priori to be strongly prognostic for survival in the present series, in which many patients lived long enough to be exposed to the risk of deaths from "natural" causes, and the proportional hazards model shows age to be the main prognostic factor for death from all causes in all stages, and sex also to be a significant factor in all of them. When causes of death were divided into those from HD and those from other causes, the model showed age to be the main prognostic factor in all stages for survival from deaths due to causes other than HD (together with sex, which was the only other significant factor). However, age was also a prognostic factor in all stages for survival from deaths due to HD. Evidently age is related both to deaths from "natural" causes and also to deaths from HD.

The effect of age on the CR rate [*Statistical Report, Table VI-11*] and RFS [*Statistical Report, Figure VII-8*] is relatively small compared to its effect upon overall survival [*Statistical Report, Figure VIII-9*] indicating that the increase in the death rate from HD in older patients is relatively small compared to the increase in the death rate from "natural" causes in these patients. The disadvantages of using age (and perhaps sex) as an indication for the use of aggressive treatment have been outlined already in the previous section on CS III-IV disease.

The estimation of the success of treatment for HD in older patients is thus prone to inaccuracy when death is included as an end point, since it is difficult if not impossible to discount those deaths which occurred from causes operative in the general population, particularly those from second cancer (and probably also those from cardiovascular disease), as some will have been due to the effects of treatment. A futher complication is provided by the relationship between age and second cancers, whose incidence was associated with older age groups, as is that of cancer in the general population. Second cancers occurred with unexpectedly high frequency in many sites in the present series [*Statistical Report, Table IX-2*]. This could be due to some innate susceptibility existing in patients with HD. However Kaldor et al., in a series of patients with testicular or ovarian cancer, together with over 28,000 patients with HD, reported unexpectedly high incidences of second cancers in all three groups, and it seems probable that the unexpected second cancers in the present series were due to late effects of treatment (Kaldor et al., 1988). Thus the use of RT was associated with an increase in the relative risk of solid tumours, compared to general population incidence rates, in most of the sites potentially submitted to RT. Bonadonna and Santoro have reported that approximately two-thirds of the solid tumours occurring in patients with advanced HD treated with RT and CT have so far occurred in the radiation field (Valagussa et al., 1988; Bookman & Longo, 1986); and Haybittle et al. reported a small but significant increase in mortality from second cancer (and also from cardiovascular disease) in a large series of patients receiving adjuvant RT for breast cancer (Haybittle et al., 1989). In addition, the high risk of acute leukaemia in the present series compared to the general population was related to treatment with CT, as well as to age, and Devereux et al., as Henry-Amar et al., found the incidence of AL in HD to be related to the amount of treatment with CT which had been received (Henry-Amar et al., 1989; Devereux et al., 1990).

Initial treatment of clinical stage I-II

The success of initial treatment in the production of complete remission in CS I-II patients was lower after the use of initial CT alone than after inital RT alone or initial RT+CT. This finding is difficult to interpret: the number of patients treated with initial CT alone was relatively small, and this treatment may have been reserved primarily for patients with poor prognosis. However one might reasonably expect that RT+CT would also be reserved for such patients. It seems probable therefore that initial CT is less successful than RT in treating clinically evident disease, and that RT is a necessary component of initial treatment for the induction of complete remission.

The RFS after initial RT+CT was consistently higher than after initial RT or CT alone. The high RFS resulting from RT+CT compared to RT alone was evidently due to the action of the CT component in preventing the relapses which frequently occur after initial RT alone in sites remote from those evident at presentation, presumably due to the growth of underdetected occult disease in areas untreated by initial RT. There appeared to be no difference in the CR rate between laparotomised and non-laparotomised patients when initial CMT was used.

It would seem that CMT is the treatment of choice, if initial treatment is to be given with curative intent. The disadvantage in Stage I-II disease of using CT "up front" for all patients is that a considerable percentage of them can be cured by initial local RT alone, since the latter produces a DFS of 30%-60% (Rosenberg, 1985; Stucliffe et al., 1985; Haybittle et al., 1985). Some patients will therefore have received CT unnecessarily, resulting in a high proportion being rendered sterile. However it is possible to reduce this proportion by appropriate choice of the particular drugs used (though the effectiveness of such non-sterilising drug combinations has yet to be proven). Chemotherapy is also associated with secondary acute leukaemia, but the cumulative incidence of this cancer was low in the present series and probably occurs mainly in patients who are resistant to initial cure of their HD (Devereux et al., 1990). Furthermore, relatively local RT fields can be used if CT is given also, thereby reducing the risk of secondary solid tumour occurring in the irradiated field, since the Pierre-et-Marie-Curie Group found no significant overall increase in DFS with wider fields using RT+CT (Zittoun et al., 1985). It is also possible that initial CT may reduce the incidence of those relapses (and deaths associated with them) which occur in areas remote from the original clinically evident sites of disease after initial RT alone, since any undetected occult disease is theoretically more amenable to treatment with CT initially when small in bulk than later at relapse.

Laparotomy

Laparotomy findings were negative in approximately two-thirds to three quarters of the patients on whom they were performed, and there appeared to be no difference between the CR rates or DFS of laparotomised and non-laparotomised patients treated with initial CMT. An appreciable number of laparotomy negative patients relapse below the diaphragm, and the procedure is associated with significant early and late morbidity, and with an immediate mortality of around 0,5%: it is also associated with deaths from late fulminant infections (Jelliffe & Vaughan Hudson, 1987). (It has been suggested that all splenectomised laparotomised patients should receive "Pneumovax" together with Penicillin daily for the rest of their lives).

Prognostic factors

The effects of any particular treatment given for HD vary widely, even if the patients to whom it is given are of the same status with respect to stage and systemic symptoms. Some achieve permanent complete remission, but others later relapse, or achieve only partial or even no remission.

It would be of obvious advantage to be able to identify at presentation the likelihood of success of a given treatment for an individual patient. Identification of patients who required only RT to their clinically evident sites of disease would obviate the use of initial CT; whilst those identified as being unlikely to benefit from standard treatment could be considered as candidates for very intensive therapy with autologous bone marrow transplant rescue.

The reasons for the varying response to treatment are uncertain. They may involve the amount of tumour present, the aggressiveness of the tumour, and possibly the resistance of the host to its own tuour. The two former factors are at present only assessable in a quasi-quantitative manner, since the estimated size of a particular nodal mass varies widely between different observers, as does the perception of the morphology of any given tumour section; and the existence of host resistance remains unproven.

Data concerning tumour bulk was not requested in the present series, due to difficulties in the standardisation of such data. Histopathological subtyping is discussed in an other chapter of the present work. The difference in RFS between the different subtypes was relatively small [*Statistical Report, Figure VII-4*], with the exception of the lymphocyte-depleted subgroup which comprises only a small proportion of patients. The prognostic value of age and sex have already been discussed. The degree of usefulness of haematological parameters in the present series has not yet been established, mainly due to the amount of missing data, and the influence of these parameters has so far been examined only individually. It may be possible on further analysis to combine these factors with other parameters, and so perhaps identify patients with a very high chance of cure on the one hand, and those with very poor chances on the other.

References

Bookman, M.A. & Longo, D.L. (1986): Concomitant illness in patients treated for Hodgkin's disease. *Cancer Treat. Rev.* 13, 77-111.
Devereux, S. et al. (1990): Leukaemia complicating treatment for Hodgkin's disease: The British National Lymphoma Investigation experience. *(Submitted for publication)*.
Haybittle, J.L. et al. (1985): Review of British National Lymphoma Investigation studies of Hodgkin's disease and development of prognostic index. *Lancet* i, 967-972.
Haybittle, J.L. et al. (1989): Postoperative radiotherapy and late mortality: Evidence from the CRC trial for early breast cancer. *Br. Med. J.* 298, 1611-1614.
Henry-Amar, M. et al. (1990): Risk of second acute leukemia and preleukemia after Hodgkin's disease: The Institut Gustave Roussy experience. In *New Aspects in the Diagnosis and Treatment of Hodgkin's Disease*, ed. V. Diehl, M. Preundschuh & M. Löffler, pp. 270-283. Recent Res. Cancer Res. vol. 117. Berlin, Heidelberg: Springer-Verlag.
Jellife, A.M. & Vaughan Hudson, G. (1987): Staging laparotomy in Hodgkin's disease. In *Hodgkin's disease*, ed. P. Selby & T.J. McElwain, pp. 160-180. London: Blackwell Scientific Publ.
Kaldor, J.M. et al. (1987): Second malignancies following testicular cancer, ovarian cancer and Hodgkin's disease: An international collaborative study among cancer registries. *Int. J. Cancer* 39, 571-585.
MacLennan, K.A. et al. (1981): The pretreatment peripheral blood lymphocyte count in 1100 patients with Hodgkin's disease: The prognostic significance and the relationship to the presence of systemic symptoms. *Clin. Oncol.* 7, 333-339.
Rosenberg, S.A. (1985): The current status of the Stanford randomized clinical trials of the management of Hodgkin's disease. In *Malignant Lymphomas and Hodgkin's disease: Experimental and Therapeutic Advances*, ed. F. Cavalli, G. Bonadonna & M. Rozencweig, pp. 281-292. Boston: Martinus-Nijhoff.
Specht, L. & Nissen, N.I. (1988): Prognostic factors in Hodgkin's disease satge IV. *Eur. J. Haematol.* 41, 359-367.

Sutcliffe, S.B. et al. (1985): Prognostic groups for management of localized Hodgkin's disease. *J. Clin. Oncol.* 3, 393-401.

Valagussa, P. et al. (1988): Hodgkin's disease and second malignancies. *Proc. Am. Soc. Clin. Oncol.* 7, 227.

Vaughan Hudson, B. et al. (1987): Selective peripheral blood eosinophils associated with survival advantage in Hodgkin's disease. (BNLI report n° 31). *J. Clin. Pathol.* 40, 247-250.

Wagstaff, J. et al. (1988): Prognostic factors for survival in stage IIIB and IV Hodgkin's disease: A multivariate analysis comparing two specialist treatment centres. *Br. J. Cancer* 58, 487-492.

Zittoun, R. et al. (1985): Extended versus involved fields irradiation combined with MOPP chemotherapy in early stages of Hodgkin's disease. *J. Clin. Oncol.* 3, 207-214.

Hodgkin's disease treatment strategy - stage I-II

R.T. Hoppe

Department of Radiation Oncology, Stanford University Medical Center, Stanford, California 94305, USA

Summary

Success in the management of stage I-II Hodgkin's disease has improved dramatically in the last three decades. These improvements are the results of the use of more careful and definitive staging, the identification of prognostic factors to assist in the selection of treatment programs, the refinement of techniques of radiation therapy, the development of effective combinations of drugs, and the careful follow up of patients to identify complications of therapy. The use of definitive stafing studies has permitted the development of our understanding of the natural history of Hodgkin's disease and the selection of appropriate treatment programs. Initially, lymphography identified a high likelihood of subdiaphragmatic disease where other clinical staging studies were negative. Later, staging laparotomy and splenectomy revealed a high risk (30%) of subdiaphragmatic disease even when all clinical staging studies where within normal limits. More recently, computerized tomographic scanning and magnetic resonance imaging have permitted careful evaluation of potential sites of disease above and below the diaphragm. The relative role of each of these staging procedures will vary from one institution to another depending upon the facilities and expertise available.

Careful staging of patients, standard application of therapy, and close follow up permits the identification of prognostic factors. In stage I-II disease, the overriding factor of importance appears to be bulk of disease. This may be measured by size of tumor masses, total volume of disease, etc. Additional biologic factors are important such as the prsence of systemic symptoms and the erythrocyte sedimentation rate (ESR). In general, the significance of prognostic factors will be greatest when the treatment is most limited. When treatments are aggressive, and cure rates high, the significance of prognostic factors may be blurred somewhat. This may account for differences in prognostic factors analysis which are reported among different institutions and cooperative groups.

The treatment of patients with stage I-II Hodgkin's disease primarily has been with radiation therapy. Careful application of this modality can result in the cure of most (75-80%) patients. The extent of radiation therapy necessary to achieve this result is dependent upon the presence of various prognostic factors. In certain situations, treatment with irradiation alone may not achieve adequat results. Patients with bulky mediastinal adenopathy, for example, are generally acknowledged to have a better outcome after treatment with combined modality therapy. The role of chemotherapy in other settings of stage I-II disease is debatable and currently being investigated by several groups.

The excellent long term survival of patients with stage I-II Hodgkin's disease permits the identification and assessment of risk of various complications of therapy. These range from minor problems such as thyroid abnormalities, to more serious difficulties such as secondary malignancies which may appear in long term follow up. In addition, there are complicated groups of psychosocial problems which are difficult to quantitate. The identification of these complications requires refinement of treatment programs and this will provide the challenge for future generations of clinical investigators.

Résumé

Les résultats de la prise en charge et du traitement des stades I-II de maladie de Hodgkin se sont considérablement améliorés en l'espace de 30 ans. Ces gains sont le fruit d'un meilleur bilan initial de la maladie, de l'utilisation de facteurs de pronostic dans le choix des traitements, l'affinement des techniques de radiothérapie, l'apparition de nouvelles chimiothérapies efficaces, ainsi que le suivi minutieux des malades permettant d'identifier les complications iatrogènes. La réalisation d'études décisives concernant le bilan initial a favorisé une meilleure connaissance de l'histoire naturelle de la maladie et permis une sélection opportune des stratégies de traitement. Initialement, la lymphographie a permis de faire le diagnostic d'envahissement sous diaphragmatique dans des cas où les investigations cliniques étaient négatives. Plus tard, la laparotomie associée à une splénectomie a montré que la probabilité d'un envahissement sous diaphragmatique était de l'ordre de 30% même lorsque les résultats des examens cliniques étaient dans la limite de la normale. Plus récemment, la tomodensitométrie et l'imagerie en résonnance magnétique ont permis l'investigation de toutes les localisations potentielles de la maladie situées de part et d'autre du diaphragme. L'utilisation de chacune de ces techniques d'évaluation est amenée à varier d'un centre à un autre en fonction des disponibilités et de l'expérience de chacun.

Un bilan initial précis, l'utilisation de techniques de radiothérapie standardisées, et un suivi étroit des malades ont permis la mise en évidence de facteur de pronostic. Dans le cas des stades I-II, le volume tumoral apparait comme le facteur pronostique le plus important. Le volume tumoral peut être évalué en mesurant la taille des masses tumorales, leur volume, etc. Les paramètres biologiques, comme la présence de signes généraux ou la vitesse de sédimentation, sont aussi des facteurs importants. En général, la valeur pronostique propre de ces facteurs est d'autant plus importante que le traitement est limité. Lorsque les traitements utilisés sont plus agressifs, et par conséquent les taux de guérison élevés, leur valeur pronostique est quelque peu atténuée. Ceci peut expliquer les différences observées entre les résultats des analyses pronostiques publiées par différentes équipes.

La première thérapeutique employée dans le cas des stades I-II de maladie de Hodgkin a été la radiothérapie. Une utilisation optimale de cette technique peut induire des taux de guérison de l'ordre de 75% à 80%. L'augmentation du nombre des volumes à irradier, nécessaire pour obtenir de tels résultats, dépend essentiellement des facteurs pronostiques. Dans certaines situations, la radiothérapie ne permet pas à elle seule d'obtenir des résultats satisfaisants. Par exemple, les malades porteurs d'importantes adénopathies médiastinales nécessitent en général d'être traités par une association radio-chimiothérapie. La place de la chimiothérapie dans le traitement d'autres catégories de patients à un stade localisé de la maladie est l'objet de controverses et est en cours d'évaluation.

Les excellents résultats quant à la survie de ces malades ont permis de mettre en évidence et de quantifier les risques iatrogènes associés à certains traitements. Les complications recensées sont variées et leur importance variable. Cela va de l'hypothyroidie biologique, considérée comme peu grave, à la survenue d'une deuxième tumeur maligne, laquelle peut ne survenir que longtemps après le diagnostic initial de maladie de Hodgkin. Les complications psychologiques existent aussi bien que leur importance soit difficile à quantifier. La réalité de ces complications implique que nous réajustions les stratégies thérapeutiques proposées, un défi que devraient relever les prochaines générations de médecins-chercheurs.

Introduction

The management of Hodgkin's disease has undergone continuous evolution in the last two decades. The application of definitive staging, initially with lymphography and later with staging laparotomy and splenectomy, has provided incites into the natural history and spread of this disease. Newer clinical staging techniques, such as magnetic resonance imaging, gallium scanning with single photon emission tomography, and ultrasound tissue characterization studies may improve further upon our ability to detect minimal disease.

Treatment programs for Hodgkin's disease have also undergone significant change. The concept of high dose extended field irradiation for curative management of patients with early stage disease is now widely accepted. Irradiation treatment has become more refined by the routine use of CT treatment planning, field simulation, custom contoured blocks, and the linear accelerator. The wide availability of physics support and quality assurance programs has made effective and safe treatment available in many communities throughout the world.

Combination chemotherapy, at first used so successfully in the management of patients with advanced disease, has now been incorporated into combined modality treatment programs for certain subgroups of patients with stage I-II disease and is being used as a single modality for limited disease in prospective clinical trials. Novel chemotherapy, with proved efficacy and potentially less toxicity is also being utilized in clinical trials for these patients.

As the treatment for Hodgkin's disease has become more successful, and large cohorts of patients have been followed for ten years or longer, the toxicities of therapy have become more apparent. These include irradiation or chemotherapy induced organ failure such as hypothyroidism, cardiac or pulmonary failure, and infertility, secondary cancers including leukemia and solid tumors, and also a complicated group of psychosocial problems.

Given the variety of potentially effective treatments for Hodgkin's disease and the differences in access to various services for both staging and treatment, it is not surprising that a number of different effective management programs have developed throughout the world. It is appropriate that different treatment strategies continue to be used, based upon local experiences. The primary concepts applicable to all patients is that they be evaluated carefully for the extent of disease at the time of presentation, that they be treated with special attention to all details of therapy, and that they be followed closely to detect recurrence of disease or complications of therapy.

Staging

Improvements in the clinical staging of Hodgkin's disease have contributed to an improved outcome of treatment. An assessment of the extent of disease permits selection of the most effective initial therapy. Clinical stage, as defined by the Ann Arbor criteria, is one of the most important prognostic factors in Hodgkin's disease (Carbone et al., 1971).

Lymphography has long been regarded as an important clinical study to obtain in newly-diagnosed patients with Hodgkin's disease. Recently, this concept has been challenged, as proponents of computerized tomographic (CT) scanning, Gallium scanning, and MRI scanning have tried to establish the superiority of these modalities. However, the lymphogram remains the most accurate study for the identification of retroperitoneal disease. In experienced hands, the study has an overall accuracy of 95% (85% sensitivity and 98% specificity) (Table 1) (Castellino et al., 1984). The lymphogram has other attributes in addition to initial staging. It provides important information for radiation therapy treatment planning and definition of treatment fields. The amount of normal tissue (e.g. kidneys and bone marrow) irradiated can be minimized when the subdiaphragmatic nodes are localized precisely. In addition, the lymphogram provides an important and easy means for follow-up evaluation after the completion of therapy, a characteristic not shared by other imaging techniques. Adequate lymphographic contrast may remain to assess the size of opacified nodes for one to three years after completion of the study. In skilled hands, repetition of the examination is not difficult.

Table 1. Hodgkin's disease : Retroperitoneal nodes - CT *vs* LAG.

	Sensitivity	Specificity	Overall accuracy
CT	13/20 (65%)	80/87 (92%)	93/107 (87%)
LAG	17/20 (85%)	85/87 (98%)	102/107 (95%)

CT : computerized tomographic scan of abdomen and pelvis; LAG : bipedal lymphogram

(From Castellino et al., 1984)

Among treating physicians there is a general consensus that lymphography continue to be performed in Hodgkin's disease. Unfortunately, younger diagnostic radiologists have not always been trained adequately to perform or interpret lymphograms and they have emphasized the use of other types of imaging studies. Regrettably, we may have to acknowledge that lymphography will be performed less universally in the initial staging of patients with Hodgkin's disease.

Disagreement continues regarding the role of laparotomy staging in Hodgkin's disease. Staging laparotomy with splenectomy was introduced at several centers in the late 1960's and became routine at many in subsequent years. At some centers, the procedure was never adopted, and at others it has been used only selectively. The role of staging laparotomy varies from one center to another based upon established programs of management for patients with different stages of disease. It may be considered as a means for identifying patients who are candidates for treatment with irradiation alone. If clinical studies were perfectly accurate in identifying patients who required systemic treatment then a staging laparotomy could not be justified. Unfortunately, clinical staging parameters cannot predict the yield of laparotomy with perfect accuracy.

In the general management of stage I-II disease, one may "understage", i.e. avoid laparotomy, and compensate by employing more aggressive initial treatment or else accept a higher initial relapse rate. Alternatively, one may use more refined clinical prognostic factors or laparotomy to tailor individual treatment programs. Despite differences in relapse risk, both policies may provide for equivalent long term survival in large cohorts of patients. For example, at the Princess Margaret Hospital in Toronto, laparotomy and splenectomy have been performed only selectively. Treatment results were compared to data from Stanford, where the procedure was performed more routinely (Bergsagel et al., 1982). The ten year freedom from relapse was approximately 50% and 67% with laparotomy performed selectively or routinely respectively. However, the long term survivals were similar (approximately 70%) in both groups.

In evaluating the efficacy of staging laparotomy, favorable prognostic groups, which have a low yield for the study, have been identified in single institutional studies as well as in the

EORTC Hodgkin's disease database (Leibenhaut et al., 1989). Favorable factors include gender (female favorable), age (younger more favorable), histology (lymphocyte predominance more favorable) and number of sites of involvement (fewer sites more favorable). Good prognostic groups, with a yield of laparotomy of less than 10%, include all women with clinical stage I disease and all men with clinical stage I disease and lymphocyte predominance histology. In addition, women with clinical stage II disease who have three or fewer sites of involvement and who are younger than 27 years old have a risk of subdiaphragmatic disease of only about 10% (Table 2). Patients with these characteristics account for about 20% of patients with CS I-II disease. In a program with selective utilization of laparotomy, the procedure may be avoided in these individuals.

Table 2. Hodgkin's disease : Yield of staging laparotomy.

Favorable Groups of Clinical Stage I-II	Yield	
CS I Female	6%	48% of all CS I patients
CS I Male; LP, IF	4%	
CS II Female ⩽ 3 sites; ⩽ 26 years old	9%	15% of all CS II patients

(From Leibenhaut et al., 1989)

In an attempt to test the question of therapeutic benefits of laparotomy, the EORTC H-2 trial was designed to randomize patients with CS I-II disease to staging laparotomy or clinical staging only. Among patients treated initially with irradiation alone, the benefit in relapse free survival in the group who had undergone laparotomy was only marginal and there was no difference in long-term survival (Tubiana et al., 1984).

In a more recent EORTC trial, the H6 study, patients with clinical stage I-II and favorable prognostic factors (one or two lymph node areas only involved **and** ESR < 50 in asymptomatic patients **or** ESR < 30 in patients with B symptoms) were randomized to staging with or without laparotomy. Treatment in the non-laparotomy group included irradiation both above and below the diaphragm. In the laparotomy group, treatment was adjusted according to histological and pathological stage. Four year results show freedom from relapse in favor of the laparotomy group ($p = 0.02$), however there is no difference in survival (Table 3) (Tubiana et al., 1989).

Prognostic Factors

Individual institutional analyses, studies of cooperative clinical groups, and the EORTC database for Hodgkin's disease indicate important prognostic factors for survival and freedom from relapse in Hodgkin's disease (Tubiana et al., 1985). These include age, gender, histology, bulk of disease, number of sites of involvement, specific sites of involvement, the presence of B symptoms, and abnormalities of the erythrocyte sedimentation rate or other biological factors.

Table 3. Hodgkin's disease : EORTC H6-F trial - 4 year results.

	# patients	Survival	FFR
No Laparotomy	118	89%	75%
		$p > .5$	$p < .02$
Laparotomy Negative : Mantle or STNI Laparotomy Positive : CMT	114	93%	85%

STNI : subtotal nodal irradiation; CMT : combined modality therapy; FFR : freedom from relapse

(From Tubiana et al., 1989)

Exactly which prognostic factors are the most important is another source of disagreement. This is probably due to different techniques of analysis, variable definitions of factors such as number of regions involved or bulky disease, and differences in the intensity of staging or type of treatment.

Age is indeniably an important prognostic factor in Hodgkin's disease, especially when the endpoint of analysis is survival. It is also an important consideration in selection of treatment programs, with special modifications being appropriate for the very young (prepubertal) and the very old. However, for the majority of patients with Hodgkin's disease, who may range in age from 15 to 50 years, it is not clear that age is an important prognostic factor independent of stage and other disease parameters that warrant special treatment considerations.

Likewise, gender may have a subtle influence on prognosis which becomes minimal when disease-related characteristics are considered. Nevertheless, gender may be helpful in planning staging procedures (as noted above) and is very important to consider when selecting a treatment program because of issues of infertility related to certain components of therapy.

Histology is a potentially important prognostic factor. It is most important with respect to the natural history of disease and in an untreated population of patients may be of supreme importance. However, in the context of management programs which include intensive staging and aggressive therapy, the prognostic import of histology is blurred somewhat in all but the largest series of patients. In addition ,many large modern series have an overwhelming majority of patients (70-80%) in the nodular sclerosis category, and almost none in the lymphocyte depleted category, especially for stge I-II. Nevertheless, considerations of histology may be helpful in choosing stage procedures, as noted above. In addition, nuances of histology, such as the subclassification of nodular sclerosis as proposed by the BNLI (British National Lymphoma Investigation) investigators, may prove to be more helpful in predicting prognosis than are more traditional concepts in histology (Bennet et al., 1983). Furthermore, as the trend develops to decrease the intensity of treatment in Hodgkin's disease (in recognition of long term complications), histology may once again prove to be a very important prognostic factor and an aid in the selection of treatment programs.

Disease-related parameters, such as stage, number of sites involved, bulk of disease, and biologic measurements of disease activity such as the erythrocyte sedimentation rate (ESR) are the most important prognostic factors in Hodgkin's disease. These factors are decisive in the selection of optimal treatment programs. The Ann Arbor staging system has withstood the test of time and remains an effective means for grouping patients according to prognosis. However, it is not perfect, its primary deficiency being its failure to consider the extent of disease in stage II. The extent of disease may be reflected by several measures including the number of regions involved, size of lymph node masses, the ESR, or various combinations of these factors (Mauch et al., 1978; Specht et al., 1988; Tubiana et al., 1989). When properly applied, these measurements enhance our ability to refine treatment programs within stage II.

Most investigators agree that bulk is an important prognostic factor in Hodgkin's disease. This has been demonstrated most convincingly for disease in the mediastinum, less so in abdominal or peripheral sites. Even in the context of bulky disease in the mediastinum, however, confusion exists because definitions of bulky disease have varied widely. Perhaps the biologically most relevant definition would be a volumetric measurement (Willett et al., 1988). However, volumetric determinations may be tedious to perform. Others have proposed surface area calculations, absolute width measurements, or ratios of mass width to intrathoracic measurements. Unfortunately, the use of different definitions hampers the comparison of treatment results between different centers. Other factors related to bulk in the mediastinum which should be considered in the selection of therapy include location within the mediastinum (upper, middle, lower) and the degree of extension to adjacent organs and tissues such as the lungs, pericardium, chest wall, and pleura.

Therapy of Stage I-II

Based upon the results which have been published in the literature, as well as the EORTC database and discussions at the Hodgkin's Disease Symposium, several generalizations may be made. Most patients with bulky mediastinal disease (defined as a maximum mediastinal mass measurement which exceeds one-third of the maximum intrathoracic diameter), may be treated most effectively with combined modality therapy. Exceptions may exist when the mass is marginal in size, superior mediastinal in location, when extralymphatic extension does not pose a serious problem, and when there has been careful CT staging to assist in the design of the radiation fields (Hoppe, 1985). In most common situations, however, single modality therapy is inadequate for the management of bulky disease and a combined modality approach is warranted (Mauch et al., 1978; Hoppe et al., 1982; Young et al., 1978).

Table 4. Hodgkin's disease : Stage II bulky mediastinum. Clinical trials.

EORTC H6-U	A.	MOPP x 3 / Mantle / MOPP x 3
	B.	ABVD x 3 / Mantle / ABVD x 3
STANFORD C4,5	A.	PAVe x 3 / Mantle / PAVe x 3
	B.	ABVD x 3 / Mantle / ABVD x 3

Although most patients with bulky mediastinal disease will be treated with combined modality therapy, questions remain regarding the selection and duration of chemotherapy, the sequence of treatment, and the irradiation dose. Clinical trials are underway to answer some of these questions (Table 4). The EORTC H6-U study compares split course MOPP plus mantle versus split course ABVD plus mantle (Tubiana et al., 1989). While the results of treatment are similar, there may be short term disadvantages of ABVD with respect to pulmonary toxicity (Cosset et al., 1989). At Stanford, an analogous trial (C4,5 study) demonstrates similar results. At the MD Anderson hospital, the efficacy of only two cycles of MOPP followed by mantle and low dose lung irradiation is being evaluated in a non-randomized study and demonstrates very encouraging short term results (Fuller et al., 1988).

The majority of patients with CS I-II disease do not have bulky mediastinal involvement. If a laparotomy has not been performed, the selection of treatment must be based upon clinical parameters. Certain combinations of clinical parameters may mandate the use of combined modality therapy. These parameters may include B symptoms, unfavorable histology, large number of sites of involvement, male gender, older age, and elevated ESR (Sutcliffe et al. 1985; Carde et al., 1988; Tubiana et al., 1989). The exact combination of factors which requires systemic management for optimal outcome differs from one report to another. In general, the greater the number of risk factors, the greater the indication for systemic treatment.

If a laparotomy has not been performed, and treatment is with irradiation alone, then the extent of irradiation has generally included both mantle and subdiaphragmatic fields (including the spleen). However, the newest trial of the EORTC, the H7-VF trial, addresses the issue of whether subdiaphragmatic irradiation is essential in the most favorable group of clinically-staged patients. While it may be possible to identify a favorable cohort of clinically-staged patients who can be treated successfully to the mantle alone, careful long term follow up will be necessary, since these patients may be the very ones who are at greatest risk for late relapse (Herman et al.. 1985).

When patients with CS I-II disease have undergone laparotomy and splenectomy (PS I-II), treatment may be assigned according to pathological stage. At many centers, treatment both above and below the diaphragm is considered routine for this group of patients. Examples of treatment outcome with this management program are summarized in Table 5. Long term survival is generally reported to be around 90% and freedom from relapse 70-80%.

Table 5. Hodgkin's disease : PS I-II / Mantle + paraaortic - 10 year results.

	# patients	Survival	FFR
EORTC H-5 trial	98	91%	70%
Joint Center	315	90%	82%
Stanford	385	87%	75%

FFR : freedom from relapse

The use of less extensive irradiation in this setting has been reported from some centers. When this policy is followed for the majority of stage I-II patients, extension of disease to sites below the diaphragm may account for more than one-third of all relapses (Verger et al., 1988). However, the failure rate may be reduced by the careful selection of patients based upon well defined favorable clinical characteristics (Fuller et al., 1988). More limited treatment in laparotomy-staged patients has also been the subject of prospective clinical trials. For example, in the EORTC H5 trial, patients with favorable characteristics (age < 40, lymphocyte predominance or nodular sclerosis histology, **and** ESR < 70) were randomized to treatment with mantle alone or mantle plus paraaortic splenic pedicle field after negative staging laparotomy. Nine year results show freedom from relapse of 70% versus 69% and survival of 91% versus 94% (Tubiana et al., 1989). Therefore, there is growing support for the concept that subdiaphragmatic treatment may be omitted in patients with favorable clinical presentations who have undergone laparotomy staging.

Other important questions regarding the management of CS I-II disease, such as the role of systemic therapy, remain unanswered. However, this is the subject of several interesting trials.

A GATLA study randomized CS I-II patients to treatment with CVPP (cyclophosphamide, vincristine, procarbazine and prednisone) chemotherapy or CVPP chemotherapy plus involved field irradiation (Pavlovsky et al., 1988). At seven years, patients treated with CVPP alone had a survival of 82% and disease free survival of 62% compared to 89% (p = 0.3) and 71% (p = 0.01) for the patients treated with CVPP plus irradiation. More detailed analysis revealed that a favorable group of patients (age ≤ 45, only one or two lymph node groups involved, **and** no bulky disease) enjoyed similar outcome, irrespective of the initial treatment approach. On the other hand, the unfavorable group (age > 45, > 2 lymph node groups **or** bulky disease) had a significantly better prognosis with combined modality therapy (survival 84%, disease-free survival 75%) than with chemotherapy alone (survival 66%, disease free survival 34%, p = 0.001).

Cimino et al. have reported the results of an Italian cooperative group study (Cimino et al., 1989). Patients with PS I-II (laparotomy staged) were randomized to treatment with either MOPP (nitrogen mustargen, vincristine, procarbazine and prednisone) alone or irradiation alone (mantle plus subdiaphragmatic fields). Treatment outcome was similar in the two groups. Despite the lack of a treatment difference, however, the authors concluded that the initial irradiation approach was preferable, since complications were more severe in the MOPP group. This underlines the importance of following long term complications as well as outcome of therapy in contemporary randomized clinical trials.

Finally, at the NCI (National Cancer Institute), patients with PS I-II Hodgkin's disease (laparotomy staged), including some with bulky mediastinal disease, were randomized to treatment with MOPP alone or irradiation alone (mantle and subdiaphragmatic field) (Longo et al., 1987). With a median follow up of 40 months, 9% of the MOPP-treated patients have relapsed and 9% have died. One-third of the irradiated patients have relapsed (p = 0.007) and 22% have died (p = 0.09).

The results of treatment with chemotherapy alone on these three trials are summarize in Table 6. This issue remains an unresolved but important question for clinical trials, and it will be essential to measure both the outcome and toxicity of therapy. This will require that large cohorts of patients be followed for extended period of time.

Table 6. Hodgkin's disease : Stage I-II / MOPP chemotherapy.

		# patients	Survival	FFR
GATLA (CVPP)	(7 yr)	142 (CS)	82%	62%
Cimino et al.	(5 yr)	44 (PS)	87%	73%
NCI	(median = 40 mo)	44 (PS)	40/44 (91%)	40/44 (91%)

CS : clinical stage only; PS : pathological staging, including laparotomy

FFR : freedom from relapse

Still another approach to the management of stage I-II Hodgkin's disease is to use less intensive chemotherapy combined with irradiation. This may take the form of fewer cycles of a standard chemotherapy, such as MOPP, or novel chemotherapy with less potential toxicity, such as VBM (vinblastine, bleomycin, and methotrexate).

Investigators from the Pierre-et-Marie-Curie Group in France have reported the use of three cycles of MOPP plus involved field irradiation in patients with CS I-II (no staging laparotomy) (Zittoun et al., 1985). Disease-free survival is a respectable 82%. The reduction of the amount of chemotherapy to only three cycles and the extent of irradiation to involved fields permits a decrease in potential long-term toxicity of therapy.

At Stanford, we have completed a trial comparing treatment with irradiation alone (mantle plus subdiaphragmatic field) versus involved field irradiation plus VBM chemotherapy in laparotomy-staged patients (C1-3 studies) (Horning et al., 1988). VBM was selected as an adjuvant therapy because all of the drugs included have single-agent efficacy in the treatment of Hodgkin's disease and none is associated with sterility or secondary leukemia. In the most recent report of this trial, patients treated with involved field plus VBM showed an improved freedom from relapse compared to those treated with irradiation alone (95% vs 70%, p = 0.10), but the survivals are similar in the two arms of the study (100% vs 97%). In a new Stanford trial, a combination of VBM chemotherapy and regional irradiation is being compared to treatment with irradiation alone in patients who have **not** undergone laparotomy staging.

Treatment strategies for stage I-II Hodgkin's disease have evolved significantly over the past 20 years. Effective treatment modalities have been identified and treatment techniques have been refined to assure an optimal outcome. These improvements have been facilitated by the use of intensive staging procedures which provided information about the natural history and spread of the disease and also by the careful conduct of prospective clinical trials by investigators around the world. Important issues regarding the refinement of treatment programs and the reduction of complications remain to be answered and will provide challenges for clinical investigators for many years in the future.

References

Bennett, M.H., et al. (1983): The prognostic significance of cellular subtypes in nodular sclerosing Hodgkin's disease; an analysis of 271 non-laparotomised cases. *Clin. Radiol.* 34, 497-501.
Bergsagel, D.E., et al. (1982): Results of treating Hodgkin's without a policy of laparotomy staging. *Cancer Treat. Rep.* 66, 717-731.
Carbone, P.P., et al. (1971): Report of the committee on Hodgkin's disease staging classification. *Cancer. Res.* 31, 1860-1861.
Carde, P., et al. (1988): Clinical stage I and II Hodgkin's disease: A specifically tailored therapy according to prognostic factors. *J. Clin. Oncol.* 6, 239-252.
Castellino, R.A., et al. (1984): Computed tomography, lymphography and staging laparotomy: correlations in initial staging of Hodgkin's disease. *Am. J. Radiol.* 143, 37-41.
Cimino, G., et al. (1989): MOPP Chemotherapy versus extented field radiotherapy in the management of pathological stages I-IIA Hodgkin's disease. *J. Clin. Oncol.* 7, 732-737.
Cosset, J.M., et al. (1989): Increased pulmonary toxicity in the ABVD arm of the EORTC H6-U trial (Abstr.) *Proc. Am. Soc. Clin. Oncol.* 8, 253.
Fuller, L.M., et al. (1988): The adjuvant role of two cycles of MOPP and low-dose lung irradiation in stage IA through IIB Hodgkin's disease: Preliminary results. *Int. J. Radiat. Oncol. Biol. Phys.* 14, 683-692.
Herman, T.S., et al. (1985): Late relapse among patients treated for Hodgkin's disease. *Ann. Intern. Med.* 102, 292-297.
Hoppe, R.T. (1985): The management of stage II Hodgkin's disease with a large mediastinal mass: A prospective program emphasizing irradiation. *Int.J. Radiat. Oncol. Biol. Phys.* 11, 349-355.

Hoppe, R.T., et al. (1982): The management of stage I-II Hodgkin's disease with irradiation alone or combined modality therapy: The Stanford experience. *Blood* 59, 455-465.

Horning, S.J., et al. (1988): Vinblastine, bleomycin, and methotrexate: An effective adjuvant in favorable Hodgkin's disease. *J. Clin. Oncol.* 6, 1822-1831.

Leibenhaut, M.H., et al. (1989): Prognostic indicators of laparotomy findings in clinical stage I-II supradiaphragmatic Hodgkin's disease. *J. Clin. Oncol.* 7, 81-91.

Longo, D., et al., (1987): Randomized trial of MOPP chemotherapy vs subtotal nodal radiation therapy in patients with laparotomy. Documented early stage Hodgkin's disease. *Proc. Am. Soc. Clin. Oncol.* 6, A812.

Mauch, P., et al., (1978): The significance of mediastinal involvement in early stage Hodglin's disease. *Cancer* 42, 1039-1045.

Mauch, P., et al. (1988): Stage IA and IIA supradiaphragmatic Hodgkin's disease: Prognostic factors in surgically staged patients treated with mantle and paraaortic irradiation. *J. Clin. Oncol.* 6, 1576-1583.

Pavlovsky, S., et al (1988): Randomized trial of chemotherapy versus chemotherapy plus radiotherapy for stage I-II Hodgkin's disease. *J. Natl. Cancer Inst.* 80, 1466-1473.

Specht, L., et al. (1988): Tumor burden as the most important prognostic factor in early stage Hodgkin's disease. *Cancer* 61, 1719-1727.

Sutcliffe, S.B., et al. (1985): Prognostic groups for management of localized Hodgkin's disease. *J. Clin Oncol.* 3, 393-401.

Tubiana, M., et al. (1984): The EORTC treatment of early stages of Hodgkin's disease: The role of radiotherapy. *Int. J. Radiat. Oncol. Biol. Phys.* 10, 197-210.

Tubiana, M., et al. (1985): A multivariate analysis of prognostic factors in early stage Hodgkin's disease. *Int. J. Radiat. Oncol. Biol. Phys.* 11, 23-30.

Tubiana, M., et al. (1989): Toward comprehensive management tailored to prognostic factors of patients with clinical stages I and II in Hodgkin's disease. The EORTC lymphoma group controlled clinical trials: 1964-1987. *Blood* 73, 47-56.

Verger, E., et al. (1988): Radiotherapy results in laparotomy-staged Hodgkin's disease. *Clin. Radiol.* 39, 428-431.

Willett, C.G., et al. (1988): Stage IA to IIB mediastinal Hodgkin's disease: Three-dimensional volumetric assessment of response to treatment. *J. Clin. Oncol.* 6, 819-824.

Young, R.C., et al. (1978): Patterns of relapse in advanced Hodgkin's disease treated with combination chemotherapy. *Cancer* 42, 1001-1007.

Zittoun, R., et al. (1985): Extended versus involved fields irradiation combined with MOPP chemotherapy in early clinical stages of Hodgkin's disease. *J. Clin. Oncol.* 3, 207-214.

The current EORTC strategy for stage I-II Hodgkin's disease

J.M. Cosset[1], J. Thomas[2], E.M. Noordijk[3]
for the EORTC Lymphoma Cooperative Group

1 *Institut Gustave Roussy, 94805 Villejuif, France*
2 *St Rafaël Ziekenhuis 3000 Leuven, Belgium*
3 *University Hospital, P.O. Box 9600, 2300 RC Leiden, The Netherlands*

The current policy of the EORTC Lymphoma Cooperative Group for stage I-II supradiaphragmatic Hodgkin disease (HD) is based on the results of the four successive trials which have been carried out by the Group from 1964 to 1988 (Carde et al., 1988; Van der Werf Messing et al., 1973; Somers et al., 1989; Tubiana et al., 1981, 1984a, 1984b, 1984c, 1985, 1986, 1989).

As for the work-up strategy, we shall only briefly consider the question of laparotomy. R. Hoppe already reported in the previous chapter the results of our successive attempts to test the therapeutic benefit of exploratory laparotomy and splenectomy in the H2, H5 and H6 EORTC controlled studies. Actually, based on these data, it was decided for the ongoing H7 trial (activated in October 1988) to give up using laparotomy in the systematic work-up of supradiaphragmatic stage I-II HD. The ongoing H7 trial is thus only dealing with *clinically staged* (CS) limited HD patients. The study aims at asking specific questions for three well defined groups of patients.

The very favourable subgroup (H7 VF)

Such a subgroup of patients is seldom individualized in the current protocols. However, most trained "hodgkinologists" recognize that there is a small subset of patients with very "benign" presentation, for whom staging and treatment can safely be limited.

Turning to the EORTC database, the Lymphoma Group tried to identify a subgroup of patients which could be safely proposed a *minimal* treatment, i.e. a mantle field irradiation *alone*. These patients would thus be spared the untoward effects of laparotomy, chemotherapy and of extended field radiotherapy. Actually, the EORTC data indicated that only a *very small* subset of patients could be proposed such a limited irradiation as the sole treatment. This subgroup is very restrictively defined, only including patients with CS I, below 40 years of age, without any systemic symptom and with ESR (erythrocyte sedimentation rate) less than 50 mm (1rst hour), of female gender, of lymphocytic predominance and nodular sclerosis and without bulky mediastinal involvement. This subgroup only represents 6% of the total number of CS I-II supradiaphragmatic HD in the EORTC experience.

These patients are therefore currently proposed a *mantle field irradiation* alone. The small number of patients to be included in this study does not permit randomization. The relapse rate is expected to be low, and these rare relapses are expected to be easily salvaged in these non aggressively treated patients. However, as emphasized above by R. Hoppe, careful *long term* follow-up is necessary, in order to detect possible *late* relapses.

The unfavourable subgroup (H7 U)

At the other end of the scale, there is a general agreement to consider that the clinical presentation of some patients is so severe that :
1) laparotomy is no more useful, since it would not change a therapy which should be aggressive anyway;
2) Chemotherapy is mandatory treatment.

The EORTC lymphoma group thus defined an "unfavourable group" which comprises about 40% of the patients. The presence of only *one* of the following prognostic factors is sufficient for a patient to be included in this group: Age over 50 years; no B symptoms with ESR > 50 (or presence of B symptoms with ESR > 30); 4 (or more) involved sites (i.e. CS II_4 or more); or bulky mediastinal involvement (M/T ratio > 0.35). For these patients, the data gathered by the EORTC as well as *by* other groups, clearly indicate that a *combination of chemotherapy and radiotherapy* is superior to radiotherapy alone for long term survival.

The question which remains is to find out what would be the "best" combination considering not only response rate, but also late toxicity (fertility, secondary leukemia, etc...). In the ongoing H7 U trial, it was decided that the following two schedules be compared:
- 6 EBVP II (a combination of Epirubicine, Bleomycine, Vinblastine and Prednisone) followed by an irradiation limited to the *initially involved fields;*
- 6 MOPP/ABV (according to the conventional scheme) followed by the same type of radiotherapy.

Relapse and survival rates, but also acute and late toxicities, are to be carefully evaluated in both arms of the trial.

The favourable subgroup (H7 F)

It includes all the patients who were not entered in the previous two groups. It represents about 54% of the patients in the EORTC experience. For this group, the analysis of the EORTC database showed a significant advantage of the chemotherapy-radiotherapy combination over radiotherapy alone in terms of *disease free survival.* However, similar -and satisfactory- long term survival rates were achieved by both modalities. Therefore only a difference in *toxicity* (mostly long-term toxicity) would result in preference given to one of these two treatment strategies.

It was thus decided for the H7 F trial to compare **a)** Subtotal nodal radiotherapy (mantle field, then paraaortic and spleen irradiation), without any chemotherapy, to **b)** 6 courses of EBVP II (see above) followed by the irradiation of the initially involved fields. Acute and late treatment toxicities are carefully and prospectively recorded in both arms of this controlled study.

Conclusion

Long term survival rates superior or close to 90% are at hand for most of the patients presenting with clinical stage I-II supradiaphragmatic Hodgkin disease. Beside the necessary efforts for improving the outcome of the few patients still failing our primary treatments, our energy should now be devoted to the reduction of long-term toxicity. The present EORTC H7 trials, which are reserving aggressive (and potentially toxic) treatment to well defined unfavourable situations, and which are trying to lighten the burden of the therapy for low risk patients, thus keeping in line with this objective.

References

Carde, P., et al. (1988): Clinical stages I and II Hodgkin's disease: a specifically tailored therapy according to prognostic factors. The 1977-1982 H5 controlled trials program. *J. Clin. Oncol.* 6, 239-252.

Somers, R., et al. (1989): EORTC lymphoma cooperative group studies in Hodgkin's disease. In *New aspects in the diagnosis and treatment of Hodgkin's disease*, ed. V. Diehl, M. Pfreundschuh & M. Löffler. Recent Results in Cancer Research, vol. 17, pp. 175-181. Berlin: Springer Verlag.

Tubiana, M., et al. (1981): Five year results of the EORTC randomized study of splenectomy and spleen irradiation in clinical stages I and II of Hodgkin's disease. *Europ. J. Cancer*, 17, 355-363.

Tubiana, M., et al. (1984a): Prognostic significance of erythrocyte sedimentation rate in clinical stages I-II of Hodgkin's disease. *J. Clin. Oncol.* 2, 194-200.

Tubiana, M., et al. (1984b): Prognostic significance of the number of involved areas in the early stages of Hodgkin's disease. *Cancer* 54, 885-894.

Tubiana, M., et al. (1984c): The EORTC treatment of early stages of Hodgkin's disease. The role of radiotherapy. *Int. J. Radiat. Oncol. Biol. Phys.* 10, 197-210.

Tubiana, M., et al. (1985): A multivariate analysis of prognostic factors in early stage Hodgkin's disease. *Int. J. Radiat. Oncol. Biol. Phys.* 11, 23-30.

Tubiana, M., et al. (1986): The contribution of clinical trials to the treatment of patients with early stages of Hodgkin's disease. *Drug Exp. Clin. Res.* 12, 105-112.

Tubiana, M., et al. (1989): Toward comprehensive management tailored to prognosis factors of patients with clinical stages I and II in Hodgkin's disease. The EORTC group controlled clinical trials: 1964-1987. *Blood* 73, 47-56.

Van der Werf Messing, B. (1973): Morbus Hodgkin's disease, stage I and II trial of the EORTC. Hodgkin's disease Symposium, Stanford University, 1972. *Nat. Cancer Inst. Monograph* 3, 381-386.

Hodgkin's disease treatment strategy, stage I-II

B. Hoerni

Fondation Bergonié, 180, Rue Saint-Génès, F-33076 Bordeaux cedex, France

My comments are based on our experience during the past two decades either in our single institution (Lagarde et al., 1988) or in a cooperative Pierre-et-Marie-Curie Group trial (Zittoun et al., 1985). We developed as soon as the late 1960's a policy of almost systematic association of chemotherapy and radiotherapy and never performed staging laparotomy. In these conditions the results obtained among our patients compare favorably with other series.

Our observations allow us to emphasize the potentially curative effect of chemotherapy alone as observed in some comparative trials or in our patients whose spleen was never removed nor irradiated but only treated with chemotherapy and who experienced no special rate of relapse. Probably these observations are due to a fairly good chemosensitivity of Hodgkin's cells and also to their small number for a given tumor mass in comparison with other tumors, since numerous non malignant cells are associated with a few cancer cells in the involved lymph nodes or other tumors. this potential efficacy of chemotherapy has to be remembered when we consider underdeveloped countries where radiotherapy facilities are not yet available (Colonna, 1985). This efficacy has also to be favorably balanced with decreased toxicity in comparison with the "old" MOPP given the development of new combinations with fewer risks of secundary leukemia or male sterility (Hoerni et al., 1988).

However, the respective roles of different kinds of radiotherapy and of different kinds of chemotherapy remain to be defined in prospective trials. Henceforth, these trials should not only study survival (relapse free or overall) but also the quality of life (Hoerni & Eghbali, 1989) on a long term basis. This quality of life depends not only on the different treatments but also on the different manner in which these treatments are given: as simply and shortly as possible, on an outpatient basis, with adjuvant measures to reduce toxicity, with continuation of professional life for the longest possible period. The characteristics of the patients play an important role for the personal evaluation of the quality of life. This allows us to suspect that in the near future treatment will be planned and schedule following the characteristics of Hodgkin's disease but also more and more following each patient's characteristics. One of the best improvements in this way would be to better evaluate the chemo-sensitivity of a given Hodgkin's mass to a given treatment depending on individualized pharmacokinetics, vascularization and size of the tumor. We may guess that according to a precisely observed response it will be possible to determine for each patient if he/she must receive more treatment to be cured or if the treatment may be alleviated without jeopardizing the chance of a cure. It seems timely to turn now to a more personalized approach of the treatment of Hodgkin's disease.

References

Colonna, P. (1985): Traitement de la maladie de Hodgkin dans les pays en voie de developpement. In *Maladie de Hodgkin,* ed. G. Hoerni-Simon & C. Gisselbrecht, pp. 157-164. Paris: Doin.
Hoerni, B., et al. (1988): Nouvelle Association d'épirubicine, Bléomycine, vinblastine et prednisone (EBVP II) avant radiothérapie dans les stades localisés de maladie de Hodgkin. Essai de phase II chez 50 malades. *Bull. Cancer* 75, 789-94.
Hoerni, B. & Eghbali, H. (1989): Quality of life during and after treatment of Hodgkin's disease. In *New aspects in the diagnosis and treatment of Hodgkin's disease,* ed. V. Diehl, M. Pfreundschuh, & M. Löffler, pp. 257-269. Berlin: Springer.
Lagarde, P. et al. (1988): Brief chemotherapy associated with extended field radiotherapy in Hodgkin's disease. Long-term results in a series of 102 patients with clinical stages I-IIIA. *Eur. J. Cancer Clin. Oncol.* 24, 1191-8.
Zittoun, R. et al. (1985): Extended versus involved field irradiation combined with MOPP chemotherapy in early clinical stages of Hodgkin's disease. A 1976-1981 trial from the Pierre-et-Marie-Curie Cooperative Group. *J. Clin. Oncol.* 3, 207-14.

Treatment of patients with clinically-staged I and II Hodgkin's disease

F.B. Hagemeister[1], L.M. Fuller[2]

1 *Department of Hematology*
2 *Department of Radiotherapy M.D. Anderson Cancer Center, 1515 Holcombe Boulevard, Houston, Texas 77030, USA*

Treatment of patients with clinically-staged Hodgkin's disease has been studied more extensively in Europe and Canada than it has in the United State. However, findings at laparotomy, treatment of patients following surgical staging, and treatment with combined modality therapy have been thoroughly explored at multiple institutions in the United States. Investigators have identified certain features as important prognostic factors and current concepts regarding management of clinically and pathologically-staged disease are changing. Current management for patients with early stages of the disease should include treatment selection based on knowledge of disease-free survival results rather than anticipated overall survival results. It appears that patients with very favorable upper torso presentations may not need a staging laparotomy and may even be treated with limited radiotherapy (Sutcliffe et al., 1985; Hagemeister et al., 1988). Alternatively, patients with favorable upper torso presentations who are staged by laparotomy may not need abdominal radiotherapy or chemotherapy to achieve good disease-free survival results (Hagemeister et al., 1982; Abrahamsen & Host, 1981). Finally, patients with either unfavorable upper torso or lower torso presentations should be treated with chemotherapy for optimal disease-free survival results ; however, only 2 to 3 cycles of chemotherapy may be necessary if the treatment plan includes radiotherapy (Ferme at al., 1984; Andrieu et al., 1980; Santoro et al., 1987; Fuller et al., 1988).

Before 1970, disease-free survival results were important to the management of the patient with Hodgkin's disease since the only effective treatment available was radiotherapy. Patients with disease progression after radiotherapy could not be salvaged prior to the development of modern chemotherapy became widely available, investigators developed combined modality programs to prevent disease progression. This eventually resulted in a focus on survival as an endpoint for determining the efficacy of adjuvant chemotherapy, since patients who received radiotherapy as initial treatment could often be salvaged with MOPP or similar chemotherapy regimens. However, more recently, investigators have again begun to focus on disease-free survival as an endpoint for determining effectiveness of response to treatment and the benefit of adjuvant chemotherapy. This renewed interest in disease-free survival as an endpoint is due in part to the fact that not all patients who are treated with salvage chemotherapy following radiotherapy survive, particularly those who have adverse factors at initial diagnosis. It has been shown that subsets of patients with lower disease-free survivals also have lower overall survival results (Hagemeister et al., 1982). Some investigators have also demonstrated that the amount of adjuvant chemotherapy that are necessary to achieve good results can be less than the amounts needed for salvage of relapsing disease (Ferme at al., 1984; Andrieu et al., 1980;

Santoro et al., 1987; Fuller et al., 1988). Finally, quality of life is closely related to disease-free survival. The threat of relapse for patients with adverse prognostic features may be a significant psychological factor after treatment with radiotherapy alone (Wasserman et al., 1987).

Another example of treatment results which influence current management has been the demonstration that patients with favorable presentations may not need abdominal radiation if they are staged by laparotomy (Sutcliffe et al., 1985; Hagemeister et al., 1988). In the past, investigators have selected specific categories of patients for staging based on treatment policies at their institutions. At some institutions, patients with all stages of disease had staging laparotomies in order to detect extent of involvement for data-gathering purposes. At other institutions, the decision to perform staging laparotomies was based on an attempt to determine whether patients with clinically-positive abdominal findings actually had disease in the abdomen, including hepatic involvement. At our institution and at some other institutions, laparotomy has been used as a mechanism for treatment selection for patients with limited disease rather than for patients with more extensive disease. At our institution, staging laparotomy results have affected our treatment decisions. Characteristics of patients with consistently negative laparotomy findings have been unilateral neck presentations located above the cricoid cartilage ; lymphocyte-predominant stage I disease and nodular sclerosing stage I disease without mediastinal involvement in women (Hagemeister et al., 1988; Leibenhaut et al., 1989). Management for such patients should be clinical staging followed by limited field radiotherapy. For patients with somewhat less favorable presentations, laparotomy can play an important role in selection treatment. Patients with small or no mediastinal involvement and no hilar adenopathy or B symptoms have very good disease-free results after treatment with radiotherapy only (Hagemeister et al., 1982). Currently, we continue to recommend laparotomy for patients with favorable presentations. These patients can be spared chemotherapy and in our experience do not need abdominal radiation.

Finally, in an adjuvant setting to radiotherapy, less chemotherapy may be as effective as more when it is given for patients with unfavorable presentations. Other investigators found that results for patients treated with 3 cycles of ABVD or MOPP followed by radiotherapy were as good as those obtained in patients treated with 6 cycles followed by radiotherapy (Valagussa, personal communication). At our institution, 2 cycles of MOPP followed by radiotherapy for patients with unfavorable upper torso presentations provides disease-free survival results which are similar to those obtained with 6 cycles of MOPP and radiotherapy for patients with similar features. Current studies are evaluating treatment of patients with clinically-staged disease with chemotherapy and radiotherapy using less toxic drugs than those in the MOPP regimen (Hoppe, personal communication; Hagemeister, unpublished data). Such treatment may give results equivalent to those achieved with MOPP followed by radiotherapy, with less toxicity.

References

Abrahamsen, A., et al. (1981): Mantle field irradiation for stages IA and IIA Hodgkin's disease. *Scan. J. Haematol.* 26, 306-310.
Andrieu, J.M., et al. (1980): Chemotherapy/radiotherapy association in Hodgkin's disease, clinical stages IA, II2A. *Cancer* 46, 2126-2130.
Ferme, C., et al. (1984): Combined modality in Hodgkin's disease: Comparison of six versus three courses of MOPP with clinical and surgical restaging. *Cancer* 54, 2324-2329.
Fuller, L.M., et al. (1988): The adjuvant role of two cycles of MOPP and low-dose lung irradiation in stage IA through IIB Hodgkin's disease: Preliminary results. *Int. J. Radiat. Oncol. Biol. Phys.* 14, 683-692.
Hagemeister, F.B., et al. (1988): Staging laparotomy: Findings and applications to treatment decisions. In *Hodgkin's Disease and Non-Hodgkin's Lymphomas in Adults and Children*, ed. LM Fuller, FB Hagemeister, M Sullivan & WS Velasquez, pp. 170-185. New York: Raven Press.

Hagemeister, F.B., et al. (1982): Stage I and II Hodgkin's disease: Involved-field radiotherapy versus extended-field radiotherapy followed by six cycles of MOPP. *Cancer Treat. Rep.* 66, 789-798.

Leibenhaut, M.H., et al. (1989): Prognostic indicators of laparotomy findings in clinical stage I-II supradiaphragmatic Hodgkin's disease. *J. Clin. Oncol.* 7, 81-91.

Santoro, A., et al. (1987): Long term results of combined chemotherapy/radiotherapy approach in Hodgkin's disease: superiority of ABVD plus radiotherapy versus MOPP plus radiotherapy. *J. Clin. Oncol.* 5, 27-37.

Sutcliffe, S.B., et al. (1985): Prognostic groups for management of localized Hodgkin's disease. *J. Clin. Oncol.* 3, 393-401.

Wasserman, A.L., et al. (1987): The psychological status of survivors of childhood/adolescent Hodgkin's disease. *Am. J. Dis. Child* 141, 626-631.

Approaches to treatment of early Hodgkin's disease at the Royal Marsden Hospital

A. Horwich

Academic Unit - Department of Radiotherapy and Oncology
The Royal Marsden Hospital and Institute of Cancer Research. Downs Road, Sutton, Surrey SM2 5PT, England

Supported by Grants from the Cancer Research Campaign

Role of laparotomy

The pattern of investigation and treatment of early Hodgkin's disease has changed at the Royal Marsden Hospital over the last 20 years. The proportion of patients staged by laparotomy was 2/107 (21%) in the era 1964-1969, 82/143 (57%) in 1970-1974, 116/139 (85%) in 1975-1980, and 14/58 (24%) in 1981-1983 (Duchesnes et al. 1989). At present, laparotomy is only rarely a component of the management strategy. This change is based firstly on the appreciation that laparotomy findings give prognostic information rather than change prognosis (Haybittle et al., 1985, Tubiana et al., 1989), secondly on the ability of non-invasive investigations to provide similar prognostic information (Horwich et al., 1986, Leibenhaut et al., 1989, Haybittle et al., 1985, Sutcliffe et al., 1985, Pavlovsky et al., 1988), thirdly on increased use of initial combination chemotherapy in early Hodgkin's disease (16/107 (15%) patients in 1964-1968, 21/143 (15%) patients in 1970-1974, 60/139 (43%) in 1975-1980 and 35/58 (60%) patients in 1981-1983), and fourthly on the inadequacy of laparotomy in excluding abdominal disease since this remains the most common site of relapse in pathological stage I and II patients treated with mantle radiotherapy (Verger et al., 1988).

The abandonment of laparotomy is based on 2 separate assumptions in different patient populations. In patients treated by radiotherapy alone the assumption is that treatment of overt recurrence outside the field is as effective as initial treatment of subclinical disease. In patients treated with chemotherapy or combined chemotherapy and radiotherapy, the assumption is that chemotherapy can deal with original subclinical disease more effectively than it can deal with overt recurrence. These apparently paradoxical viewpoints can only be compatible if one recognize the heterogeneity of early Hodgkin's disease such that a conservative management approach can be correct for patients with biological determinants of good prognosis since these determinants will indicate successful treatment of radiation recurrence, whereas the patient with poor prognosis disease merits initial aggressive therapy with both chemotherapy and radiotherapy despite the increased toxicity of this approach. Within this framework, the role of laparotomy is to improve definition of the good prognosis group with the benefit restricted to a reduction of recurrence rather than an impact on overall survival.

Definition of good and poor prognostic groups in early Hodgkin's disease

Retrospective analyses have helped to define presentation prognosis factors relevant to the risk of having a positive laparotomy (Brada et al., 1985), recurrence of Hodgkin's disease (Horwich & Peckham, 1987) and overall survival (Horwich et al., 1986). To define the group whose recurrence after radiotherapy can easily be treated, the most appropriate analysis is of overall survival. Analyses from different centres and cooperative groups are in broad agreement over which presentation factors confer an adverse prognosis (Sutcliffe et al., 1985, Haybittle et al., 1985, Horwich et al., 1986, Tubiana et al., 1984). However, it is only a relatively small proportion of patients who have adverse features such as systemic symptoms, bulky mediastinal disease, lymphocyte depleted histology or >3 nodal sites involved and this has weakened the power of the analyses and led to a variation in the definition of the good prognostic subgroup. The Royal Marsden Hospital study of 398 adults with clinical stage I or II Hodgkin's disease found on univariate analyses that age over 70 years, male sex, lymphocyte depleted histology, systemic symptoms, bulky mediastinal disease and erythrocyte sedimentation rate >40 mm/1st hr were significant adverse factors (Horwich et al., 1986). The prognostic model (Table 1) was based on multiple factor regression analysis of survival of patients treated between 1970-1979 and identifies adverse groups with a 5 year survival probability of 78-84%, and the good prognosis group with 5 year survival probability of 92%.

Table 1. Prognosis of CS I & II Hodgkin's disease[a] (Royal Marsden Hospital)

	Definition of Group	Predicted 5 year survival
A. One of :	Age > 60 years L.D. histology > 3 sites MT ratio > 1/3 Systemic symptoms	78%
B. Two of :	ESR > 40 Male sex 3 sites M.C. histology	84%
C.	Neither A or B	92%

[a] *Data from Horwich et al. 1986*

It should be emphasized that this approach was based on analysis of overall survival and as argued above, a better method of defining a group to be managed by clinical staging and by relatively limited extent of radiation fields, might be based on an analysis of the probability of salvage of relapse after radiotherapy and an important project for the EORTC Symposium database will be the investigation of this group directly.

Discussion

It would be desirable to define the patient groups who could be managed by clinical staging rather than by laparotomy, and also by limited field radiotherapy (involved field or mantle field or inverted Y field) rather than total nodal irradiation. Despite sophisticated prognostic factor analyses laparotomy data indicate that limited field radiotherapy will fail to treat subclinical extension of Hodgkin's disease in 5%-50% of cases, as revealed both in previous publications (Brada et al., 1986, Verger et al., 1988) and in the EORTC Symposium database. The basis of this management should be a high probability of salvage and furthermore it is important that the patient has a good insight into the rationale of the conservative treatment approach and will therefore reliably attend for regular and close follow-up. A problem of this approach is the prolonged pattern of relapse after treatment of clinical stage I and II Hodgkin's disease. Our analysis of timing of relapse in 432 patients treated between 1964 and 1983 revealed a 15.7% actuarial risk of late relapse more than 3 years after treatment (Duchesne et al. 1989). Late relapse was commoner after radiotherapy than after combined modality therapy. Thus it is also important that conservative management be associated with prolonged follow-up. The benefit to the patient of conservative management is the avoidance of the toxicities of laparotomy (Green et al., 1983, Feld and Sutcliffe, 1987), of extended field radiotherapy, (Green et al., 1987, Smith et al., 1989, Gallez-Marchal 1984, Cola & Hanks 1988) or of chemotherapy, especially infertility and leukaemogenesis (Colman et al., 1988, Henry-Amar et al., 1985).

The model illustrated in Table 1 allows selection of the adverse subgroup (A & B) in whom it is logical to develop programmes of combined radiotherapy and chemotherapy whereas in Group C low toxicity programmes should be investigated such as mantle field radiotherapy alone, or Vinblastine, Bleomycin, Methotrexate (VBM) + involved field radiotherapy (Horning et al., 1988).

In the poor prognosis patient group the aim of future management should be the reduction of recurrence and mortality from Hodgkin's disease using combined modality therapy (Horwich & Peckham 1987). In this context it is necessary to establish the optimal chemotherapy schedule and the role of high dose chemotherapy, the optimal extent of radiation fields, and the appropriate sequencing of the two treatment modalities. Though randomised studies have failed to detect a survival benefit from combined modality therapy there is evidence from stage III Hodgkin's disease to support this approach (Brada et al., 1989) and relapse analysis illustrates improvement in control of both local disease and dissemination (Table 2).

Table 2. Stage III Hodgkin's disease: Patterns of relapse

Treatment group	% relapsing at involved site	new site
Radiotherapy	10 %	51 %
Chemotherapy	21 %	26 %
Combined modality	5 %	23 %

[a] and not previously irradiated
Data from Brada et al., 1989.

References

Brada, M., et al. (1989): Stage III Hodgkin's disease - long term results following chemotherapy, radiotherapy and combined modality therapy. *Radiother. Oncol.* 14, 185-198.

Brada, M., et al. (1986): Clinical presentation as a predictor of laparotomy findings in supradiaphragmatic stage I and II Hodgkin's disease. *Radiother. Oncol.* 5, 15-22.

Cola, L.P., et al. (1988): complications from large field intermediate dose infradiaphragmatic radiation: An analysis of the pattern of care outcome studies for Hodgkin's disease and seminoma. *Int. J. Radiat. Oncol. Biol. Phys.* 15, 29-35.

Colman, M., et al. (1988): Second malignancies and Hodgkin's disease. The Royal Marsden Hospital Experience. *Radiother. Oncol.* 3, 229-238.

Duchesne, G., et al. (1989): Changing patterns of relapse in Hodgkin's disease. *Br. J. Cancer* 60, 227-230.

Feld, R., et al. (1987): *Immune deficiency and infectious complications of Hodgkin's disease*, pp. 301-338. Oxford: Blackwell Scientific Publication.

Gallez-Marchall, D., et al. (1984): Radiation injuries of the gastrointestinal tract in Hodgkin's disease: the role of exploratory and fractionation. *Radiother. Oncol.* 2, 93-99.

Green, D.M., et al. (1983): Staging laparotomy with splenectomy in children and adolescents with Hodgkin's disease. *Cancer Treat. Rev.* 10, 23-28.

Green, D.M., et al. (1987): The effect of mediastinal irradiation on cardiac function in patients treated during childhood and adolescence for Hodgkin's disease. *J. Clin. Oncol.* 5, 239-245.

Haybittle, J.L., et al. (1985): Review of British National Lymphoma Investigation studies of Hodgkin's disease and development of prognostic index. *Lancet* i, 967-972.

Henry-Amar, M. (1988): Quantitative risk of second cancer in patients in first complete remission from early stages of Hodgkin's disease. *NCI Monogr.* 6, 65-71.

Horning, S.J., et al. (1988): Vinblastine, bleomycin and methotrexate: an effective adjuvant in favorable Hodgkin's disease. *J. Clin. Oncol.* 6, 1822-1831.

Horwich, A., et al. (1986): An analysis of prognosis factors in early stage Hodgkin's disease. *Radiother. Oncol.* 7, 95-106.

Horwich, A., et al. (1987): Combined chemotherapy and radiotherapy in the management of adult Hodgkin's disease: indications and results. In *Hodgkin's Disease*, ed. P. Selby & T.J. McElwain, pp. 250-268. Oxford: Blackwell Scientific Publications.

Leibonhaut, M.H., et al. (1989): prognostic indicators of laparotomy findings in clinical stage I-II supradiaphragmatic Hodgkin's disease. *J. Clin. Oncol* 7, 81-91.

Pavlovski, S., et al. (1988): Randomised trial of chemotherapy versus chemotherapy plus radiotherapy for stage I-II Hodgkin's disease. *J. Nat. Cancer Inst.* 80, 1466-1473.

Smith, L.M. (1989): results of a prospective study evaluating the effects of mantle irradiation on pulmonary function. *Int. J. Radiat. Oncol. Biol. Phys.* 16, 79-84.

Sutcliffe, S.B., et al. (1985): prognostic groups from management of localised Hodgkin's disease. *J. Clin. Oncol.* 3, 393-401.

Tubiana, M., et al (1981): Five-year results of the EORTC randomised study of splenectomy and spleen irradiation in clinical stages I and II of Hodgkin's disease. *Eur. J. Cancer* 17, 355-363.

Tubiana, M., et al. (1989): Toward comprehensive management tailored to prognostic factors of patiens with clinical stages I and II in Hodgkin's disease. The EORTC lymphoma Group Clinial Trials: 1964-1987. *Blood* 73, 47-56.

Verger, E., et al. (1988): Radiotherapy results in laparotomy staged Hodgkin's disease. *Clin. Radiol.* 39, 428-431.

Hodgkin's disease treatment strategy in stage I-II according to socio-economic status and therapeutic ressources

S. Pavlovsky

Department of Onco-haemotology, Instituto de Investigaciones Hematologicas «Mariano R. Castex». Academia Nacional de Medicina, J.P. de Melo 3081, Buenos Aires, Argentina

Dr. R. Hoppe has made an excellent update of the staging strategy, prognostic factors and therapy of stage I-II.

Prognostic factors in early stage of Hodgkin's disease varied in different countries according to race and socio-economic status of the population, but also within countries(Hu et al., 1988). Incidence of mixed cellularity, presence of B-symptoms and bulky disease were more frequently found in patients from hispanic origin.

We agree with Dr. Hoppe that lymphogram remains the most accurate investigation for the identification of retro-peritoneal disease. Also it is much less expensive than CAT scan or MNR imaging and can be done in any place with only the use of standard X-ray. The importance of the lymphogram to follow the evolution during and after therapy for one to three years is not always mentioned as Dr. Hoppe did and provide a cheapest way to monitor the follow-up of retro-peritoneal lymph nodes.

There is a general agreement that optimal treatment for patients with bulky disease, B-symptoms, unfavourable histology, large number of site of envolvement is combined modality therapy. The type and amount of chemotherapy as well as the size and dose of radiation therapy varied among groups without apparent major difference in relapse free survival and survival.

Most of the centers in Latin America and probably of numerous countries in Africa and Asia are lacking well equiped radiotherapy facilities (Pavlovsky & Litvak, 1984). Several factors related to radiotherapy treatment have been recognized associated with higher incidence of recurrence such as part-time practice, inadequate margins in the treatment technique, treatment machinery (< 80 cm ^{60}Co), and lack of treatment simulation (Hanks at al., 1983).

The use of combined modality treatment in unfavorable prognosis stage I-II tends to obscure the effect of inadequate technology for radiation therapy and results are similar in several studies all around the world.

The major field of controversies remains in patients with stage I-II with favorable prognosis. At the Stanford University Medical Center, the Joint Center for Radiation Therapy in Boston, and in many other places, where are large and well equiped therapy facilities, policy of staging laparotomy and splenectomy is currently used and radiation therapy treatment assigned according to pathological stage. Long-term survival rate reported by this group and mentioned in Table 5 by Dr. Hoppe is about 90%, and freedom from relapse rate 70-80%.

Unfortunately most of the patients with Hodgkin's disease all around the world have not the chance to be treated in this kind of cancer centers reporting treating patients according to the strategy of Stanford, several of the factors related to the recurrence of disease are present and results are poor. Also only excellent results with radiotherapy from large centers are published.

In our group (GATLA) (Pavlovsky et al., 1988) we have explored in a randomized study the use of chemotherapy alone versus chemotherapy plus radiation therapy in stage I-II of Hodgkin's disease. Throught our results emerge that unfavorable stage I-II, that are those with > 45 years of age, more than two lymph nodes areas involved, or the presence of bulky tumor, had better disease-free survival (75% versus 34%) and overall survival (84% versus 66%) at 84 months when treated with combined modality treatment than with chemotherapy alone. The difference in disease free survival was highly significant ($p=0.001$, Table 1).

Table 1. Percentage of complete remission, disease-free survival, and overall survival according to treatment arm and prognostic group at 84 months.

Prognosis	CVPP				CVPP + RT			
	No of patients	CR (%)	At 84 mo FDS (%)	SV (%)	No of patients	CR (%)	At 84 mo DFS (%)	SV (%)
Favorable	82	88	77	92	91	97	70	91
Unfavorable	60	82	34*	66	44	86	75*	84
Total	142	85	62@	82	135	93	71	89

CR: complete remission; DFS: disease free survival; SV: overall survival.
Reproduced from J. Natl. Cancer Inst. (1988) 80, 1466-1473.
* $p = 0.001$.   @ $p = 0.01$.

However patients with favorable prognosis had similar rate of disease free survival (70% versus 77%) and survival (91% versus 92%) at 84 months whenever treated by combined modalities or chemotherapy alone. The results of the group with favorable prognosis clinically staged treated with chemotherapy alone are similar to those reported by the EORTC, the Boston group and the Stanford group for patients pathologically staged.

The high rate of sterility in men is a major concern of the use of chemotherapy. However, if the rate of relapse using only radiotherapy is high, most of patients will eventually need chemotherapy. Also several studies have shown that about 50% of male patients were fonctionally in a subfertile state at time of diagnosis and no information is available on how many of them will recover normal spermatogenesis.

The EORTC data base have shown that not one patient that remain in first complete remission in spite of the treatment strategy done, have secondary leukemia. For this reason if we have successfull long term disease free survival with a particular therapy will be of little concern the possibility of developing leukemia.

It can be concluded that general agreement is: for patients with unfavorable prognosis stage I-II, the combined modality therapy is the treatment of choice. Patients with favorable prognosis treatment should be tailored according to the resources of expertise of the Institutions. Probably radiotherapy alone in pathological staged patients including mantle and subdiaphragmatic fields; chemotherapy alone or less intensive chemotherapy with irradiation to the involved fields in clinical stage, are equivalent in providing excellent disease free survival and survival.

References

Hu, E., et al. (1988): Third-World Hodgkin's disease at Los Angeles County-University Southern California Medical Center. *J. Clin. Oncol.* 6, 1285-1292.

Pavlovsky, S. & Litvak, J. (1984): Multidisciplinary consideration of cancer in Latin America. *Int. J. Radiat. Oncol. Biol. Phys.* 10, 77-79.

Hanks, G.E., et al. (1983): Patterns of care outcome studies. Results of the National Practice in Hodgkin's disease. *Cancer* 51, 569-573.

Pavlovsky, S., et al. (1988): Randomized trial of chemotherapy versus chemotherapy plus radiotherapy for stage I-II Hodgkin's disease. *J. Nat. Cancer Inst.* 80, 1466-1473.

Treatment strategy in Hodgkin's disease stages I-II : the Finsen Institute approach

L. Specht, N.I. Nissen

Department of Haematology, Rigshospitalet, 9 Blegdamsvej, DK-2100 Copenhagen, Denmark

In the treatment of Hodgkin's disease both megavoltage radiotherapy and combination chemotherapy are effective. As regards the treatment of early stage disease a crucial question is whether patients should initially be treated with both modalities or whether radiotherapy should be applied alone with combination chemotherapy reserved for relapse. This question has been addressed in some 20 randomized trials in Europe and America. All these trials have shown a significant improvement in relapse free survival in the group treated initially with both modalities. However, owing to the effectiveness of chemotherapy salvage of relapse after radiotherapy alone, no significant improvement in overall survival has yet ensued. Three possible explanations for this may be conceived. First, contrary to what one would expect, there may, in fact, be no improvement in survival to be gained by preventing a relapse after radiotherapy. Secondly, it may be that remissions induced by chemotherapy after radiotherapy relapse will after all prove less durable, and, hence, with even longer observation time a difference may indeed emerge. The third possible explanation is that, because survival is so high (about 90% long term survival), the improvement in survival one may realistically expect from the addition of combination chemotherapy to the initial treatment (probably a 10-15% reduction in number of deaths) could not be expected to emerge from any single one of these trials, because each contains, at the most, only a few hundred patients.

An improvement in survival of the above mentioned size would, however, still be worth establishing, certainly in groups of patients with poor prognostic characteristics. In order to obtain a sufficiently large patient material to shed light on this problem a metaanalysis of all the randomized trials of radiotherapy alone vs. radiothrapy plus combination chemotherapy in early stage Hodgkin's disease has been initiated in collaboration with the Clinical Trial Service Unit in Oxford, England. Most trialists approached in connection with this project have agreed to participate. Hopefully, this metaanalysis will conclusively establish if, and by how much, we can expect to improve survival by adding chemotherapy to the initial radiotherapy treatment.

The current treatment policy at the Finsen Institute is to administer radiotherapy alone to good prognosis patients, and to give combined modality treatment to poor prognosis patients. The separation into good and poor prognosis patients is arbitrary and based on the relapse frequency considered acceptable in patients treated with radiothrapy alone (about 25%). The most accurate predictor of relapse has in our patient material proved to be an estimate of the total tumour burden (Specht et al., 1988). In the future it is intended to apply this prognostic method when determining which treatment the individual patient is to receive. Alternatively, one might use prognostic factors which are closely correlated with tumour burden, such as size of mediastinal involvement or number of involved regions.

Another crucial question with regard to the management of early stage disease is whether or not to use exploratory laparotomy with splenectomy in the staging work-up. For a patient with an established high tumour burden the result of the splenectomy would not influence treatment strategy, since such a patient would receive combined modality treatment in any case. We therefore did not perform splenectomies except in patients with low tumour burdens, who might be referred to radiotherapy treatment alone. Even in these cases it is uncertain whether splenectomy is of any real value with regard to eventual survival. This problem is closely related to the question whether the prevention of relapse after radiotherapy by adding combination chemotherapy to the initial treatment does in fact improve survival. Only if this is so the information may not be sufficient in these patients with a relatively low risk of relapse to outweigh the risks of the operation. As outlined above, this question awaits further clarification, and for the time being we adhere to the policy of performing splenectomy in patients who are candidates for radiotherapy alone.

New approaches to the treatment of early stage Hodgkin's disease include combination chemotherapy alone, which has been tried in a few trials with varying results (Pavlovsky et al., 1988; Chimiono et al., 1989; O'Dwyer et al., 1985); less intensive chemotherapy used in combination with radiotherapy (Horning et al., 1988); and less extensive radiotherapy combined with chemotherapy (Zittoun et al., 1985; Rosenberg & Kaplan, 1985; Jones et al., 1982). All of these concepts are potentially interesting and may prove superior to present standard treatment. However, as long term results of these new approaches are still unavailable we feel that they should only be applied in controlled clinical trials. As standard tratment we adhere to mantle field irradiation, in good prognosis patients supplemented by irradiation to para-aortic nodes, in poor prognosis patients supplemented by six cycles of MOPP. To the rare patients with infradiaphragmatic presentation irradiation is administered to an inverted Y-field, with no further treatment in good prognosis patients, but supplemented by six cycles of MOPP in poor prognosis patients.

Refereneces

Cimino, G., et al. (1989): MOPP chemotherapy versus extended-field radiotherapy in management of pathological stages I-IIA Hodgkin's disease. *J. Clin. Oncol.* 7, 732-7.

Horning, S.J., et al. (1988): Vinblastine, bleomycin, and methotrexate: An effective adjuvant in favorable Hodgkin's disease. *J. Clin. Oncol.* 6, 1822-31.

Jones, S.E., et al (1982): Conclusions from clinical trials of the Southwest Oncology Group. *Cancer Treat. Rep.* 66, 847-53.

O'Dwyer, P.J., et al. (1985): Treatment of early stage Hodgkin's disease: A randomized trial of radiotherapy plus chemotherapy versus chemotherapy alone. In *Malignant Lymphoma and Hodgkin's Disease: Experimental and Therapeutic Advances*, ed. F. Cavalli, G. Bonadonna & M. Rozencweig, pp. 329-336. Proceedings of the Second International Conference on Malignant Lymphomas, Lugano, Switzerland, June 13-16, 1984. Boston: Martinus Nijhoff.

Pavlovsky, S., et al. (1988): Randomized trial of chemotherapy plus radiotherapy for stage I-II Hodgkin's disease. *J. Natl. Cancer Inst.* 80, 1466-73.

Rosenberg, S.A. & Kaplan, H.S. (1985): The evolution and summary results of the Stanford randomized clinical trials of the management of Hodgkin's disease: 1962-1984. *Int. J. Radiat. Oncol. Biol. Phys.* 11, 5-22.

Specht, L., et al. (1988): Tumor burden as the most important prognostic factor in early stage Hodgkin's disease. Relations to other prognostic factors and implications for choice of treatment. *Cancer* 61, 1719-27.

Zittoun, R., et al. (1985): Extended versus involved fields irradiation combined with MOPP chemotherapy in early clinical stages of Hodgkin's disease. *J. Clin. Oncol.* 3, 207-14.

Hodgkin's disease treatment strategy – stage I-II

B. Vaughan Hudson

British National Lymphoma Investigation. Middlesex Hospital, Mortimer Street, London W1N 8AA, England

Introduction

Stage I/II is often referred to as "localised disease", implying that it is confined to the site or sites in which disease is clinically evident at presentation. However after initial local treatment with radiotherapy to these sites alone, disease later reappers in many patients in other additional sites (notably elsewhere in the lymphatic chains, in bone, etc.), even though disease has been eradicated in its original presenting site. Consequently the disease free survival (DFS) resulting from initial treatment with local radiotherapy (RT) is relatively low. Thus after initial involved field RT, Fuller and Hutchinson 1982, Rosenberg 1985, Sutcliffe et al. 1985, and the BNLI (Haybittle et al., 1985) found DFS lying in the 30%-60% range at 10-14 years after treatment of clinically or pathologically staged I/II patients.

Initial chemotherapy

The success of combination chemotherapy (CT) in the form of MOPP and MOPP-like combinations in salvaging these failures resulted in the use of initial CT alone by some groups for I/II disease. Mandelli et al. reported a DFS of 68% at 4 years after initial MOPP, and Pavlovsky et al. found a DFS of 62% at 7 years after initial CVPP.

Initial combined modality therapy

In contrast to these results of the use of RT or CT alone in the initial treatment of I/II HD, reports of the use of both RT and CT, given as initial combined modality therapy (CMT), show 78% - 89% relapse free survival rates (Workshop Statistical Report, Tables VII-7 to VII-9). It would appear that it is necessary to use both modalities initially if the cure rate from initial treatment is to be maximised.

Although initial CMT produces a higher DFS than initial RT or CT given alone, it does not appear to produce a higher overall survival (Workshop Statistical Report, Tables VIII-7 to VIII-9). However it is possible that only poor risk subgroups benefit from initial CT, and that such benefit is masked by patients whose survival is unaffected. In a randomised BNLI trial of I/II A patients with poor prognostic characteristics in which patients were randomised to initial RT or initial CT, almost all failures to initial treatment in the CT arm have been in sites of clinically evident disease at presentation so far, whereas in the arm they have been in areas remote from such sites. BNLI data also shows that initial MOPP, given to stage I/II patients with B-symptoms, has resulted not only in markedly and significantly fewer relapses in areas other than the original clinically evident sites of presentation, but also in significantly fewer deaths following such relapses, than initial RT (mantle/total nodal irradiation). These patients were not randomised, but the group receiving RT had a potentially more favourable prognosis, since it contained a much higher proportion of laparotomised patients together with a lower proportion of patients with poor prognosis nodular sclerosing histology.

It appears that some patients have occult ("micrometastatic") disease at presentation which remains untreated by initial local RT, and that chemotherapy is more effective in treating such disease if given initially when it is undetectably small in volume than if given later at relapse when it has grown sufficiently bulky to be evident clinically.

Long term effects of chemotherapy

It was evident from the Workshop that several groups have divided their I/II patients retrospectively into those having a good and those having a poor chance of survival on the basis of various prognostic factors, and given more aggressive treatment, including CMT, to their "high risk" patients. However it appeared from the Symposium that some clinicians were unwilling to add initial CT to initial RT without firmer evidence that it does in fact improve overall survival. prognostic factors are imprecise, and it is inevitable that some patients will receive chemotherapy, which is prone to cause sterility and secondary leukaemia, unnecessarily. However sperm banking is available for some males, an sterility is related to the particular drugs used. In addition, the cumulative incidence of secondary leukaemia is low in Hodgkin's disease [2.2% at 15 years (Workshop Statistical Report, part IX); 1.7% at 15 years (BNLI, paper awaiting publication)], and is associated in many patients with heavy pre-treatment for resistant disease from which they would have eventually died (BNLI, ibid).

Long term effects of radiotherapy

It appears to be usual for patients to be treated with relatively wide field radiotherapy if RT is used alone as initial treatment. The use of radiotherapy was associated with an increase in relative risk compared to general population incidence rates for solid tumours in most of the sites potentially submitted to radiation therapy in the present analysis (Workshop Statistical Report, part IX), and Bonadonna and Santoro have found that so far approximately two-thirds of the solid tumours which occurred in patients with advanced disease treated by CT and RT occurred in the radiation field (Bookman & Longo, 1986; and Valagussa et al., 1988). Haybittle et al., 1989, reported a small but significant increase in mortality from second malignancies (mostly solid tumours) and from cardiovascular disease in patients treated with adjuvant radiotherapy for breast cancer. It would therefore seem advisable to limit radiotherapy fields whenever possible.

Efficacy of salvage therapy

The overall survival of I/II patients who failed to achieve permanent complete remission from their initial treatment was poor: most of those who did not achieve complete remission died or only 50% of those who relapsed remain alive (Workshop Statistical Report, part VIII). BLNI data shows that for I/II A patients receiving second line treatment after first line failure from local or mantle RT, the overall survival at 15 years after failure was approximately two-thirds (65%) at 15 years for those patients who achieved complete remission (CR) to their second line treatment, and was less than 6% at 10 years for those who failed to obtain CR to their second line treatment: almost all of the deaths were associated with Hodgkin's disease. Thus probably virtually none of those patients who failed to achieve CR from their second line treatment were cured. There were thus only two opportunities for cure; from the indication of CR by first line (initial) treatment, or from its induction by second line (i.e. first salvage) treatment. It is therefore important to achieve permanent complete remission from initial treatment, since there is no guarantee that "salvage" therapy will do so.

Measurement of initial treatment success

The measurement of initial treatment success poses a number of problems, as was evident from the Workshop discussion. Relapse free survival (FRS) gives no indication of the percentage of patients achieving complete remission; patients who achieve CR may have a low relapse rate but this is not an indication of successful treatment if hardly any patients achieved CR. Overall survival (OS) measures the success not only of initial treatment, but also of the salvage therapy given to those in whom it was unsuccessful. Disease free survival is a measure of the success of initial treatment alone, but like OS, is affected by deaths due to causes other than Hodgkin's disease. This is of advantage insofar as it takes deaths related to treatment into account (including unexpected second malignancies); the disadvantage, which it shares with OS, is that it includes deaths unrelated to HD which also occur in the general population. This is of minor importance if the patients in question are all young, but is important if appreciable numbers of them are in their fifties, sixties, or even seventies or more, as occurs in multicentre studies. Thus it is meaningless to attempt to compare different groups' treatments if the age ranges of the patients to whom they have been given are widely different.

Assessment of new treatment regimes

As the EORTC analysis shows, relapses continue for up to 16 years after initial treatment (Workshop Statistical Report, Table VII-22), and the cumulative incidence of deaths due to solid tumours possibly caused by treatment is still increasing at 20 years (Workshop Statistical Report, Figure IX-1).

Thus the results of any new treatment will tend to show relatively high (and hence encouraging) DFS and OS over its first few years, since patients will not have been exposed to the full time of attrition, and assessment of its efficacy is therefore difficult if not impossible in the early years.

It may be necessary for twenty years to pass before an initial treatment can be assessed definitively.

References

Bookman, M.A. & Longo, D.L. (1986): Concomitant illness in patients treated for Hodgkin's disease. *Cancer Treat. Rev.* 13, 77-111.
Fuller, L.M. & Hutchison, G.B. (1982). Collaborative clinical trial for stage I and II Hodgkin's disease: significance of mediastinal and nonmediastinal disease in laparotomy - and non laparotomy - staged patients. *Cancer Treat. Rep.* 66, 775-787.
Haybittle, J.L., et al. (1985). Review of British National Lymphoma Investigation studies of Hodgkin's disease and development of prognostic index. *Lancet* i, 967-972.
Haybittle, J.L., et al. (1989). Postoperative radiotherapy and late mortality: evidence from the CRC trial for early breast cancer. *Br. Med. J.* 298, 1611-1614.
Mandelli, F., et al. (1986): Evaluation of therapeutic modalities in the control of Hodgkin's disease. *Int. J. Radiat. Oncol. Biol. Phys.* 12, 1617-1620.
Pavlovsky, S., et al. (1988): Randomised trial of chemotherapy versus chemotherapy plus radiotherapy for stage I-II Hodgkin's disease. *J. Natl. Cancer Inst.* 80, 1466-1473.

Rosenberg, S.A. (1985): The current status of the Stanford randomised clinical trials of the management of Hodgkin's disease. In *Malignant lymphomas and Hodgkin's disease: Experimental and therapeutic advances,* ed. F. Cavalli, G. Bonadonna & M. Rozencweig, pp. 281-292. Boston: Martinus Nijhoff.

Sutcliffe, S.B., et al. (1985): prognostic groups for management of localised Hodgkin's disease. *J. Clin. Oncol.* 3, 393-401.

Valagussa, P., et al. (1988): Hodgkin's disease and second malignancies. *Proc. Am. Soc. Clin. Onc.* 7, 227.

Advanced Stage Hodgkin's Disease

Maladie de Hodgkin : stades disséminés

Prognostic factors of stage III and IV Hodgkin's disease

M. Löffler[1], D.O. Dixon[2], R. Swindell[3]

1 Biometric Division, Medical University Clinic, 5000 Köln 41, Federal Republic of Germany
2 Department of Biomathematics, University of Texas, M.D. Anderson Cancer Center, Houston TX 77030, USA
3 Biometric Division, Christie Hospital and Holt Radium Institute, Manchester M20 9BX, England

Summary

A multivariate analysis for prognostic factors in stage III and IV Hodgkin's disease (HD) was performed with respect to complete remission, relapse-free survival, disease specific survival and overall survival. From 20 participating centres, 5,217 patients were registered in the international database. The data showed a certain degree of heterogeneity in treatment types, treatment period, and histological subtyping. For complete remission age, systemic symptoms, erythrocyte sedimentation rate (ESR), and serum albumin were prognostic factors in stage III; age and topography of disease location in stage IV. For relapse-free survival age was prognostic in stage IIIA, IIIB and IV; number of lymph node areas involved was prognostic in stage IIIA; male gender and mediastinal involvement were prognostic in stage IIIB. Of relapsing patients after complete remission, 50% died within 5 years, mostly of disease progression.

With respect to disease specific survival stage, systemic symptoms, age, gender (only in stage IV) and histology were prognostic factors. In addition, the number of lymph node areas involved appeared prognostic in stage IIIA.

On the basis of these analyses it can be concluded that stage IV is a fairly homogenous disease with respect to complete remission, relapse-free survival and survival, while stage III is a fairly heterogenous disease. Biological parameters (ESR, serum albumin) and spread of disease (number of lymph node areas, mediastinal involvement) play a role. In general the prognostic relevance of the classical prognostic factors such as age, gender, stage, systemic symptoms and histology is confirmed, but additional factors appear to be valuable.

Résumé

Une analyse pronostique multivariée prenant comme critères successifs la réponse initiale, la survie sans récidive, la survie sans maladie, et la survie globale, a été réalisée sur les stades III et IV de maladie de Hodgkin. La série étudiée rassemblait 5217 cas issus de 20 centres ayant participé à l'élaboration d'une base de données. Les résultats ont mis en évidence une certaine hétérogénéité des données en ce qui concerne les traitements, la période pendant laquelle les malades avaient été traités, et le type histologique. Les facteurs pronostiques de la réponse au traitement initial étaient, pour les stades III, l'âge, les signes généraux, la vitesse de sédimentation (VS) et le taux d'albumine sérique. Pour les stades IV étaient pronostiques l'âge et la topographie initiale des lésions. Pour la survie sans récidive, l'âge était pronostique dans les stades IIIA, IIIB et IV; les nombre d'aires ganglionnaires envahies était pronostique dans les stades IIIA; enfin le sexe masculin et l'envahissement médiastinal étaient pronostiques dans les stades IIIB. Parmi les malades ayant rechuté, 50% sont morts dans les 5 années suivant la rechute, la majorité d'entre eux d'évolution.

En ce qui concerne la survie sans maladie, le stade, les signes généraux, l'âge, le sexe (pour les stades IV uniquement) et l'histologie étaient pronostiques. De plus, le nombre d'aires ganglionnaires envahies était pronostique dans les stades IIIA.

Ces résultats font apparaître une relative homogénéité des stades IV en ce qui concerne la réponse au traitement, la survie sans récidive et la survie globale. Au contraire, les stades III apparaissent comme une maladie beaucoup plus hétérogène. Les paramètres biologiques (VS, albumine sérique) ainsi que la dissémination de la maladie (nombre d'aires ganglionnaires envahies, envahissement médiastinal) semblent jouer un rôle. En général, la valeur pronostique des paramètres classiques comme l'âge, le sexe, le stade, les signes généraux et l'histologie est confirmée. Toutefois d'autres paramètres apparaissent comme pouvant avoir un intérêt.

Introduction

History and Rationale

Hodgkin's disease (HD) has become a fascinating disease in haemato-oncology because of its potential curability. This has raised the question of finding the best compromise between a tendency to increase treatment intensity in order to achieve a high cure rate and a tendency to reduce treatment intensity in order to minimize long term sequelae. The selection of treatment strategies is complicated by the large variety of therapeutic options (e.g. drug combinations, radiotherapy techniques). In addition the disease is by no means homogeneous and many attempts have been undertaken to rank and predict its prognosis for a given patient in order to select an appropriate treatment.

<u>**Classical (Ann Arbor)**</u>

Age
Sex
Stage
Histology
Systemic Symptoms

<u>**New**</u>

Number of Lymph Node Areas
Mediastinal Tumor
Erythrocyte Sedimentation Rate
Serum Albumin
Alkaline Phosphatase
Tumor Burden

Table 1. Prognostic factors previously claimed for overall survival (Multivariate analysis).

The twenty year old Ann Arbor staging system relies on anatomical localisation of the disease which proved to be correlated to prognosis. The definition of stages reflects the availability of the two therapeutic principles at hand: local *vs* systemic, i.e. radio- *vs* chemotherapy. The Ann Arbor system is complemented by a histopathological grading system (Rye classification) which provides additional independent information about the disease malignancy. The definition of systemic symptoms was a first step to introduce a parameter on disease activity. Besides that it is well known that age and sex play a role in prognosis. This set of five parameters can be called the classical prognostic factors for Hodgkin's disease (Table 1).

In the last years new factors have been claimed to play a role and to present additional independent information at least for some subsets of patients. Among them were anatomical parameters like the number of lymph node areas involved (Tubiana et al., 1985), the size of mediastinal mass (Lee et al., 1980; Fuller et al., 1980) and tumour burden (Specht et al., 1988a; Specht et al., 1988b), but also parameters believed to relate to disease activity like erythrocyte sedimentation rate (ESR), serum albumin (SA), haemoglobin (Hb), and alkaline phosphatase (AP) (Haybittle et al., 1985; Tubiana et al., 1985; Gobbi et al., 1986; Vaughan Hudson et al., 1986; Gobbi et al., 1988; Löffler et al., 1988). Most of them have been obtained in exploratory analyses of small studies and up to now there is no common view on the relevance of these factors.

During an international symposium on HD in 1987 in Köln (West Germany) a workshop was dedicated to an attempt to define a consensus about the relevant prognostic factors for the selection of 'risk adapted' treatment (Diehl et al., 1989). It became evident that a part of the controversy resulted from conclusions drawn from inadequate sample sizes and that the statistical analyses used were not directly comparable (different models). It was therefore suggested to make an effort to pool data from many available data bases and to perform a common statistical analysis of the combined material (Diehl et al., 1989; Löffler et al.; 1989). The initiative was taken up by the EORTC. The results of this exceptional international collaboration are presented in this volume.

Objective of the joint analysis

The objective of the joint analysis was to assess the relevance of parameters commonly used in the management of HD with respect to treatment response and prognosis. The idea was *i)* to collect data about individual patients treated according to established study protocols; *ii)* to request data on patient characteristics, on the details of staging, on the type of treatment, the success of treatment, date of relapse and death, and the causes of death; and *iii)* to perform a multivariate analysis for prognostic factors. It was recognized from the outset that many factors influenced the treatment assignments of the patients reported in the database, so that simple comparisons of outcomes according to treatment would be inappropriate. Instead the main purpose of the joint study was to facilitate better design of future treatment studies by giving indications for selecting patients and stratification variables. Further aims were to recommend reporting procedures for publications, to give suggestions for new staging criteria in Hodgkin's disease and to identify good or poor risk groups of patients for whom less or more intensive treatment should be recommended. Some but not all of these aims were achieved, and it will become evident, that the data base has to be extended and explored further in the future.

Results

Description of the data set

From 20 participating centres, 14,308 evaluable patients were registered to the database. Of these 5,217 (35.5%) were stages III and IV. Only about 6 % were treated in the 1960s. Most of the patients (57%) were treated in the 1970s and 37% in the 1980s [*Statistical Report, Table II-1*]. It should be noted that the percentage of patients registered in stage III and IV varies between 10% and 60% for individual centres reflecting the fact that some of the centres had a

	CS III (n=3,347) 64%	CS IV (n=1,870) 36%
Age (mean)	36 yrs	39 yrs
Systemic Symptoms	53%	78%
Mediast involvement	56%	59%
E-disease	7%	19%
Bone Marrow	2%	23%
ESR ($\geq$50mm)	48%	64%
AP ($\geq$75% Quantile)	25%	50%
Serum Alb ($\leq$25% Quantile)	23%	46%
Hb ($\leq$60 mmol/l)	25%	45%

Table 2. Clinical stages III and IV. Initial patient characteristics.

	CS III (n=1,318)	CS IV (n=327)
PS I	4%	-
PS II	17%	5%
PS III	68%	14%
PS IV	11%	80%

Table 3. Pathological stage after staging laparotomy.

greater emphasis on recruiting patients for radiotherapy and others more for chemotherapy [*Statistical Report, Table I*]. This indicates the possibility of selection effects. The biggest cohorts were reported from the British National Lymphoma Investigation, Southwest Oncology Group and Stanford University.

With respect to the initial characteristics of the patients nothing unexpected was found [*Statistical Report, Table II-1*]. Stage IV patients seemed to be slightly older, had more systemic symptoms than stage III and more extranodal disease (Table 2). There was a difference between stage III and IV for the various biological parameters ESR, AP, SA, and Hb.

It is noteworthy that these biological parameters were pairwise correlated and that all of them had significant correlation with systemic symptoms [*Statistical Report, Table IV-6*]. This is schematically summarized in Figure 3 (positive correlation: +, negative correlation: -). Here the question arises whether the systemic symptoms classification could possibly be replaced by a set of more objective parameters. This question was not assessed in the present analysis but can possibly be answered by a further analysis of the data.

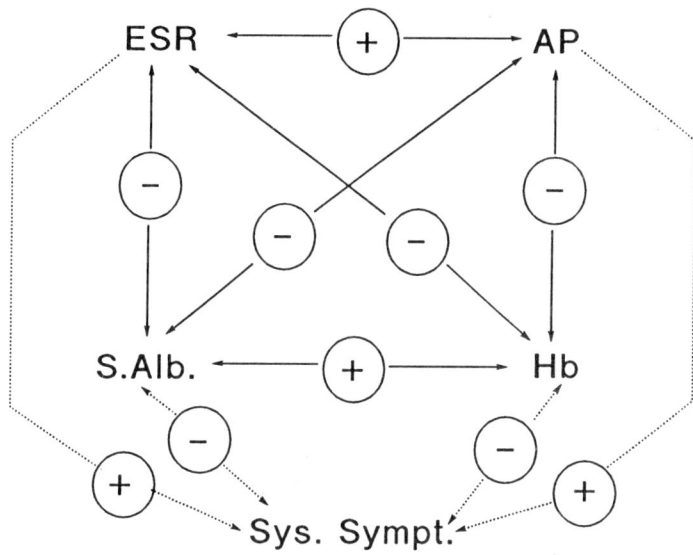

Figure 3. *Correlations of biological parameters.*

Sources of heterogeneity

Besides the selection problem mentioned above there are some additional sources of heterogeneity, three of which deserve particular mentioning.

The first is the composition of the clinical stages. It is important to note that the prognostic factor analysis is performed for clinical stage (CS) rather than pathological stage (PS). As a matter of fact only 1,318 patients (39.4%) of CS III and 327 (17.5%) of CS IV were laparotomized. If laparotomy was performed in clinical stage III about 68% were indeed PS III, 11% were PS IV, and 21% were PS I or II (Table 3). In contrast clinical stage IV was

Stage III	1960s	1970s	1980s
LP	8.5	6.2	4.4
NS	46.8	54.1	58.4
MC	35.0	33.0	30.4
LD	3.7	4.3	2.8

Stage IV	1960s	1970s	1980s
LP	3.2	4.0	2.7
NS	33.9	50.9	61.3
MC	40.3	30.9	24.9
LD	16.1	10.3	5.5

Table 4. Changes in the relative proportion (%) of histologic subtypes over time.

Treatment	1960s	1970s	1980s
Lap	15	53	22
RT alone	62	21	6
CT alone	8	36	54
RT+CT	20	40	39

(Rest unspecified)

Table 5. Changes in relative proportion (%) of treatment types over time for CS III.

indeed a PS IV in 80% of the cases. This indicates that the CS III is a fairly heterogenous disease compared with CS IV.

A second source of heterogeneity is a considerable change in the frequency of histopathological diagnosis. Over the last 20 years the nodular sclerosis subtype was diagnosed more frequently in both stages while mixed cellularity and lymphocyte depletion were less frequently diagnosed in stages IV (Table 4, derived from Statistical Report, Table II-1). Although one cannot exclude a real shift of diagnostic subtypes in the spectrum of the disease it is believed that the changes are most likely due to a change in diagnostic histopathological criteria. It is likely that pathologists have slowly changed the borderline towards non-Hodgkin lymphomas and T-cell lymphomas.

Thirdly, within the last 20 years there was a considerable shift in initial treatment types in particular for stage CS III [*Statistical Report, Table III-1*]. While laparotomy was quite rare in the 1960s it became more frequent in the 1970s apparently following the Ann Arbor recommendations. But recently laparotomy has become less popular presumably due to the more extended use of polychemotherapy (Table 5).

The change of treatment strategies is also apparent. While radiotherapy alone was the standard treatment for CS III in the 1960s it has become rare nowadays. Instead combined modality treatment has slowly increased but in over half of the patients no radiotherapy and only chemotherapy treatment is given. In stage IV pure chemotherapy makes up 68% of all initial treatments in the 1980s, the rest being combined modalities.

Treatment	III	IV
Lap + RT	13%	1%
no Lap + RT + CT	22%	21%
no Lap + CT	30%	58%
Lap + CT	10%	13%

Type of CT:

MOPP like (eg. MOPP, LOPP, MVPP, CVPP)	83%
Adriamycin containing (eg. ABVD,	4%
Alternating (M/A)	13%

Table 6. Clinical stages III and IV. Initial treatment types.

Table 6 summarizes the composition of different treatment types in the material. It is particularly important to mention that among the chemotherapies over 80% were MOPP-like regimens and 13% were alternating regimens with MOPP and adriamycin-containing

CSIII		<50	≥50 yrs
Systemic Symptoms	A	86	80
Age	B	77	69

(ESR)
(S. Albumin)

CSIV		<50	≥50 yrs
Age	one side	76	65
Topography	both sides	65	52

Table 7. Complete remission rates (%) by stage and major prognostic factors (Logistic regression).

	Relative Risks		
Factors	CS III A	CS III B	CS IV
Age	1.4[b]	1.7[a]	1.8[a]
Sex (female)	-	0.7	-
No. LN areas	1.4[c]	-	-
MT	-	1.3	-

Table 8. Prognostic factors for RFS in clinical stages III and III. Proportional hazards model stratified for type of treatment, treatment period, and laparotomy *(a: age > 60; b: age >50; c: 4 lymph node areas involved or more)*.

SV-Rate (%)	CSIIIA	CSIIIB	CSIV
5 yr	55	55	41
10 yr	42	42	23

Causes of death (%)	CSIIIA	CSIIIB	CSIV
HD	79	78	73
2⁰Neopl.	5	6	3
Other	16	16	24

Table 9. Survival after relapse by clinical stage and presence or absence of B symptoms.

combinations. Other chemotherapies are rare. Thus any conclusions with respect to chemotherapy hold primarily for MOPP-like regimens (i.e. MOPP, C-MOPP, LOPP, MVPP, CVPP).

Treatment Results and Prognostic Factors

Laparotomy

The results of laparotomy have already been mentioned in Table 3. There is considerable interest in knowing whether one can identify a subset of CS III patients who are indeed not PS III but PS I or II. Although the stepwise logistic regression analysis yields several prognostic factors for laparotomy, a more detailed analysis shows that the predictive value is limited. For CS III patients there is no group for which one can predict a PSI-II with a probability of more than 0.42 on the basis of non-invasive procedures [Statistical Report, Table V-11]. On the other hand about 27% of all CS I-II patients were PS III [Statistical Report, Table III-1], but there was no reasonable way to predict this for an individual patient. Only the subset of CS I-II with more than 4 lymph node areas involved and negative mediastinal involvement seems to have a probability of more than 0.5 of being PS III or IV [Statistical Report, Table V-6]. The only reasonable predictibility could be found for the large group of CS III patients with LP-NS subtype. They rarely are PS IV [Statistical Report, Tables V-8 & V-10]. This result, however, is clinically not very relevant. Consequently there is no real relevant prognostic factor to predict outcome of laparotomy for CS III and IV patients.

Prognostic Factors for Complete Remission

The overall complete remission rates are 87% for CS IIIA, 76% for CS IIIB and 63% for CS IV [Statistical Report, Tables VI-6 to 9] with little change between the 1970s and 1980s. There is, however, a certain indication that combined modality treatment was more effective than chemo- or radiotherapy alone [Statistical Report, Tables VI-7 & VI-9]. One should treat this observation with extreme caution, because a selection of patients could have allocated a bad prognostic group to the pure chemotherapy treatments rendering the comparison unfair. Here more detailed statistical analyses are necessary.

Table 7 summarizes the prognostic factors for complete remission according to stage and major prognostic factors for patients in whom staging laparotomy was not performed [Statistical Report, Tables VI-16 & VI-17]. Their complete remission rates are 79% for stage III and 63% for stage IV. For CS III systemic symptoms and age are significant prognostic factors and have considerable discriminating value. Young patients without systemic symptoms had a complete remission rate of 86% and old patients with systemic symptoms had a complete remiossion rate of 69%. In addition, there was an indication that high ESR rate and low SA are prognostic factors for CR. However, one should treat this observation with some caution, because of the large amount of missing data so that the result may not be absolutely reliable. With respect to clinical stage IV, age and topography were the only significant prognostic factors with disease in young patients restricted to one side of the diaphragm being the most favourable with a complete remission rate of 76% and old patients with extended desease having a complete remission rate of 52% [Statistical Report, Tables VI-16 & VI-17].

Prognostic Factors for Relapse Free Survival (RFS)

The first observation is that RFS shows considerable improvement from the 1960s to the 1970s, but hardly any change from the 1970s to the 1980s [Statistical Report, Figure VII-13]. It is important to note that the curves show a plateau, starting about 6 to 8 years after treatment, indicating that cure of the disease is practically achieved by this time, although there are occasional relapses even over 10 years after remission [Statistical Report, Table VII-22].

Looking for the possible reasons of this time trend one gets the impression that it is primarily related to the historical change of the type of treatment with pure radiotherapy being less effective than combined modality treatment and pure chemotherapy. Therefore the prognostic factor analysis was undertaken using models stratified for the initial type of treatment (radiotherapy, chemotherapy, combined treatment), treatment period (1960s, 1970s, 1980s) and in addition for laparotomy (done, not done).

The significant prognostic factors for RFS are listed in Table 8, giving the relative risks. High age, above 50 or 60, was associated with an increased risk in all stages ranging between 1.4-1.8. Female gender was a favorable prognostic factor for clinical stage IIIB (relative risk below 1.0). The number of lymph node areas involved was an adverse prognostic factor for clinical stage IIIA, while mediastinal involvement was an adverse factor for CS IIIB (small and large M/T ratios were not distinguished). Histology, topography, or biological parameters did not appear as prognostic factors for RFS.

Of course, the question is how serious a relapse may be. To get an impression one can look at the survival after relapse [*Statistical Report, Figure VIII-17*].

Within five years about half of the CS III and IV patients, who relapsed for the first time, die, and within ten years only about 20-40% survive (Table 9). Looking for the causes of death it is evident that Hodgkin's disease is the prominent reason and secondary neoplasia play a minor role. Other causes of death make up between 16% and 24%. Thus it appears evident that achievement of continuing complete remission is an important therapeutic aim for these stages, and that a relapse is associated with a fairly unfavourable prognosis.

Relative Risk

Factors		HD-Deaths only			Death from all causes		
		CSIIIA	CSIIIB	CSIV	CSIIIA	CSIIIB	CSIV
Age	60+	2.5	3.0	2.1	4.2	4.0	2.9
	50-59	–	1.6	1.6	2.8	2.2	1.9
	40-49	–	–	–	1.8	1.7	1.4
Sex(male)		–	–	1.4	1.4	–	1.4
Histology	LD	2.4	1.6	–	–	–	–
	MC	1.5	–	–	–	–	–
	not NS	–	–	1.5	–	–	1.4
No. Lymph Node Areas		1.4	–	–	1.4	–	–

Table 10. Prognostic factors for survival in clinical stages III and IV. Proportional hazards model stratified for type of treatment, treatment period, and staging laparotomy.

Prognostic Factors for Survival

Within the last 20 years, there was an improvement in overall survival for stages III and IV [*Statistical Report, Figure VIII-12*]. The difference is about 10% to 15%, the majority being evident between the 1960s and 1970s.

In order to perform a prognostic factor analysis for survival a proportional hazards model was used, stratified again for treatment type, treatment period and laparotomy.

In Table 10 the results of the prognostic factor analysis for survival are shown where deaths from HD only and from all causes are considered. With respect to HD death only it is evident that higher age groups have a higher risk in all stages, female gender is favorable in stage IV, and in all stages a significant contribution by histological subtypes is found, in particular by the lymphocyte depleted form. In stage IV the nodular sclerosis subtype is favourable. A large number of lymph node areas involved is an unfavourable prognostic factor in CS IIIA. Biological parameters did not appear as significant prognostic factors for SV.

Having given the prognostic factor analysis for survival in CS III and IV separately one should mention that if one takes all the stages CS I-IV together, stage and systemic symptoms are also prognostic factors. This confirms in general the classical prognostic factors, established almost two decades ago as mentioned in Table 1.

With respect to death from all causes age and sex are the prominent prognostic factors but the number of lymph node areas plays a role in stage CS IIIA (Table 10).

It is instructive to inspect a series of overall curves, to illustrate the relevance of the prognostic factors mentioned. For CS III-IV patients the sex difference is not very dramatic. Survival rates differ by not more than 10% [*Statistical Report, Figure VIII-13*].

The survival differences for histological types are more prominent with the lymphocyte depleted form being particularly unfavourable. The various other groups (NS, LP, MC) behave similarly with MC being at the lower end of the spectrum [*Statistical Report, Figure VIII-4*].

The curves showing survival by stage indicate that CS IIIA is more different from CS IIIB than CS IIIB is from stage IV. The CS IIIA group seems to parallel the CS IB-IIB group [*Statistical Report, Figure VIII-6*].

The most dramatic prognostic factor, however, is age [*Statistical Report, Figure VIII-9*]. One finds a very clear monotonic reduction of survival with higher age. This reduction is far more than should be expected by the natural aging process in these age groups. In particular the survival curves for older patients decline rapidly in the beginning. The problem with age, however, is, that it is a difficult parameter to interpret because it is not a parameter of the disease. On the other hand it may have an influence on the disease progression, on treatment tolerance (reduced dose or dose intensity), and on the predisposition for secondary neoplasia. The difficulty is that all these components can not be clearly distinguished. In any case, however, the enormous divergence of the curves in particular in the initial years after start of treatment raises the question of an appropriate 'age adapted' treatment. This discussion should be facilitated by a more detailed analysis for prognostic factors restricted to the old age group, which was not yet performed.

Prognostic Factors for Late Deaths

Having mentioned above that relapses become rare after 6 to 8 years, one might expect the overall survival curves (including death of any cause) to show only a slow decline according to the natural aging process. As a matter of fact the decline is considerably steeper. What is behind the late deaths?

Although the cause of death was not broken down in the statistical report for CS III and IV separately, one can get good insight by looking at the data for the complete set of CS I-IV (Table 11) [*derived from Statistical Report, Table VII-22*].

Of the patients with a failure of the initial treatment 83% died within 10 years and they mostly died of HD. Of the patients who had a complete remission and then relapsed, 50% died within 10 years, most of them of HD (see also Table 9). Patients in a continuous complete remission also died. The figure amounts to 12% within 10 years. Of these patients a third died of secondary neoplasia and 14% of treatment related sequelae. Only about half died of other causes which may mostly be related to the natural aging process. The cumulative incidence of death from second neoplasia was over 10% after 20 years in the cohort which achieved an initial complete remission [*Statistical Report, Figure IX-3*]. Therefore it is evident that one has to think of treatment strategies to reduce long term sequelae for those patients likely to achieve continuous complete remission, while this aim is less important for patients likely to relapse. As it is shown in a more detailed report in this volume [*Statistical Report, part IX*], the most outstanding prognostic factors for secondary neoplasia in patients achieving complete remission are age and treatment types (MOPP for leukemia, total nodal irradiation for solid tumors). High age was associated with relative risks of over 10 indicating a considerably increased sensitivity of old patients for mutagenic events.

Initital treatment success	10yr Death Rate	HD	Treatment	2^0 Malignancy	Intercurrent Disease
No CR	83%	85%	5%	2%	7%
CR > Relapse	51%	81%	3%	8%	7%
Cont. CR	12%	—	14%	32%	53%

Table 11. All stages. Causes of death.

Summary of Prognostic Factors and Conclusions

Table 12 summarizes the analysis of the prognostic factors for CS III-IV. Age is a prognostic factor for all endpoints and all stages. The other prognostic factors differ for endpoints and stages considered. Most of them are classical; however with respect to complete remission rates there is an indication that biological parameters (ESR, SA) play a role. With respect to RFS and survival the extent of disease in CS III, measured by the number of lymph node areas involved and the mediastinal involvement are relevant. For CS IV only a few disease related parameters like topography for complete remission and histology for survival play a role.

From the above analysis one can draw the following conclusions for CS III-IV:

1. For survival the classical prognostic factors age, stage, sex, systemic symptoms and histology were confirmed. In addition the number of lymph node areas involved plays a role.
2. With respect to complete remission and relapse free survival CS IV is a fairly homogeneous disease.
3. With respect to complete remission, RFS and survival CS III is a fairly heterogeneous disease. Biological parameters play a role for complete remission and spread of disease (mediastinal involvement, number of lymph node areas) for RFS and survival.
4. Of the patients relapsing after complete remission 50% die within 5 years, mostly of HD.
5. Of the patients in continous complete remission 12% die within 10 years, 30% of them from second malignancies.

Discussion

With respect to clinical consequences this analysis suggests that CS III defines not a very uniform cohort of patients. Consideration of additional staging parameters for the spread and activity of the disease should be helpful. Prognosis of a very limited IIIA disease appears to be very different from a IIIB disease with many locations involved. For stage IV addition of new staging parameters does not seem to add much to the predictability of prognosis. With respect to the bad prognosis after relapse therapeutic intention should aim at achieving continuous complete remission from the beginning. This implies selection of treatments which are effective in primary therapy. Although worries about long term sequelae are reasonable they should play a less prominent role for the majority of CS III-IV patients. This may be differentfor CS I-II. For CS III-IV patients cure of HD remains the primary aim. But it is noted that the therapeutic interval between undertreatment and overtreatment appears fairly narrow with the regimens used.

	CS III	CS IV
CR	Age Sys. Symptoms [ESR, SA]	Age Topography
RFS	Age Sex Sys. Symptoms No. LN Areas Med. involvement	Age
SV	Age Sys. Symptoms Histology No. LN Areas	Age Histology Sex

Table 12. Prognostic factors in clinical stages III and IV. Summary.

The role of biological parameters as prognostic factors needs further investigation. On one hand the parameters are not routinely measured in all institutions. This could cause an ascertainment bias if it was measured only in patients where some other problem was noted. On the other hand for recent patients the parameters are more likely to be observed but the follow up time may be too short to see noticable effects. Thus further prospective accumulation of these data is necessary.

Age was the major prognostic factor for all endpoints. Its validity is, however, difficult to interpret in terms of an independent parameter characterizing the disease. Although age may influence the biology of the disease (e.g. reduced immune competence to control it) it may also be related to a reduced tolerance of aggressive treatment. This could have resulted in a reduced dose or dose intensity for old patients, diminishing their chance to eliminate the tumour. In addition old patients seem to be more sensitive to mutagenic events and more frequently acquire second neoplasia (e.g. reduced repair capacity). It is clear that more detailed statistical analysis is needed to separate the contribution of these effects to prognosis. Nevertheless it might be recommendable to take particular care of the old HD patient. The development of tolerable but highly effective treatments appears to be the primary aim for this cohort of patients.

With respect to reporting treatment results of CS III and IV patients the above analysis suggests that reports should include a breakdown of the results for biological parameters, for the number of lymph node areas and in particular for age (if possible in groups of 10 year intervals). In the design of new randomized trials stratification for age is highly recommended.

Although the above analysis was successful in identifying significant prognostic factors suggesting some deterministic components in the course of the disease, the stochastic character of the process is still dominant. As summarized in Tables 8 and 10 the relative risks identified rarely exceeded 2 and mostly were smaller. This implies that the deterministic components though present are not overwhelming. On the other hand one has to keep the composition of the data material in mind. It is heterogeneous with respect to patient selection, to staging procedures and treatment strategies and it is complicated by missing values (particularly for the biological parameters). In addition the use of the proportional hazards model implies some assumptions which are at least debatable. The assumption of proportionality of prognostic factors in all strata and over such a long time as 20 years and the assumption that prognostic factors are independent of the choice of treatment must be considered as a severe model limitation. It will be a task of future analyses to apply statistical tools which require less strict assumptions. Recent developments of new statistical methodology and computer algorithms, such as recursive partitioning (Davis & Anderson, 1989), should be applied. Taken together it becomes obvious that the above analysis could only detect the 'top of the iceberg' of the underlying prognostic factor structure. Data structure and the statistical methodology used present limitations which may cloud the real value of prognostic factor found and which may explain why others remained below detection levels.

There are several suggestions for further analysis, partly technical and partly clinical. Technically one question is whether the model of analysis was correct. It will be necessary to check the proportional hazard assumptions, and to check for possible interactions between different prognostic factors or between prognostic factors and treatment. Furthermore it will be important to examine additional endpoints and see whether they are more sensitive than complete remission and RFS. We propose in particular an endpoint that quantifies the failure of primary treatment to achieve cure such as i.e. time to treatment failure (Dixon et al., 1987; Löffler et al., 1988a; Löffler et al., 1988b). Failure is defined as being any of the following: no complete remission at the end of primary treatment, relapse, death of any cause if not preceded by progression or relapse. This endpoint is particularly useful in a disease where cure is the intent of primary treatment.

With respect to clinical perspectives, one may investigate the possibility of replacing the often subjective feature, systemic symptoms, by one or more laboratory variables. Furthermore we have not fully exploited the possibility of identifying subgroups for either less intensive or more intensive or differently designed treatments, e.g. the groups for which radiotherapy is sufficient, the groups which need high dose chemotherapy plus autologous bone marrow transplantation, and the prognostic factors for old patients. Finally, we have to think about procedures to allow some type of treatment comparison, which was so far excluded from the analysis. In the database there was a suggestion that chemotherapy alone (mostly MOPP) was less effective in complete remission, RFS and survival of CS III and IV than combined modality treatment. These topics make a point for a further expansion and use of the database which in our mind has already proven valuable and instructive.

Acknowledgements

We like to thank Walter Gregory (London), Michel Henry-Amar (Villejuif), Dirk Hasenclever and Michael Pfreundschuh (Köln), and Lillian Fuller and Frederic Hagemeister (Houston) for valuable discussion and Stephan Gontard (Köln) for help with the manuscript.

References

Davis, R.B., et al. (1989): Exponential survival statistics. *Medicine* 8, 947-961.
Diehl, V., et al. (1989): *New aspects in diagnosis and treatment of Hodgkin's disease*.ed. V. Diehl, M. Pfreundschuh & M. Löffler, 283 p. Recent Results in Cancer Research 117. Berlin: Springer Verlag.
Dixon, D.O., et al. (1987): Reporting outcome in Hodgkin's disease and lymphoma. *J. Clin. Oncol.* 5, 1670-1672.
Fuller, L.M., et al. (1980): Evaluation of the significance of prognostic factors in stage III Hodgkin's disease treated with MOPP and Radiotherapy. *Cancer* 45, 1352-1364.
Gobbi, P.G., et al. (1986): Prognostic significance of serum albumin in Hodgkin's disease. *Haematologica (PAVIA)* 71, 95-102.
Gobbi, P.G., et al. (1988): Hodgkin's disease prognosis: A directly predictive equation. *Lancet* i, 675-679.
Haybittle, J.L., et al. (1985): Review of British national lymphoma investigation studies of Hodgkin's disease and development of prognostic index. *Lancet* i, 967-972.
Kaplan, H.S., et al. (1980): Prognostic significance of mediastinal involvement in Hodgkin's disease treated with curative radiotherapy. *Cancer* 46, 2403-2409.
Löffler, M., et al (1988a): Prognostic risk factors in advanced Hodgkin's disease. *Blut* 56, 273-281.
Löffler, M., et al (1988b): Probleme der Konzeption und auswertung von therapiestudien bei lanser behandkungsdauer; Mittler CR-rate un langer überlebensdauer In *Proceedings of the 30.GMDS Annual Meeting*, H.K. Selbmann. Berlin: Springer-Verlag.
Löffler, M., et al. (1989): Risk factor adapted treatment of Hodgkin's lymphoma: Strategies and perspectives - report of the German Hodgkin study group. In *New aspects in diagnosis and treatment of Hodgkin's disease*, ed. V. Diehl, M. Pfreundschuh & M. Löffler, pp. 142-162. Recent Results in Cancer Research 117. Berlin: Springer Verlag.
Pocock, S.J. (1983): *Clinical trials: A Practical approach*. New-York: John Wiley & Sons.
Specht, L., et al (1988a): Prognostic factors in Hodgkin's disease stage III with special reference to tumor burden. *Eur. J. Haematol.* 41, 80-87.
Specht, L., et al (1988b): Prognostic factors in Hodgkin's disease stage IV. *Eur. J. Haematol.* 41, 359-367.
Tubiana, M., et al. (1985): A Multivariate analysis of prognostic factors in early stage Hodgkin's disease. *Int. J. Radiat. Oncol. Biol. Phys* 11, 23-30.
Vaughan Hudson, B., et al (1987): Systemic disturbance in Hodgkin's disease and its relation to histopathology and prognosis (BNLI Report n° 30). *Clin. Radiol.* 38, 257-26.

The treatment of advanced Hodgkin's disease : strategy

P. Carde[1], D.E. Bergsagel[2], N.I. Nissen[3], A. Hagenbeek[4]

1 Institut Gustave-Roussy, 94805 Villejuif Cedex, France
2 The Princess Margaret Hospital, 500, Sherbourne Street, M4X 1K9 Toronto, Canada
3 Rigshospitalet, 9 Blegdamsvej, 2100 Copenhagen Denmark
4 Dr Daniel den Hoedklinick, Groene Hilledijk 301, 3075 EA Rotterdam, The Netherlands

Summary

This paper first reviews the current therapeutic strategies for advanced Hodgkin disease (HD), and second considers whether the prognostic factors identified for the Workshop series will permits the identification of groups of patients with reduced chances of achieving a complete response (CR) and increased risk of relapsing from a CR, following current primary therapy.

Three hypotheses to explain the improved results of treating HD patients with alternating MOPP/ABVD are examined. The first suggests that alternating non-cross resistant drug combinations delays the onset of drugs resistance and this improves the results over that achieved with either regimen alone. The second holds that MOPP and ABVD have the same overlapping activity for most of their curative potential, but each regimen retains marginal, independent activity at one end of the spectrum. The third hypothesis is that the improved results with MOPP/ABVD occurs because ABVD is more effective than MOPP. The preliminary results of the CALGB trial of MOPP vs ABVD vs MOPP/ABVD suggest that the third hypothesis is correct. These observations, taken together with the evidence that ABVD is less myelotoxic, retains fertility and is less leukemogenic than MOPP, suggest that ABVD should be the basic primary chemotherapy for patients with advanced HD.

Age is the major factor predicting a CR and relapse-free survival in patients with advanced HD; older patients have a lower CR rate and relapse more frequently than younger patients. The maintenance of high dose-intensity, especially during the early courses of primary chemotherapy for advanced HD, and the achievement of CR within 3 to 5 courses of MOPP, have an important influence on relapse-free survival. MOPP chemotherapy leads to cumulative myelotoxicity and is poorly tolerated, especially by older patients. ABVD is better tolerated and may permit the delivery of higher dose-intensity chemotherapy to older patients.

Much improvement is required in the treatment of advanced HD, for only 50% of these patients achieve prolonged relapse-free survival. In devising improved strategies for therapy we must recognize that older patients do not tolerate aggressive therapy well and discover more effective, better tolerated drugs and biological response modifiers, or agents, such as haemopoietic growth factors, which may allow older patients to tolerate higher dose-intensity chemotherapy.

Résumé

Cet article passe d'abord en revue les différentes stratégies thérapeutiques actuelles de la maladie de Hodgkin, puis discute les facteurs pronostiques mis en évidence par la population de patients étudiés lors du Workshop, pour en isoler des groupes de patients à haut risque d'échecs en terme de rémission complète et de rechute après le traitement initial.

L'amélioration des résultats par une alternance de MOPP et d'ABVD en comparaison avec le MOPP seul, suscite trois hypothèses qui sont successivement examinées. La première suggère que l'alternance de chimiothérapie sans résistance croisée théorique retarde la survenue des résistances aux drogues et explique ainsi l'amélioration des résultats par rapport à ceux que peut espérer l'une des deux associations isolées. La seconde fait l'hypothèse que le MOPP et l'ABVD ont, pour l'essentiel de leur pouvoir curateur, une activité superposée et identique, mais que chaque association possède, à une extrémité du spectre, une activité marginale indépendante. Dans la troisième hypothèse, c'est parce que l'ABVD est plus efficace que le MOPP, que l'association MOPP-ABVD est supérieure. Un certain nombre d'observations et le fait que i) l'ABVD soit moins myélotoxique, ii) préserve la fertilité chez l'homme comme chez la femme, et iii) soit moins leucémogène que le MOPP, suggèrent que l'ABVD pourrait être la chimiothérapie de base pour les patients porteurs de maladie de Hodgkin étendue.

L'âge est le facteur prédictif principal de l'entrée en rémission complète et de la survie en première rémission complète chez les patients porteurs de maladie de Hodgkin étendue, les sujets les plus âgés ayant les moins bons résultats. Le maintien d'un rythme d'administration élevé des drogues, en particulier au cours des premiers cycles de chimiothérapie et l'obtention rapide d'une rémission complète apparente dans les 3 à 5 premiers cycles de MOPP influencent de façon déterminante la survie en première rémission complète. Le MOPP entraîne une toxicité médullaire cumulative et il est mal toléré en particulier par les patients les plus âgés. L'ABVD est mieux toléré et peut permettre l'administration de doses de chimiothérapie plus élevées par unité de temps chez les patients plus âgés.

Beaucoup de progrès sont nécessaires dans le traitement des maladies de Hodgkin étendues, car seulement 50 % des patients peuvent jouir d'une rémission prolongée. En mettant au point de nouvelles stratégies de traitement, nous devons prendre en considération que les patients les plus âgés ne tolèrent pas bien les traitements agressifs et rechercher des drogues à la fois plus efficaces et mieux tolérées. Certains modificateurs de la réponse biologique ou des agents comme les facteurs de croissance hématopoïétiques, pourraient permettre aux patients les plus âgés de tolérer correctement la chimiothérapie administrée à plus haute dose.

Introduction

The term "advanced" Hodgkin's disease covers a broad spectrum, ranging from groups with good prognostic features, who enjoy prolonged progression-free survival following treatment, to those who do not achieve a complete remission with their initial therapy. Advanced HD includes patients with nodal disease on both sides of the diaphragm (Stage III), and those with organ involvement (Stage IV), without systemic manifestations of fever, night sweats and weight loss (A), or with these features (B). Clinically staged (CS) patients with IIIA through IVB HD form the broad group; the Workshop data indicate that over 50% of these patients died within 10 years of initial diagnosis. Chemotherapy plays a major role in the treatment of advanced HD, but there have been few attempts to develop special treatment strategies for different pronostic groups. Some patients with good prognosis advanced HD may be overtreated with the current prescription of six courses of MOPP, ABVD or alternating MOPP/ABVD, while others do poorly, and require a new approach.

This paper will first review the current therapeutic strategies for newly diagnosed advanced HD, relapses being covered in another article (Burgers, present issue). A guiding principle has been to achieve the highest possible complete remission (CR) rate as the first step towards curative therapy (De Vita, 1988). In the Workshop series, 42% and 44% in CS IIIB and IV respectively of the patients who achieved a CR after MOPP-like CT relapsed. Two questions arise. First, can the risk of failure or relapse be reduced by such approaches as improved compliance to chemotherapy (CT), use of new drug combinations, alternating non cross-resistant cycles, adjuvant radiation therapy, high-dose chemotherapy, maintenance chemotherapy, or biological response modifiers? Second, can the patients at high risk of CR failure or relapse be identified?

The second intention is to investigate whether the prognostic factors identified in the series of over 4000 cases of advanced HD in the Workshop series will permit, as anticipated (Löffler et al., 1989) the identification of groups of patients with an increased risk of relapse and who would require a new treatment strategy.

We do not intend to draw any firm conclusions, but rather to indicate the directions to be investigated in the development of new therapeutic strategies for HD. Firm recommendations will have to await the demonstration of significant advances by well-designed clinical trials.

1. Yielding a higher complete response rate

The achievement of a CR is considered to be the corner stone of curative chemotherapy for advanced HD (De Vita et al., 1979; De Vita, 1988). We will consider some of the factors that can affect the CR rate. The Workshop series revealed that combination chemotherapy achieved a CR rate of 56% in Stage IV and 65% in Stage IIIB.

1.1. Type and administration of induction chemotherapy

1.1.1. MOPP : MOPP was the first successful drug combination used in the treatment of advanced HD (De Vita et al., 1970), and most of the patients evaluated in the Workshop series were so treated. The large, single institution NCI study (De Vita et al., 1980; Longo et al., 1986) reports excellent results for MOPP in the treatment of HD. In stage IV, there was a 77% CR rate and for those who achieved a CR, the relapse free survival (RFS) at 5 years was 65%. Further, at 5 years 56% of the patients enjoyed freedom from progression (FFP), and if only deaths from HD are counted, 57% of the patients were alive at 5 years. No derived regimen was unanimously called superior to MOPP (Nissen et al., 1979).

1.1.2. Drug dosing : Compliance with recommended doses and the schedules of administration were of major importance for the achievement of CR in 132 patients treated with MOPP at Stanford (Carde et al., 1983). In this retrospective study it was difficult to identify how much different factors, such as the general status of the patient, the biologic characteristics of the disease, defective myelopoiesis, a deficient immune response, and the failure to achieve CR. B symptoms were the only other independent prognostic factor, aside from variables in dose and schedule, which influenced the chance of achieving a CR. The mean total dose and the delivery rate dose intensity were important for all drugs in the MOPP combination, aside from prednisone. Moreover, compliance was especially important during the first 3 cycles. These findings have been confirmed in other retrospective studies with MOPP and similar regimens (Green et al., 1980; De Vita et al., 1987). In the NCI series, investigators were unable to evaluate the effect of variations in drug doses, because a special effort was made to maintain the drug doses as high as possible. Nevertheless, the dose of vincristine was found to be one of the most important variables for survival, even in the NCI series (Longo et al., 1986). This was also observed in a prospective EORTC evaluation of MOPP in the treatment of HD (submitted for publication). The importance of maintaining high-dose intensity has also been established for ABVD and for MOPP alternating with ABVD (Bonadonna et al., 1986).

1.1.3. Number of cycles : Continuing MOPP beyond 6 to 8 cycles did not translate into improved CR rates (De Vita et al., 1980). In a 12-year update of a National Cancer Institute of Canada trial of MOPP alone versus 3 courses of MOPP followed by radiation to involved sites (Bergsagel et al., 1980; Yelle et al., 1987; Yelle, 1988), a significant interaction between age and treatment was uncovered. Patients under the age of 30 tolerated more than 3 courses of MOPP well, achieving CR status and long-term survival. Those over the age of 30 did not tolerate more than 3 courses of MOPP well. The dose intensity of MOPP had to be reduced markedly after the first 3 courses of MOPP and the frequency of relapse and death from HD was significantly greater in patients older than 30 years.

The NCI policy of administering cycles of induction MOPP until a CR is achieved, and then adding 2 more, with a minimum of 6, has proven to be safe (Young et al., 1973). Two arguments favor this flexible approach to induction therapy. First, increasing the number of cycles of induction MOPP does not increase the proportion of CRs or improve survival (Bergsagel et al., 1980; Bloomfield et al., 1982), and continuing MOPP as maintenance therapy has not been beneficial (Canellos et al., 1983). During the Workshop, Nissen recalled that patients randomized to receive 12 cycles of MOPP fared worse than those treated with 6 cycles in the CALGB study (Bloomfield et al., 1982). Second, increasing the cumulative dose of CT increases the risk of a second malignancy (Henry-Amar, 1989).

1.1.4. Alternating non cross-resistant regimens : There is little doubt that alternating MOPP/ABVD results in a superior CR rate and FFP, as compared to the initial use of MOPP alone. In a recent update of 88 HD patients treated in Milan since 1974, the 9 year FFP was 63% for MOPP/ABVD and 36% for MOPP (p=0.008) and survival was respectively 60% vs 58% (Valagussa et al., 1989). A previous report had indicated that MOPP/ABVD achieved higher CR rates and FFP particularly in patients with the poorer prognosis factors such as older age, bulky disease, systemic symptoms and nodular sclerosis histology (Bonadonna et al., 1986). At least three other studies have confirmed the superiority of alternating schedules over MOPP alone or its derivatives: the ECOG (Glick et al., 1988), CALGB (Canellos et al., 1988) and EORTC (Somers et al., 1988) studies all suggest the same trend. In addition, a number of other studies are underway (Rosenberg et al., 1985; Löffler et al., 1988).

The mechanism responsible for the improved results of treating HD with MOPP/ABVD is a key question because the strategy to be followed in the clinical application of this observation is critically dependent on the mechanism of action. Three hypothetical mechanisms of action and the resulting treatment strategies are explored in Table 1.

Table 1. Strategies resulting from different mechanisms of MOPP/ABVD superiority over MOPP

Hypothesis	% range of activity of CT regimens	Strategy
1/ Enhancement (Goldie-Coldman)	MOPP alone = 50 ABVD alone = 50 MOPP/ABVD = 130	Investigate improve alternating regimens
2/ Addition of marginal independent effects	MOPP alone = 115 ABVD alone = 115 MOPP/ABVD = 130 each with 100 overlapping and 15 independent effects	Give up alternation Delete and replace overlaping drugs
3/ Superiority of ABVD which also carries all the potential of MOPP	MOPP alone = 100 ABVD alone = 130 MOPP/ABVD = 130	Drop MOPP and improve ABVD

The first hypothesis is that the use of two non-cross resistant CT regimens results in enhancement and an improved result over that achieved with either CT regimen alone. The hypothesis is based on the theory of spontaneous mutations leading to drug resistance that may be overcome by the early application of all available effective drugs (Goldie et al., 1982). The mathematical rationale of this theory is supported by the results of treating animal tumours and by the observation that in the Milan trials ABVD/MOPP was more effective in the treatment of poor-prognosis patients and reduced the incidence of early progression. However, this hypothesis has been criticized on a theoretical basis (Green, 1989) and has not been confirmed in other solid tumours or lymphomas. If this hypothesis were to be validated, other drug alternations should be investigated. As an example, the MOPP/ABV hybrid scheme (Connors et al., 1987), where dacarbazine has been deleted and the dose of adriamycin increased, is being compared to MOPP/ABVD by the National Cancer Institute of Canada Clinical Trials Group. Other examples are the comparison LOPP/EVAP to LOPP alone by the BNLI and the comparison of MOPP/ABVD/RT to MOPP/ABV/CAD/RT at Memorial Sloan Kettering Cancer Center in New-York (Straus et al., 1989).

The second hypothesis is that MOPP and ABVD have the same overlapping spectrum of activity for most of their curative potential, but each regimen retains marginal, independent activity at one end of its spectrum. If this hypothesis is correct, the improved performance of MOPP alternating with ABVD would only reflect the addition of two independent effects. It is of interest that the benefit of alternating MOPP and ABVD is lost when the two combinations are administered in a sequential manner. This observation suggests that MOPP and ABVD do not have marginal, independent activity. However, the failure of sequential MOPP and ABVD to be as effective as alternating MOPP/ABVD could also be explained by the reduced dose intensity associated with the sequential scheme. The administration of several courses of MOPP in a row does lead to cumulative myelotoxicity, while less cumulative toxicity is associated with ABVD. Several groups have observed, but not fully reported, that MOPP alternating with ABVD is better tolerated than MOPP alone (Bonadonna et al., 1986; Canellos et al., 1988; Somers et al., 1988), and this resulted in improved drug delivery rates in HD patients treated with alternating MOPP/ABVD in the CALGB and EORTC studies. If the hypothesis of the addition of independent, marginal activity for MOPP and ABVD could be proven, then attempts to improve treatment should be through the deletion of drugs which are only weakly active or associated with undesirable toxicity, and the substitution of new drugs with more attractive characteristics.

The third hypothesis is that the superiority of MOPP/ABVD reflects that ABVD is more effective than MOPP. This hypothesis is supported by the observations that the results of ABVD plus irradiation tended to be somewhat better than MOPP plus irradiation in the treatment of early stage HD in Milan (Valagussa et al., 1989) and in the results of the H6 EORTC trial (unpublished data). The only prospective trial testing this hypothesis is the CALGB study of MOPP alone vs ABVD alone vs alternating MOPP/ABVD (Canellos et al., 1988); it was updated during the Workshop by J.R. Anderson. The preliminary results indicate that the CR rates and failure-free survival (FFS) rates at 3 years are significantly better for the ABVD and MOPP/ABVD groups, as compared to the MOPP group. The fact that the preliminary results with ABVD are equivalent to those achieved with MOPP/ABVD suggest that this third hypothesis may be correct. If this proves to be true we should drop MOPP and its derivatives, and investigate drug regimens modified from ABVD, with higher anthracycline dosage, such as EBVP from EORTC, or with additional, drugs e.g. EVAP from BNLI, or CAVPE from GATLA.

1.1.5. New drugs. A number of "new" drugs have been tested in patients with relapsing HD, but no drug with obvious superior activity has been identified. However, drugs with mechanisms of action which are different from the widely used alkylating agents, vinca alcaloids and doxorubicin, should be considered for inclusion in front-line regimens. The podophylotoxin derivatives, which inhibit topoisomerase II, should be considered because of their activity at conventional and higher doses (Jagannath et al., 1986a; Jagannath et al., 1989). High-dose cytosine arabinoside (Brandwein et al., 1989; Hiddeman et al., 1989) and platinum derivatives (Brandwein et al., 1989) may also prove to be useful. A second source of progress may come from the use of cytokines and haemopoietic growth factors which are now becoming available.

1.1.6. Consolidation radiotherapy. Adjuvant RT has not resulted in improved survival (Coltman, 1980; Rosenberg et al., 1985; Horwich et al., 1987; Sutcliffe et al., 1987; Raemekers et al., 1989), although a lower relapse rate within the irradiated field has been observed (Bergsagel et al., 1980; Bloomfield et al., 1982). The SWOG 7808 study, discussed during the symposium, demonstrated that low-dose involved field irradiation converted 88% of PRs following treatment with MOP-RAP into CRs (Fabian et al., 1989). The presence of more than minimal residual disease reduced the PR conversion rate and the 4-year failure-free rate. The effect of adjuvant RT on the patients achieving CRs in this study has not been reported yet. No advantage for adjuvant RT was observed in the ECOG study comparing BCVPP with BCVPP + RT (Glick et al., 1988). The EORTC has designed another randomized trial (# 20884) to assess the role of adjuvant RT following MOPP/ABV. The HD-3 german trial compares RT consolidation to continued COPP/ABVD (Löffler et al., 1988). The Canadian study (Bergsagel et al., 1980; Yelle et al., 1987; Yelle, 1988) reported by Bergsagel during the Workshop, emphasized that RT was poorly tolerated following more than 3 courses of MOPP, especially by older patients. However at Stanford University, the results of an alternating CT/RT combination compared favorably with alternating CT (Hoppe et al., 1989). An increased risk of death from toxicity and second malignancies over that observed with chemotherapy alone has not been observed during the first 10 years following combined modality therapy (Prosnitz et al., 1988; Van Rijswijk et al., 1987; Ticker et al., 1988), but the late increase in second solid tumors observed between 10 and 25 years may change this assessment (Henry-Amar, 1988; Workshop statistical report, part IX).

2. Forecasting and evaluating the response

2.1. Identification of patients unlikely to reach a complete remission

These patients need alternative approaches. The Workshop data reveal that 70% of CS III and 56% of CS IV patients achieved a CR following initial combination CT. Stepwise logistic regression included in the model the main following characteristics: sex, age, mediastinal adenopathy, histological subtype, extra nodal disease, systemic symptoms and the number of involved lymph node areas. It demonstrated that for CS III patients, age greater than 50 ($p=0.004$) and the presence of B symptoms ($p<0.001$) were associated with a lower CR rate. For CS IV patients, after treatment with MOPP-like CT two characteristics predict for a lower CR rate: age over 50 ($p<0.001$) and involved nodes on both sides of the diaphragm ($p<0.001$) (Table 2). In these 40 to 60% of the patients where biological data were recorded, ESR over 50 ($p<0.001$) and serum albumin <25th percentile ($p<0.01$) also predicted for a low CR rate in CS III. The Workshop data (Table 2 and Figure 1) allow the recognition of a subset of 25% of the patients with CS IV (1470 cases) who have no more than 48% chances to reach CR after treatment with MOPP or MOPP-like chemotherapy. The two groups demonstrated respectively 48% and 63% CR, 57% and 65% 10-year RFS, 17% and 41% 10-year FFP and 19 and 48% 10-year S. Refined prognostic criteria should identify a similar percentage of patients at even higher risk of failure.

2.2. Evaluating the risk of relapse

For patients who achieve a CR, remissions which persist beyond 2 years tend to be stable, for the relapse-free survival (RFS) plateau around 60%. Late relapses of HD do occur, but account for a drop of only 5% (a decline in RFS from 65% to 60%) between the 6th and 20th year. Most relapses occur within the first 24 months after therapy is completed. It should be noted that the continued excess death rate in HD patients during long term follow-up results largely from cardiovascular disorders and second malignancies, rather than from HD.

Table 2. Identification of major classical, and newer adverse prognostic factors for achievement of complete remission (CR) and for relapse-free survival (RFS) in CR's. *Workshop and literature data. Multivariate analysis for stage IV.*

Factor related to	CR	RFS (in CR's)	Reference
Literature data	B symptoms	Histology; B sympt.	NCI (De Vita 1980)*
	B symptoms; MOPP dose	Marrow involv.	Stanford (Carde 1983)
		ESR; alk. phosph.	German Group (Löffler 1989)
Workshop data CS IV patients treated with MOPP	Age > 50 **and** infradiaphragmatic nodes (21% of patients)	Age > 60 only	
Newer factors	Early response	Time to CR	Créteil (Kuentz 1983) NCI (Longo 1986) EORTC (Somers 1988)
		Sex; lymphocytopenia**	Danish Group (Specht 1988)

* *univariate analysis;* ** *significance not achieved*

The factors associated with an increased risk of relapse from CR are shown in Table 2. A univariate analysis of NCI data found that nodular sclerosis histology and the presence of B symptoms were associated with increased relapses (De Vita et al., 1980) and a review of the Stanford data showed that marrow involvement predicted early relapse (Carde et al., 1983). The German Group (Löffler et al., 1989) found that an elevated erythrocyte sedimentation rate and increased serum alkaline phosphatase were associated with early relapse.

Analysis of the Workshop data on CS III and IV HD, employing stepwise logistic regression, and using the prognostic factors listed earlier for the attenment of a CR in the model, revealed that only age greater than 60 (18% of patients) was associated significantly with an increased risk of relapse. This risk of relapse was associated with decreased survival (5-year survival = 26% *vs* 60% and 10-year survival = 12% *vs* 47%).

The histological subtypes of nodular sclerosis appears to be an important prognostic factor in the BNLI series (Mac Lennan, present issue) but this subtyping has to be applied and confirmed in other settings. Other parameters, such as the Ki 67 "proliferation antigen" (Grogan et al., 1988) karyotypic abnormalities, gene or oncogene rearrangements and labelling indices, are of interest but more information is required before their role can be evaluated. Discussions during the Workshop brought up the role of sex and lymphopenia. This later factor has been elegantly related to tumour burden (Specht et al., 1988). However, here again, statistical significance for lymphopenia as a prognostic factor was not achieved when only CR patients were considered. It is of interest that many common prognostic factors are shared in HD for achieving a CR and survival and that the attainment of a CR itself is the most potent factor for predicting the survival of HD patients (De Vita et al., 1980).

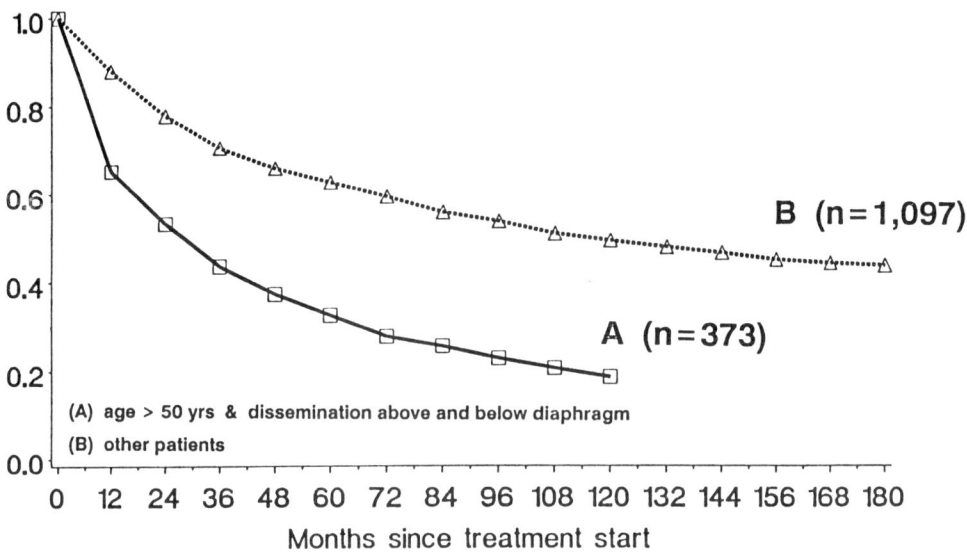

Figure 1. *Overall survival of the patients with clinical stage IV Hodgkin's disease according to the presence of the 2 factors predicting for chances to enter a complete remission: age >50 years and nodal dissemination above and below the diaphragm. At 5 years: 33% versus 63%; at 10 years 19% versus 48%.*

2.3. Treatment-related variables

Treatment-related variables such as the time to CR and dose intensity, have also been found to influence DFS.

2.3.1. Importance of time to CR : Kuentz and coworkers were the first to show that the response to initial chemotherapy is a powerful prognostic factor (Kuentz et al., 1983). They found that HD patients who achieve a CR following the first three cycles of MOPP survive significantly longer than those who did not. The latest analyses of the NCI MOPP experience (Longo et al., 1986) noted that patients receiving higher doses of vincristine achieved a higher CR rate and survived longer, and those entering CR prior to the 6th cycle had significantly longer remissions than those requiring more cycles. It has been suggested that the poor results of MOPP in Milan, as compared to the NCI, could be related to lower dose intensity in Milan, as reflected by a delayed median time to CR of 5 months in Milan *vs* 2 months at the NCI (De Vita et al., 1987). Moreover, in a prospective EORTC study designed for this purpose, Somers and coworkers reported that HD patients who were in CR after 4 courses of chemotherapy had an improved DFS at 4 years as compared to those who did not (FFP 80% vs 62%, $p<0.001$ in an updated analysis, and overall survival $p<0.001$) (Somers et al., 1988). Conversely, the type of chemotherapy (MOPP *vs* MOPP/ABVD) had less influence on FFP at 6 years ($p<0.02$) and on survival ($p = 0.09$).

2.3.2. A number of biological markers have been related to the pattern of response in HD patients and may prove to be useful in predicting relapse in patients considered to be in clinical CR. The erythrocyte sedimentation rate (ESR) is certainly easy to follow and a rising or oscillating ESR following the completion of therapy has recently been shown to predict relapse in patients with early stage HD (Friedman et al., 1988). Serum LDH and β-2 microglobulin have also been reported to be useful (Swan et al., 1988). Perhaps the most promising line of investigation has to do with relating variations in the blood levels of the soluble Hodgkin-related antigen, gp 80, to the status of the disease (Pfreundschuh et al., 1989).

2.3.3. Patients with residual masses following the completion of therapy must be followed closely, although most will do well (Thomas et al., 1988). Gallium-67 scans may help to detect active residual disease (Weiner et al., 1989). Immunoscintigraphy, using monoclonal antibodies to Hodgkin-related antigens, is addressing the same question (Carde et al., 1989). Magnetic resonance imaging provides useful information about marrow and skeletal lesions, but is less helpful in the evaluation of the more frequent mediastinal lesions.

3. Preventing relapse

In the Workshop series, around 40% of CS III and IV HD patients who achieved a CR with initial therapy administered after 1970, have relapsed. Most of these relapses occurred within the first 5 years. A number of approaches can attempt to prevent these relapses.

3.1. Adjuvant radiation therapy

Adjuvant radiation therapy as discussed earlier, has reduced the risk of relapse in the irradiation field, but not in distant sites, and overall survival was not improved.

3.2. Maintenance chemotherapy

Maintenance chemotherapy has been tested in a number of trials (for reviews see Coltman, 1980; Longo et al., 1982; Canellos et al., 1983). The addition of maintenance chemotherapy has failed to prolong CRs or to reduce the fraction of patients who relapse (Young et al., 1973; Carde et al., 1983; Hancock et al., 1989.

3.3. The application of high-dose, marrow-ablative chemotherapy followed by autologous bone marrow transplantation

The application of high-dose, marrow-ablative chemotherapy followed by autologous bone marrow transplantation (ABMT) in the treatment of HD patients who had not responded to primary induction therapy, or who were refractory to two or more chemotherapy regimens, resulted in complete remissions in close to 50%. About one half of the CRs (about 25% of the total) are expected to enjoy long term disease-free survival (Armitage et al., 1989). This approach is very aggressive, requiring long periods of hospitalization and resulting in toxic deaths in about 10%. A similar approach, using peripheral stem cell harvest, has recently been attempted through GM-CSF stimulation (Gianni et al., 1989). The role of high-dose CT and ABMT has been tested primarily in younger patients (median = 26 years old in Jagannath et al., 1989). It is known that patients who have never responded to primary induction chemotherapy are not good candidates (Jagannath et al. 1986b), and patients with advanced disease and poor marrow reserve may not be considered. High-dose chemotherapy and ABMT has not been tested as primary therapy for patients considered to be a high risk of early relapse following more conventional therapy. This will have to wait until the role of this approach in the treatment of relapses has been better defined, and the criteria for identifying patients with untreated HD who are at high risk of relapse are more refined and useful. The only factor which identifies CS IV patients with a high risk of relapse, in the Workshop series, is age greater than 60 years (Table 2) and these patients have not been candidates for high-dose chemothearpy and ABMT.

3.4. Biological response modifiers

New approaches are required to increase and prolong the CRs in advanced HD patients. Trials of biological response modifiers and haemopoietic growth factors are of great interest. Apart from a negative levamisole trial from the Memorial Sloan Kettering Cancer Center (Straus, 1986), almost no trial have been run in HD. Hodgkin and Reed-Sternberg cells secrete more and different cytokines (CSF, IL-1, rosette-inhibitive factor, etc.), as compared to other lymphomas (Stein et al., 1989). The fact that Hodgkin and Reed-Sternberg cells carry receptors for IL-2, and that IL-2 has been reported to induce growth in HD cell lines (Kalle et al., present issue) will warn investigators of possible adverse effects of this cytokine in HD patients.

4. Tailoring strategy to prognostic factors

It is difficult to design treatment strategies based on prognostic factors for advanced HD because the prognostic factors are limited to age and the presence of nodal involvement on both sides of the diaphragm for the attainment of a CR and because the only factor predicting relapse is older age (Table 2). For advanced HD, at the difference of localized HD, no

Table 3. Strategies for stepping forward in advanced Hodgkin's disease

	Younger	Elder
Low-risk	Basis: ABVD Investigate: no long-term toxic drugs Randomized trials	Basis: ABVD Investigate: any effective drug, haemopoietic GF Randomized/phase II trials

Intermediate	Basis: MOPP/ABVD
	Investigate: new effective drugs
	    selective RT
	    haemopoietic GF
	    BRMs
	    consolidation high dose CT + ABMT
	Phase II or pooled with younger high-risk group
		Basis: ABVD
		Investigate: new tolerable drugs
		    haemopoietic GF
		    BRMs
		
		Phase II or pooled randomized with elder low-risk group

High-risk	Investigate: intensive induction CT
	    consolidation high-dose CT + ABMT
	    RT/CT alternations
	    haemopoietic GF
	Phase II trials
		Basis: ABVD
		Investigate: new effective drugs
		    RT/CT alternations
		    haemopoietic GF
		
		Phase II trials

ABVD : adriamycin, bleomycin, vinblastine, dacarbazine
MOPP : mechlorethamine, vincristine, procarbazine, prednisone
BRMs : biological response modifiers
GF : growth factor
RT : radiotherapy

treatment desescalation in view of lesser late toxicities can be considered a this time. A risk of lower RFS cannot be accepted. Such an approach can be foreseen only after that some other prognostic factors than age are identified. This should permit to stratify low, intermediate and high-risk groups in young (<40 years) and older patients and to adapt the treatment intensity. Suggestion is made here to re-run the analyses of the Workshop data set in this perspective, considering selected time periods and treatment categories. Table 3 provides an attempt of such a prognosis-adapted strategy. For the present time, the limited number of factors influencing the response to treatment and DFS for patients with advanced HD does not provide guidance in designing treatment strategies, but does force us to recognize the overriding importance of age as a prognostic factor.

Older patients do not tolerate MOPP chemotherapy well, or the addition of radiation therapy following MOPP. A study by the National Cancer Institute of Canada Clinical Trials Group demonstrated that the dose intensity of vincristine and procarbazine during courses 3 to 6 of MOPP had to be reduced more markedly in patients over the age of 30, as compared to those with younger age (Yelle, 1988). As mentioned previously, the administration of ABVD is associated with less cumulative haematologic toxicity, and may allow for increased dose intensity.

The preliminary results of the CALGB trial comparing MOPP vs ABVD and MOPP/ABVD indicate that the CR rates and failure-free survival at 3 years are significantly better for ABVD and MOPP/ABVD groups, as compared to the MOPP group (Canellos et al., 1988). Furthermore, the results with ABVD alone appear to be as good as with alternating MOPP/ABVD. These observations, together with the evidence that ABVD therapy is less suppressive of fertility and less leukemogenic (Valagussa, 1989) suggest that ABVD should become the basic primary chemotherapy for advanced Hodgkin disease in all age groups. ABVD may prove to be better tolerated than MOPP by older patients.

Although adjuvant radiation therapy has not been shown to improve survival, it has been reported to reduce nodal recurrences in the irradiated field (Bergsagel et al., 1980; Bloomfield et al., 1982) and may have a role in the management of special problems such as large mediastinal masses.

Major improvements are required in the treatment of advanced HD since only 50% of these patients achieve prolonged relapse-free survival following current primary therapy. We need new agents with increased activity against Hodgkin's disease, which are well tolerated by older patients. Preference should be given to agents with new mechanisms of action, and those that enhance the activity of other drugs or interfere with the development of drug resistance. In this respect, the report that cyclosporin A has shown some activity in the treatment of patients with relapsed Hodgkin's disease is of interest (Zwitter et al., 1987; Zwitter, 1988). The use of haemopoietic growth factors may permit an increase in the dose intensity of chemotherapeutic regimens and result in an improved CR rate and relapse-free survival; this would be most helpful in the treatment of older patients. The development of new knowledge regarding the factors which regulate the growth, development and spread of Hodgkin's disease infiltrates will lead to new approaches to treatment with biological response modifiers.

Aknowledgments to R. Somers for his fruitful remarks and to D.E. Bergsagel, J. Raemekers, M. Henry-Amar and J.M. Cosset for their comments about this article; to the contributors of the Workshop data set; to the pool dactylographique of the Institut Gustave Roussy for their skilfull typing assistance.

REFERENCES

Armitage, J.O. et al. (1989): Bone marrow transplantation in the treatment of Hodgkin's lymphoma: problems, remaining challenges and future prospects. *Rec. Res. Cancer Res.* 52, 246-253.

Bergsagel, D.E. et al. (1980): Trial of MOPP alone versus MOPP and radiotherapy for advanced Hodgkin's disease. *Proc. Am. Soc.Clin. Oncol.* 464, C-570.

Bloomfield, C.D. et al. (1982): Chemotherapy and combined modality therapy for Hodgkin's disease: a progress report on Cancer and Leukemia Group B studies. *Cancer Treat. Rep.* 66, 835-846.

Bonadonna, G. et al. (1986): Alternating non-cross-resistant-combination chemotherapy or MOPP in Stage IV Hodgkin's disease. A report of 8-year results. *Ann. Intern. Med.* 104, 739-746.

Brandwein, J.M. et al. (1989): DHAP chemotherapy for relapsed Hodgkin's disease. *Proc. Am. Soc. Clin. Oncol.* 8, 265.

Canellos, G.P. et al. (1983): Chemotherapy in the treatment of Hodgkin's disease. *Sem. hematol.* 20, 1-24.

Canellos, G.P. et al. (1988): MOPP vs ABVD vs MOPP alternating with ABVD in advanced Hodgkin's disease: a prospective randomized CALGB trial. *Proc. Am. Soc. Clin. Oncol.* 7, 230.

Carde, P. et al. (1983): A dose and time response analysis of the treatment of Hodgkin's disease with MOPP chemotherapy. *J. Clin. Oncol.* 1, 146-153.

Carde, P. et al (1989): Rabiolabeled monoclonal antibodies against Reed-Sternberg cells for in vivo imaging of Hodgkin's disease by immunoscintigraphy. In *New aspects in the diagnosis and treatment of Hodgkin lymphoma*, ed. V. Diehl, M. Pfreundschuh & M. Löffler, pp. 101-111. Recent Results in Cancer Research 117. Berlin: Springer-Verlag.

Coltman, C.A. (1980): Chemotherapy of advanced Hodgkin's disease. *Sem. Oncol.* 7, 155-173.

Connors, J.M. et al. (1987): MOPP/ABV hybrid chemotherapy for advanced Hodgkin's disease. *Semin. Hematol.* 24, 35-40.

De Vita, V.T. Jr. et al. (1970): Combination chemotherapy in the treatment of advanced Hodgkin's disease. *Ann. Intern. Med.* 73, 881-895.

De Vita, V.T. Jr. et al. (1980): Curability of advanced Hodgkin's disease with chemotherapy. Long-term follow-up of MOPP treated patients at the National Cancer Institute. *Ann. Inter. Med.* 92, 587-595.

De Vita, V.T. Jr. et al. (1987): The chemotherapy of lymphomas: Looking back, moving forward. The Richard and Hinda Rosenthal Foundation Award lecture. *Cancer Res.* 47, 5810-5824.

De Vita, V.T. Jr. (1988): On the value of response criteria in therapeutic research. *Bull. Cancer* 75, 863-869.

Fabian, C. et al. (1989): Efficacy of low dose involved field (LDIF) XRT in producing and maintaining CR following PR induction with MOP-BAP chemotherapy in Hodgkin's disease, results of South West Oncology Group Study 7808. *Proc. Am. Soc. Clin. Oncol.* 8, 253.

Friedman, S. et al. (1988): Evolution of erythrocyte sedimentation rate as predictor of early relapse in post-therapy early stage Hodgkin's disease. *J. Clin. Oncol.* 6, 596-602.

Gianni, A.M. et al. (1983): Granulocytherapy in the treatment of Hodgkin's disease. *Sem. Hematol.* 20, 1-24.

Gianni, A.M. et al. (1989): Granulocyte-macrophage colony stimulating factor to harvest circulating haemopoietic stem cells for autotransplantation. *Lancet* ii, 580-585.

Glick, J. et al. (1988): A randomized ECOG trial of alternating MOPP-ABVD vs BCVPP vs BCVPP plus radiohterapy (RT) for advanced Hodgkin's disease (HD). *Proc. Amer. Soc. Clin. Oncol.* 7, 223.

Goldie, J.H. et al. (1982): Rationale for the use of alternating non cross-resistant chemotherapy. *Cancer Treat. Rep.* 66, 439-449.

Green, J.A. et al (1980): Measurement of drug dosage intensity in MVPP therapy in Hodgkin's disease. *Br. J. Clin. Pharmacol.* 9, 511-514.

Green, J.A. (1989): After Goldie-Coldman. Where now? *Eur. J. Cancer Clin. Oncol.* 25, 913-916.

Grogan, T.M. et al. (1988): Independent prognostic significance of a nuclear proliferation antigen in diffuse large cell lymphomas as determined by the monoclonal antibody Ki-67. *Blood* 71, 1157-1160.

Hancok, B.W. et al. (1989): For the BNLI. The British National Lymphoma Investigation study of Leukeran, Oncovin, Procarbazine, Prednisolone/Etoposide, Vinblastine, Adriamycin, Prednisolone (LOPP/EVAP) in advanced Hodgkin's disease. *Proc. Am. Soc. Clin. Oncol.* 8, 262.

Henry-Amar, M. (1988): Quantitative risk of second cancer in patients in first complete remission frome early stages of Hodgkin's disease. *NCI Monogr.* 6, 65-72.

Henry-Amar, M. et al. (1989): Risk of secondary acute leukemia and preleukemia after Hodgkin's disease. The Institut Gustave-Roussy experience. In *New aspects in the diagnosis and treatment of Hodgkin lymphoma,* ed. V. Diehl, M. Pfreundschuh & M. Löffler, pp. 270-283. Recent Results in Cancer Research 117. Berlin: Springer-Verlag.

Hiddemann, W. et al. (1989): Treatment of refractory Hodkin's disease with high-dose cytosine arabinoside and mitoxantrone in combination. *Proc. Amer. Soc. Clin. Oncol.* 8, 277.

Hoppe, R.T. et al. (1989): Current Stanford clinical trial for Hodgkin's disease. In *New aspects in the diagnosis and treatment of Hodgkin lymphoma,* ed. V. Diehl, M. Pfreundschuh & M. Löffler, pp. 182-190. Recent Results in Cancer Research 117. Berlin: Springer-Verlag.

Horwich, A. et al. (1987): Combined chemotherapy and radiotherapy in the management of adult Hodgkin's disease: indications and results. In *Hodgkin's disease,* ed. P. Selby & T.J. McElwain, pp. 250-268. Oxford: Blackwell Scientific Publications.

Jagannath, S. et al. (1986a): High-dose Cyclophosphamide, Carmustine and Etoposide and autologous bone marrow transplantation for relapsed Hodgkin's disease. *Ann. Intern. Med.* 104, 163-168.

Jagannath, S. et al. (1986b): Prognostic factors predicting for response to high dose chemotherapy and autologous bone marrow transplantation (ABMT) for relapsed Hodgkin's disease. *Blood* 68 (1), 274a.

Jagannath, S. et al. (1989): Cis-platinum plus high dose cyclophosphamide, carmustine, etoposide (CBVP) and autologous bone marrow transplantation in relapsed Hodgkin's disease. *Proc. Amer. Soc. Clin. Oncol.* 8, 273.

Kuentz, M. et al. (1983): Early response to chemotherapy as a prognostic factor in Hodgkin's disease. *Cancer* 52, 780-785.

Löffler, M. et al. (1989): Risk factor adapted treatment of Hodgkin's lymphoma: strategies and perspectives. In *New aspects in the diagnosis and treatment of Hodgkin lymphoma,* ed. V. Diehl, M. Pfreundschuh & M. Löffler, pp. 142-162. Recent Results in Cancer Research 117. Berlin: Springer-Verlag.

Longo, D.L. et al. (1982): Chemotherapy for Hodgkin's disease: the remaining challenges. *Cancer Treat. Rep.* 66, 925-936.

Longo, D.L. et al. (1986): Twenty years of MOPP therapy for Hodgkin's disease. *J. Clin. Oncol.* 4, 1295-1306.

Nissen, N. et al. (1979): A comparative study of a BCNU-containing 4-drug program versus MOPP versus 3-drug combinations in advanced Hodgkin's disease. A cooperative study by the Cancer and Leukemia Group B. *Cancer* 43, 31-40.

Pfreundschuh, M. et al. (1989): Clinical significance of soluble Hodgkin-related antigen in the sera of patients with Hodgkin's lymphoma. *Proc. Amer. Soc. Clin. Oncol.* 8, 273.

Prosnitz, L.R. et al. (1988): Combined modality therapy for advanced Hodgkin's disease: 15-year follow-up data. *J. Clin. Oncol.* 6, 603-613.

Raemaekers, J.M.M. et al. (1989): Prospective randomized controlled trial of adjuvant involved field radiotherapy after MOPP/ABV hybrid chemotherapy in advanced Hodgkin's disease. EORTC and Pierre et Marie Curie Groups Protocol, n° 20884.

Rijswijk, V. et al. (1987): Major complications and causes of death in patients treated for Hodgkin's disease. *J. Clin. Oncol.* 5, 1624-1633.

Rosenberg, S.A. et al. (1985): The evolution and summary results of the Stanford randomized clinical trials of the management of Hodgkin's disease. *Int. J. Radiat. Oncol. Biol. Phys.* 11, 5-22.

Somers, R. et al. (1988): MOPP vs alternating 2 MOPP/2 ABVD in advanced Hodgkin's disease (HD). *Proc. Amer. Soc. Clin. Oncol.* 7, 236.

Specht, L. et al. (1988): prognostic factors in Hodgkin's disease stage IV. *Eur. J. Haematol.* 41, 359-367.
Stein, H. et al. (1989): Immunology of Hodgkin and Reed-Sternberg cells. In *New aspects in the diagnosis and treatment of Hodgkin lymphoma*, ed. V. Diehl, M. Pfreundschuh & M. Löffler, pp. 14-26. Recent Results in Cancer Research 117. Berlin: Springer-Verlag.
Straus, D.J. (1986): Strategies in the treatment of Hodgkin's disease. *Sem. Oncol.* 13 (5), 24-26.
Straus, D.J. et al. (1989): Results and prognostic factors following optimal treatment of advanced Hodgkin's disease. In *New aspects in the diagnosis and treatment of Hodgkin lymphoma*, ed. V. Diehl, M. Pfreundschuh & M. Löffler, pp. 191-196. Recent Results in Cancer Research 117. Berlin: Springer-Verlag.
Sutcliffe, S.B. et al. (1987): Treatment of Hodgkin's disease. *Clin hematol.* 1, 109-141.
Swan, F. et al. (1988): Beta-2-microglobulin and lactic acid dehydrogenase as prognostic indicators for patients with intermediate grade lymphoma. *Proc. Amer. Soc. Clin. Oncol.* 7, 243.
Thomas, F. et al. (1988): Thoracic CT scanning follow-up of residual mediastinal masses after treatment of Hodgkin's disease. *Radioth. Oncol.* 11, 119-122.
Tucker, M.A. et al. (1988): Risk of second cnt development of acute non lymphocytic leukemia in patients treated for Hodgkin's disease. *Int. J. Cancer* 42, 252-255.
Valagussa, P. et al. (1989): 9-year results of two randomized studies with MOPP and ABVD in Hodgkin's disease: multiple regression analysis. *Proc. Amer. Soc. Clin. Oncol.* 8, 250.
Weiner, M. et al. (1989): Gallium-67 scans as an adjunct to clinical restaging in pediatric patients with Hodgkin's disease. *Proc. Amer. Soc. Clin. Oncol.* 8, 278.
Yelle, L. et al. (1987): For the HD1 Subcommittee, National Cancer Institute of Canada Clinical Trials Group. Trial of chemotherapy and radiotherapy in advanced Hodgkin's disease (Abstract). *Clin. Invest. Med.* 10, B81.
Yelle, L. (1988): A cooperative clinical trial comparing MOPP alone versus MOPP followed by radiation in stage IIIB or IV Hodgkin's disease. NCIC Trial HD1 (Thesis). Kingston, Ontario: Department of Medicine at Queen's University.
Young, R. et al. (1973): Maintenance chemothearpy for advanced Hodgkin's disease in remission. *Lancet* i, 1339-1343.
Zwitter, M. et al. (1987): Cyclosporine may alleviate B symptoms and induce a remission of heavily pretreated Hodgkin's disease: a preliminary report. *Ann. Intern. Med.* 106, 843-844.
Zwitter, M. (1988): On the potential role of cyclosporin in the treatment of lymphoproliferative diseases. *Leukem. Res.* 12, 243-248.

Management of progression/relapse in clinical stages III-IV Hodgkin's disease: classical radio-chemotherapy?

J.M.V. Burgers

Department of Radiotherapy, The Netherlands Cancer Institute, Plesmanlaan 121, 1066 CX Amsterdam, The Netherlands

Summary

Clinical stage III-IV of Hodgkin's disease comprises about 25% of the total patient group. According to several authors primary chemotherapy, with or without radiotherapy, results in disease-free survival of 50%-70%. Therefore one-third to one-half of the patients in this stage need second line treatment.

Progression can take place during the first months of chemotherapy, usually with a very agressive clinical picture with nodal and extranodal disease. Other patients start to respond to chemotherapy, but show increase of the lesions again before the first line treatment can be completed. Next to these progression patients are the early relapses where first line treatment is administered according to plan, but, within 18 months of the start of treatment Hodgkin's disease has recurred. These patients have a worse prognosis than those who recur after a longer disease-free period, i.e. more than 18 months after the start of treatment. Most recurrences are in previously involved nodal areas. In the EORTC material this was the case in 11/27 progressions and 22/36 relapses. Only a few of these relapsed only in areas that were irradiated.

Reports in the literature concern patient groups of varying composition as regards original stage, early relapse/progression, number of relapses, proportion of extranodal involvement. After second line chemotherapy, a 5-year survival of 25% is reported. In a few series of selected patients who had chemotherapy and radiotherapy a higher figure was reported. In the material of the Netherlands Cancer Institute, a 40% 5-year survival rate was observed. When these data are split for early and late relapses, a 20% 5-year survival rate is reached for the early relapses and 56% for the late relapses, while the 2-year survival figures are 40% and 80% respectively.

In the series where chemotherapy and radiotherapy are both given, the survival figures are somewhat higher, although this may be a matter of selection. As most recurrences are in sites well amenable to irradiation, such as nodal areas, bone lesions, and to a certain extent, lung involvement, combined modality treatment schedules should be extensively investigated.

Résumé

Les stades cliniques III et IV représentent environ 25 % de la population atteinte par la maladie de Hodgkin. Selon plusieurs auteurs, la chimiothérapie de première intention, associée ou non à une radiothérapie permet d'obtenir des taux de survie sans récidive ni métastase de l'ordre de 50% à 70 %. Il en résulte que ces malades nécessitent un traitement de seconde intention dans 30% à 50 % des cas. Les progressions peuvent survenir pendant les premiers mois de la chimiothérapie, présentant souvent un aspect clinique très agressif avec localisations ganglionnaires et viscérales. Certains malades réagissent d'emblée favorablement à la chimiothérapie, puis manifestent une augmentation des lésions initiales avant la fin du traitement de première intention. Parallèlement, il existe un groupe de malades avec rechutes précoces. Ceux-ci ont pu être traité selon le protocole prévu, mais ont présenté une récidive de la maladie dans un délai inférieur à 18 mois à partir du début du traitement. Ces malades ont un plus mauvais pronostic que celui des malades qui récidivent plus tardivement.

La plupart des récidives sont situées dans les aires ganglionnaires qui étaient précédemment envahies. C'est ce qui a été observé pour 11/27 des progressions et 22/36 des rechutes des malades traités par l'OERTC. Seuls quelques-uns d'entre eux ont rechuté en territoire irradié. Les groupes de malades cités dans la littérature sont hétérogènes quant au stade initial, les progressions ou rechutes précoces, le nombre de rechutes et la proportion d'envahissement extraganglionnaire. Généralement les taux de survie à 5 ans après chimiothérapie de deuxième intention sont de l'ordre de 25 %. Dans quelques séries de malades ayant été traités par association chimiothérapie et radiothérapie des taux plus élevés ont été rapportés. Dans l'expérience du Netherlands Cancer Institute, le taux de survie à 5 ans est de 40 % pour l'ensemble des malades. Il est de 20 % pour les malades avec rechute précoce alors qu'il atteint 56 % pour le groupe de malades avec rechute tardive. Pour ces deux groupes, les taux de survie à 2 ans sont respectivement de 40 % et 80 %.

Dans les séries comprenant des malades traités par chimiothérapie et radiothérapie, les taux de survie sont un peu plus élevés, mais ceci peut être la conséquence d'un biais de sélection. Comme la plupart des rechutes sont localisées dans des régions accessibles à un traitement par irradiation, comme le sont les aires ganglionnaires, les lésions osseuses, et dans une certaine mesure les envahissements pulmonaires, il semble justifié que des protocoles de traitement associant radiothérapie et chimiothérapie soient entrepris et testés de manière prospective.

The great advances made in the last twenty years in the treatment of Hodgkin's disease have applied to all stages. Nevertheless, a small proportion of patients are still dying of the disease, mainly among those who present with advanced disease in clinical stage III or IV, which is about one quarter of the total number of patients (Burgers et al., 1988; present statistical report on Treatment Strategy in Hodgkin's Disease, 1989). Patients in stage III have usually extensive disease with 4 or more lymph node regions involved (present statistical report). Extranodal extension in stage IV is most frequent to liver, lung, bonemarrow or bone. General symptoms may occur and the erythrocyte sedimentation rate (ESR) is often high. Advanced stage does not occur more often at advanced age. About 35% of patients is over 40 years and 20% is over 50 years of age at the time of presentation (present statistical report). In discussions of optimal treatment strategies other prognostic factors are also mentioned, such as bulky disease and histological subtype. The question of how to treat patients in advanced stages by chemotherapy or by combined modality treatment programs is not settled. There is a wide choice in chemotherapy schedules and in radiotherapy plans. Points to be considered in radiotherapy planning are:
1. Treatment of involved lymph node regions, or, more limited, only regions with bulky disease, or, more extensive, total nodal plus spleen irradiation;
2. Treatment of involved organs, such as lung in case of extension into lungs from mediastinal masses, or when malignant pleural effusion is present, further radiation of the liver and of bone lesions;
3. Which dose to apply to each region in case of complete, partial or no remission.

A number of studies have reported long term results of chemotherapy or combined modality treatment as first treatment for advanced disease or recurrence after primary radiotherapy (Table 1). The EORTC series (Somers et al., 1988) applies to patients in clinical stage IIIB and IV only. In this study patients were treated with MOPP or MOPP/ABVD and limited radiotherapy if in partial remission after 4 courses of chemotherapy or with initial bulky disease. The 5-year disease-free survival is 55%. We have therefore to conclude that the problem of the best management of relapse applies to between one-third and one-half of the patients presenting in clinical stage III and IV.

Table 1. Hodgkin's disease: First line chemotherapy with or without radiotherapy

		Number of patients	RFS (5-yr)	S (5-yr)	Deaths not related to disease progr.
Longo	(1986)[1]	198	68%	60%	(28%)
Prosnitz	(1988)[2]	184	70%	75%	(27%)
EORTC	(1988)[3]	192	55%	68%	

[1] pathological stage: 28; previous radiotherapy: 32; includes IIB
[2] pathological stage: 60; previous radiotherapy: 82; 22% aged 40 years or more
[3] clinical stage IIIB and IV only

What is the clinical picture that such a patient presents? Roughly we can discern three entities for whom the further course of disease is quite different (Table 2).

Table 2. Hodgkin's disease clinical stage III-IV: Relapse, time-interval

1- Progression:	- immediately, with practically no response (Ia) - during initial treatment after response (Ib)
2- Early relapse:	- within 1 year of end of treatment or 18 months from start of treatment - moderate condition, DD: slow response/side effects - bulky lesions, accelerated ESR - multiple sites, extranodal sites
3- Relapse after interval:	- more than 1 year after end of treatment - normal activity and limited extent of lesions

The most agressive type of Hodgkin's disease takes the form of progressive lesions within the first 2 to 3 months of chemotherapy, after a slight improvement at the start of treatment (Ia). Other patients show progression of lesions during the initial planned course of chemotherapy after initial improvement and/or a period of stable disease (Ib). These patients are usually in good condition and an early switch to combined modality treatment can be considered.

The second entity is formed by the group of so called "early relapses" which are generally defined as taking place within 1 year after chemotherapy, or within 18 months from the start of treatment. While some patients have enjoyed a period of well being, others also included in this group, form the category of patients who, after the end of treatment, do not recover well, complain of fatigue and malaise, keep an elevated ESR and continue to have liver function and chest X-ray abnormalities. For these patients it is difficult to say whether a slow response is taking place, whether side effect of treatment are the cause of the problems, or whether a disease recurrence is round the corner. The decision between "further treatment now" or "await events" is difficult.

The third entity comprises the patients who are cured after full delivery of the primary treatment plan. A complete remission is reached with disappearance of all signs and symptoms, recovery of general condition and the patient has resumed his normal work and lifestyle. At routine check up either new nodes are found, or an elevated ESR or general symptoms lead to further investigations. After adequate restaging a new treatment plan is made which according to the situation, may consist of radiotherapy or chemotherapy or both. The next aspect of disease presentation at the time of relapse concerns the site of the lesion(s) in relation to the original disease extent. It has been pointed out before (Young et al., 1978) that recurrence often occurs in nodal sites which might have contained bulky disease and which were not irradiated before.

In the EORTC stage IIIB-IV Hodgkin's disease trial mentioned above, a special study was made of the timing of relapse and its location. From 196 registered patients, 85 progressions/relapses were recorded. Of these 39 occurred during the initial planned chemotherapy and were coded as progression. Forty-six patients relapsed after treatment and, of these, 21 occurred within 18 months of start of treatment (early relapses), and 25 occurred later. For 63 of these 85 patients, information were available on the localisation of the progressing (27) or relapsing (36) lesions (Table 3).

Table 3. Sites of relapse in EORTC trial on clinical stage III-IV Hodgkin's disease (1981-86)

Progressions	Relapses
11 isolated nodal	22 isolated nodal[1]
5 lung/bone + nodal	6 lung/bone + nodal
3 bonemarrow	4 isolated organs
8 multipl˜ nodal + extranodal	4 multiple nodal + extranodal
27	36

[1] 3 in irradiated areas (20 Gy) only

Both for progressing and relapsing patients recurrence isolated in nodal sites only was most frequent, in 11/27 and 22/36 patients respectively. Nodal recurrence together with a lung or bone lesion(s) occurred in a further 5 and 6 patients respectively. Only 6 of these 28 nodal relapses had had radiotherapy to part or all of those nodal areas, while only three of these recurrences were in irradiated sites only. Lung lesions were usually associated with previous mediastinal involvement. Among patients with progression, only very few had had radiotherapy and 2 out of 11 recurred in irradiated sites.

In both groups, few recurrences occurred in previously uninvolved areas, usually adjacent to previously involved sites. An important proportion of patients who progressed (8/27) presented with multiple nodal and extranodal relapses, located in bonemarrow (4), liver (3), spleen (2), lung (2), cord (2) and bone (1). For relapsing patients this was a smaller proportion (4/36) with extranodal recurrences in liver (3), lung (2) and 1 in bonemarrow, bone, spleen, brain and skin respectively.

Before deciding on the treatment strategy of a patient with recurrent disease, the condition of the patient has to be evaluated. The bonemarrow reserve may be diminished by the previous treatment, particularly for the 20% of patients above 50 years of age. Residual damage of the first treatment may be present. Neuropathy and impaired fertility may not much influence the treatment stragegy, but heart, lung or liver damage are to be taken into account when planning further chemotherapy or radiotherapy. Also concomitant disease may be the cause of lung, or liver damage. Further kidney function, endocrine status (diabetes mellitus!) and cardio-vascular situation are also to be taken into account. Impairment of any of these functions increases the chance that the patient in the phase of bonemarrow depression is unable to adequately manage an infection with the risk of sepsis and sudden death.

When evaluating published reports on treatment results of either "classical radio-chemotherapy" or "modern ablative methods" it is important to be aware of these aspects, which influence the selection for each treatment schedule. Also the proportion of patients with aggressive disease, such as progression during first treatment, and original stage of the disease has to be taken into account.

The most important results of second line treatment published are cited in Table 4 including complete remission rates and proportions of patients remaining free from progression.

Table 4. Hodgkin's disease relapsing after MOPP: Second line chemotherapy

	Number of patients	CR	FFP (2-yr)	S (2-yr)	S (5-yr)	% early
Santoro (1982) ABVD	54	59%	36%	58%	32%	100%[1]
Tannir (1983) ABDIC	34	35%	22%	50%	25%	100%
Harker (1984) ABVD, B Cave	106	41%	33%	56%	24%	62%
Hagemeister MIME (1987)	47	23%		50% (1 yr)		70%[2]

[1] 11 patients received radiotherapy
[2] 53% second relapse
early = within 18 months from treatment start

For the sake of comparison, also the 2-year and 5-year survival, as an objective measure of effect have been deducted from the published curves.

Santoro (Santoro et al., 1982), from the Milano group, published a 32% 5-year survival with ABVD, in MOPP relapsing patients; radiotherapy was added in 11 of 54 of those patients. Tannir (Tannir et al., 1983) from Houston reported on 34 patients treated with ABDIC with a 25% 5-year survival after a longer median follow up. In the report from Harker (Harker et al., 1984) from Stanford, 2 patient groups are combined having had second line treatment with either ABVD of B-Cave, with a comparable 5-year survival of 24% but possibly a lower proportion of patients in early relapse, that is within 18 months of start of first treatment. The report of Hagemeister (Hagemeister et al., 1987) from Houston, mentioning third line chemotherapy with MIME, is added to this table; only a 1-year survival figure of 50% is available.

More recently, results of radiotherapy or combined modality treatment with chemotherapy and radiotherapy have been published by Mauch (Mauch et al., 1987) from Boston, by Fox (Fox et al., 1987) from Tucson and by Roach (Roach et al., 1987) from Stanford (Table 5).

Table 5. Hodgkin's disease relapsing after MOPP: second line radiotherapy with or without chemotherapy

	Number of patients	CR	FFP (2-yr)	S (2-yr)	S (5-yr)	% early
Mauch[1] (1987) 35–40 Gy	19		66%	90%	69%	68%
Fox[2] (1987) 17–50 Gy	17	88%	35%	75%	58%	76%
Roach[2] (1987)	13	93%	46%	75%	–	54%
Young (1982) MOPP/ABVD + 20 Gy	28	50%		65%	40%	*

[1] nodal only
[2] including lung RT (12), liver RT (3), bone RT (2)
early = within 18 months from treatment start
* heavily pre-treated

These patients were identified in the files of the radiotherapy department and must have been selected in the sense of having disease in areas where adequate doses of radiotherapy were still possible. Nevertheless the proportion of patients with early relapses as defined above was comparable to that in Harker's series. In this small patient group, the 5-year survival was around 60 to 70%, a figure which should stimulate further investigation of this treatment approach. Earlier Young (Young et al., 1982) from the Memorial Sloan Kettering Cancer Institute in New York reported a subgroup of heavily pretreated patients who received MOPP-ABVD followed by low dose radiotherapy 20 Gy to areas of bulky disease. This resulted in a 5-year survival of 40% for 28 patients.

In the EORTC stage IIIB-IV Hodgkin disease trial, questionnaires concerning the treatment were answered for 27/39 progressions and 36/46 relapses. Usually further chemotherapy was given, mostly with MOPP; ABVD and M-Cave CEC were also used. In 21 patients out of 63 (27+36) radiotherapy was given after chemotherapy, while in 4 cases radiotherapy only was given at the time of first relapse. High dose chemotherapy with ABMT was given in 5 patients. In this group the 2-year survival rate is 70% with a disease-free survival rate at 2 years equal to 75%.

At the Netherlands Cancer Institute, we have recently studied 63 clinical stage III and IV patients who were primarily treated in the years 1979-1986 with chemotherapy and iceberg radiotherapy to originally bulky or slowly regressing areas. Among these patients, 31 had a progression or relapse, 15 within 18 months after the start of treatment and 16 at a later interval. Retreatment was usually with chemotherapy and further radiotherapy where possible. For those 31 patients the 5-year survival rate is 40% (Table 6).

Table 6. Relapse in advanced Hodgkin's disease

	Number of patients	CR	FFP (2-yr)	S (2-yr)	S (5-yr)	
Netherlands Cancer Institute series CT +/- RT (1989)	31		47%	56%	40%	50% "early"
Carella (1988) CBV + ABMT	50	48%	50%			68% "early"
Jagannath (1989) CBV + ABMT	61	46%	45%	55%		multiple relapse or progression
Yahalom (1988) TLI + CV + ABMT	14	78%	64%[1]			multiple relapse or progression

[1] *median FU 14 months*
early = within 18 months from treatment start

In Fig. 1 the survival is separated for late and early relapses. At 2-years the survival rates are equal to 80% and 40% respectively, while at 5-years they are 56% and 21%.

In Table 6, data from two recent reports of treatment results after intensive chemotherapy with bonemarrow transplant support, from Carella (Carella et al., 1988) from Italy and Jagannath (Jagannath et al., 1989) from Houston and Omaha are included.

Five-year survival figures are not yet available. The 1-2 year freedom from progression is around 50%. Jagannath mentions that 30/61 patients had progressing disease in an area previously irradiated. The small series of Yahalom (Yahalom et al., 1988) concerns patients who had no radiotherapy prior to a second or later relapse. Total lymphoid irradiation was given with booster doses in the areas of active disease before the program of high dose chemotherapy and bonemarrow transplant support. With a short follow-up the complete remission rate is at the promising level of 64%.

In all the reports mentioned, patients in relapse after a longer disease-free interval do better than those with early relapse. In the few groups where radiotherapy was added to second line treatment, survival results seem to be somewhat better. According to the EORTC data, most later relapses are in nodal areas that were not previously irradiated, indicating that tolerance for further irradiation after induction chemotherapy should be available.

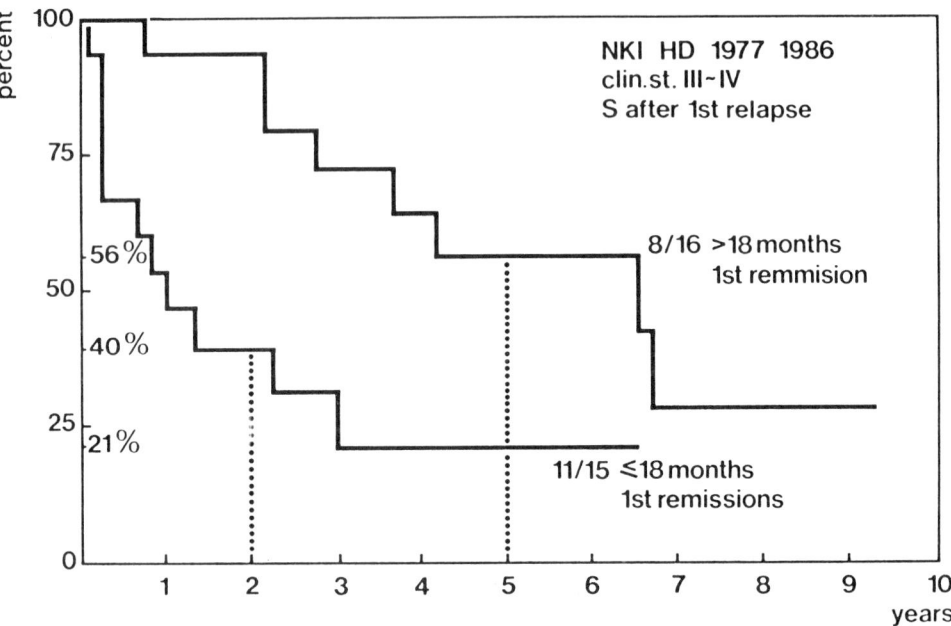

Fig. 1: *Netherlands Cancer Institute series: Survival for 31 clinical stage III-IV patients who relapsed after primary chemotherapy, according to interval from first treatment (more or less than 18 months). Retreatment was with chemotherapy combined with radiotherapy where feasible, and in 5 cases with radiotherapy alone.*

Also bone lesions, if not too many, are usually well amenable to radiation treatment. However treatment of lung lesions, the other frequent extranodal site of relapse, is hampered by the limited tolerance of normal lung. Lung relapses are often associated with initial mediastinal involvement. Irradiation of the lung, even if lung infiltration was not evident, together with the mediastinum after initial chemotherapy, should be considered.

For patients with progression or early relapses, the outlook is still grim. Some of these patients scarcely respond to any of the available chemotherapy schedules, while having widespread nodal and extranodal disease. A possibility to identify these patients very early, for instance with modern histological and immunological techniques, would allow the institution of a treatment program with a changeover in chemotherapy schedules before resistance has become apparent.

The subgroup who responds to first line chemotherapy for 3-4 cycles before some lesions progress again, should be the subject of further collaboration between radiotherapists and chemotherapists. Nodal lesions, bone lesions and possibly lung lesions could be amenable to an adequate dose of adjuvant radiotherapy, while the patient has no more B-symptoms, sufficient bonemarrow, and time to combat his lesions serially. The new approaches of hyperfractionated radio-therapy to extensive areas as reported by Yahalom, should also receive further attention.

The patients in clinical stage IIIB and IV of Hodgkin's disease who relapse, are at high risk. The possible contribution of radiotherapy could take many forms in relation to dose, number of areas to be treated, number of fractions per day and fraction size, and several other aspects. Combined planned management of these patients by chemotherapist and radiotherapist together needs more support and intensive investigation.

Conclusion

Classical treatment for patients with Hodgkin's disease relapsing after chemotherapy can reach a 30-60% 5-year survival rate. For patients who progress during treatment or have an early relapse within 18 months of the start of treatment, the projected 5-year survival rate varies from 15-30%. For patients for whom it has been possible to give radiotherapy, the treatment results are somewhat better. The possible contribution of radiotherapy in the management of both late and early relapses should therefore be further investigated, as most relapse sites are in previously involved nodal areas. Also in conjunction with modern ablative chemotherapy schedules for aggressive Hodgkin's disease, radiotherapy in one of its different forms might have a place.

Acknowledgement

Thanks are due to the radiotherapy and medical staff of the Netherlands Cancer Institute for the collaborative effort in treating these patients. I want to acknowledge in particular the inspiring cooperation with Dr. R. Somers. Also I want to thank Dr. M. Henry-Amar and Mrs. M. Tarayre (Institut Gustave Roussy) for making available the data from the EORTC trial.

References

Burgers, J.M.V., et al. (1988): Hodgkin's Disease: influence of age on prognosis. *Ned. Tijdschr. v. Geneesk.* 132, 1354-1357.
Carella, A.M., et al. (1988): High dose chemotherapy with autologous bone marrow transplantation in 50 advanced resistant Hodgkin's disease patients: an Italian Study Group report. *J. Clin. Onc.* 6, 1411-1416.
Fox, K.A., et al. (1987): Radiation therapy salvage of Hodgkin's Disease following chemotherapy failure. *J. Clin. Onc.* 5, 38-45.
Hagemeister, F.B., et al. (1987): MIME chemotherapy (Methyl-GAG, Ifosfamide, Methotrexate, Etoposide) as treatment for recurrent Hodgkin's Disease. *J. Clin. Onc.* 5, 556-561.
Harker, W.D., et al. (1984): Combination chemotherapy for advanced Hodgkin's Disease after failure of MOPP: ABVD and B-CAVe. *Ann. Int. Med.* 101, 440-446.
Jagannath, S., et al. (1989): Prognostic factors for response and survival after high dose Cyclophosphamide, Carmustine, and Etoposide with autologous bone marrow transplantation for relapsed Hodgkin's Disease. *J. Clin. Onc.* 7, 179-185.
Longo, D.L., et al. (1986): Twenty years of MOPP therapy for Hodgkin's Disease. *J. Clin. Onc.* 4, 1295-1306.

Mauch, P., et al. (1987): Wide field radiation therapy alone or with chemotherapy for Hodgkin's Disease in relapse from combination chemotherapy. *J. Clin. Onc.* 5, 544-549.

Prosnitz, L.R., et al. (1988): Combined modality therapy for advanced Hodgkin's Disease: 15 year follow up data. *J. Clin. Onc.* 6, 603-612.

Roach III, M., et al. (1987): Radiotherapy with curative intent: an option in selected patients relapsing after chemotherapy for advanced Hodgkin's Disease. *J. Clin. Onc.* 5, 550-555.

Somers, R., et al. on behalf of the EORTC Lymphoma Cooperative Group and the Groupe Pierre et Marie Curie (1988): MOPP vs. alternating 2 MOPP/2 ABVD in advanced Hodgkin's Disease (HD). *Proceedings of the 24th annual meeting Am. Society of Clin. Oncology,* 7: 236 (914).

Santoro, A., et al. (1982): Salvage chemotherapy with ABVD in MOPP resistant Hodgkin's Disease. *Ann. Int. Med.* 96, 139-143.

Tannir, N., et al. (1983): Long term follow up with ABDIC salvage chemotherapy of MOPP resistent Hodgkin's Disease. *J. Clin. Onc.* 1, 432-439.

Wagener, D.J.Th., et al. (1983): Sequential non-cross-resistant chemotherapy regimens (MOPP and CAVmP) in Hodgkin's Disease stage IIIB and IV. *Cancer* 52, 1558-1562.

Yahalom, J., et al. (1988): Accelerated hyperfractionated total lymphoid irradiation (TLI), Etoposide and high-dose Cyclophosphamide followed by autologous bone marrow transplantation for patients with relapsed and refractory Hodgkin's Disease. *Int. J. Radiat. Oncol. Biol. Phys.* 15, sup. 1, 168.

Young, C.W., et al. (1982): Multidisciplinary treatment of advanced Hodgkin's Disease by an alternating chemotherapeutic regimen of MOPP/ABVD and low-dose radiation therapy restricted to originally bulky disease. *Cancer Treat. Rep.* 66, 907-914.

Young, R.C., et al. (1978): Patterns of relapse in advanced Hodgkin's Disease treated with combination chemotherapy. *Cancer* 42, 1001-1007.

The place of bone marrow transplantation in the treatment of patients with Hodgkin's disease

J.O. Armitage

Department of Internal Medicine, University of Nebraska Medical Center, 42nd and Dewey Avenue Omaha, Nebraska 68105, USA

Summary

Bone marrow transplantation is an increasingly utilized treatment modality in the management of patients with Hodgkin disease. Although the majority of the patients who develop Hodgkin disease are cured through the use of radiotherapy and/or chemotherapy, as many as one-third of patients failed these treatments. The majority of patients who fail a front line chemotherapy regimen cannot be cured with further applications of traditional therapy. However, there are a few exceptions to this rule. For example, patients who have a very long initial remission with a front line chemotherapy regimen can achieve prolonged second remission approximately 30-40% of the time. Also, occasional patients have localized relapses after chemotherapy. Although these patients are rare, they can some times be cured with extended field radiation therapy. Unfortunately, most patients swith Hodgkin disease who fail front line chemotherapy regimens do not fit into either of these groups. When salvage chemotherapy regimens are administered at traditional doses, the results have been disappointing. Perhaps the most favorable sithation is the use of ABVD in patients who fail MOPP. A summary of a fairly large number of patients treated in this way suggests that the long-term disease-free survival rate is not in excess of 10%. Both allogeneic and autologous bone marrow transplantation have been utilized to treat patients with relapsed Hodgkin disease. Allogeneic bone marrow transplantation has been used only rarely. The few cases reported in the literature have found a high treatment related death rate and approximately 30% long-term, disease-free survivors. Autologous transplantation has been utilized much more frequently. Several hundred patients have been reported in the literature and Hodgkin disease has become one of the most frequent indications for the use of autologous bone marrow transplantation. Approximately 50% of patients undergoing autologous bone marrow transplantation for Hodgkin disease have achieved a complete remission and about 30% of all patients treated have been long-term, disease-free survivors. As might be expected, patients treated early in the course of their disease (i.e. with less previous chemotherapy regimens and a good performance status) have had better results.

At the present time, the major unresolved issues in the use of autologous bone marrow transplantation in the treatment of patients with Hodgkin disease relate to the optimal high dose therapy regimen and the preferred timing of the treatment. Identification of the best treatment regimen will require prospective, comparative trials that have not yet been organized. At the present time, I believe that patients with Hodgkin disease who fail high quality primary chemotherapy regimens should be offered bone marrow transplantation as one of their therapeutic considerations. Delaying the treatment until after patients have failed multiple salvage chemotherapy regimens increases the toxicity of this treatment approach and decreases the chances that it will be successful. To identify the best way to utilize bone marrow transplantation in the treatment of Hodgkin disease will require prospective clinical trials in which major groups of investigators throughout the world participate.

Résumé

La greffe de moëlle osseuse est une modalité de plus en plus utilisée parmi dans le traitement de la maladie de Hodgkin. Bien que la majorité des malades soit guérie par radiothérapie et/ou chimiothérapie, ces traitements conduisent à des échecs pour encore un tiers de ces malades. La majorité des malades pour lesquels la chimiothérapie de première intention est inefficace ne peuvent non plus être guéris par la poursuite d'un traitement classique. Il y a cependant quelques exceptions à la règle. Par exemple, des malades ayant une longue rémission initiale avec une chimiothérapie de première intention peuvent obtenir une seconde rémission prolongée dans 30 à 40% des cas. Par ailleurs, certains malades présentent des rechutes locales après chimiothérapie. Bien que ces cas soient rares, il peuvent parfois être guéris par radiothérapie étendue. Malheureusement, la plupart des malades pour lesquels une chimiothérapie de première intention aboutit à un échec n'entrent dans aucun de ces groupes. Dans les cas où une chimiothérapie de rattrapage a été administrée à doses classiques, les résultats ont été décevants. La situation la plus favorable est peut-être celle dans laquelle on utilise l'ABVD chez des malades chez lesquels le MOPP a été un échec. Les résultats sur un assez grand nombre de malades traités ainsi semblent montrer que le taux de survie sans rechute à long terme ne dépasse pas 10%. L'allogreffe et l'autogreffe de moëlle osseuse ont été utilisées pour traiter les malades en rechute. L'allogreffe a été rarement utilisée. Les quelques cas décrits dans la littérature ont présenté un taux de décès élevé lié au traitement et un taux de survie sans rechute à long terme d'environ 30%. L'autogreffe a été utilisée beaucoup plus fréquemment. Plusieurs centaines de cas ont été rapportés dans la littérature et la maladie de Hodgkin est devenu l'une des maladie pour laquelle l'autogreffe de moëlle est le plus fréquemment indiquée. Environ 50% des rémissions complètes ont été obtenues chez des malades traités par autogreffe de moëlle. 30% de l'ensemble de ces malades sont en vie sans rechute à long terme. Bien entendu, chez les malades traités tôt dans l'évolution de la maladie (par exemple avec un minimum de chimiothérapie et un bon "performance status") on a obtenu de meilleurs résultats.

Actuellement, les problèmes importants et non résolus dans l'utilisation de l'autogreffe de moëlle pour le traitement des malades atteints d'une maladie de Hodgkin concernent le protocole de conditionnement optimal et la recherche du meilleur moment pour l'administration du traitement. Des études prospectives et comparatives, non encore entreprises, seront nécessaires pour identifier le meilleur protocole thérapeutique. Aujourd'hui, j'estime que l'autogreffe de moëlle devrait être prise en considération comme l'un des choix thérapeutiques pour les malades pour lesquels une bonne chimiothérapie de première intention a été un échec. En en retardant l'application après de multiples échecs de chimiothérapies de rattrapage successives, on en augmente la toxicité tout en diminuant ses chances de réussite. La recherche d'une utilisation optimale de la greffe de moëlle dans le traitement de la maladie de Hodgkin nécessitera la réalisation d'essais thérapeutiques comparatifs auxquels devront participer les équipes ayant le plus d'expérience à travers le monde.

Introduction

Bone marrow transplantation is an increasingly utilized treatment modality in the management of patients with hematological malignancies. Bone marrow transplantation offers one way to circumvent treatment resistance by increasing the dose of available cytotoxic agents and radiotherapy while ameliorating myelotoxicity by infusion of hematopoietic stem cells. One would expect this treatment approach to be effective in some patients if a dose response to therapy exists. Fortunately, this appears to be true in Hodgkin disease.

Bone marrow transplantation, whether with autologous, allogeneic, or syngeneic hematopoietic stem cells, is being done more frequently each year (Armitage et al., 1986). It is anticipated that this year 2,000 autologous bone marrow transplants, and approximately 3,000 allogeneic transplants will be performed. Patients with Hodgkin disease have been treated very frequently with bone marrow transplantation - particularly autologous bone marrow transplantation - in the last few years (Gorin et al., submitted). The remainder of this manuscript will review the timing of bone marrow transplantation in Hodgkin disease, the relative merits of allogeneic and autologous transplantation, and the results to date.

Bone marrow transplantation versus other forms of salvage therapy

Patients with Hodgkin disease who present with localized disease and are treated only with radiotherapy have a comparatively good outlook after relapse. These patients respond to combination chemotherapy regimens at least equally to patients who present with more advanced disease and are treated initially with chemotherapy (DeVita et al., 1980). However, patients who fail a combination chemotherapy regimen - either with primary drug resistance or relapse from complete remission - have a much poorer outlook.

There are two subgroups of patients with relapsed Hodgkin disease who deserve special recognition. The first of these are patients who have a long initial remission and then relapse. Data from the National Cancer Institute suggest that when these patients are treated initially with MOPP and relapse late, they are very likely to respond favorably to the reinstitution of MOPP (Fisher et al., 1979). Approximately 90% of patients will enter another remission and one-third or more will have durable second remissions. One other subgroup that deserves special recognition are patients treated initially with combination chemotherapy but who have a localized relapse. These patients are occasionally able to be salvaged by extended field radiation therapy (Mauch et al., 1987; Roach et al., 1987; Fox et al., 1987).

Unfortunately, most patients with Hodgkin disease who fail combination chemoherapy regimens do not fit into either of these groups. A wide variety of treatment regimens have been utilized in these patients. Perhaps the most favorable situation is the use of ABVD in patients who fail MOPP. The largest reported series of such patients was from Milan (Santoro et al., 1982). Although these patients had a good chance to attain another remission, only 22% of the group had durable remissions. Most series of patients treated with ABVD after failing MOPP have had less good results (Krikorian et al., 1978; Sutcliffe et al., 1979; Clamon et al., 1978). As would be expected, patients who fail more than one combination chemotherapy regimen and then are treated with an alternate salvage chemotherapy regimen have an even worse outlook. Thus, there is a need for better treatment approach in patients with relapsed Hodgkin disease.

Which type of hematopoietic stem cells is best?

Allogeneic and autologous bone marrow transplantation have different advantages. Autologous bone marrow transplantation has no risk of graft-versus-host disease and almost all patients could receive this treatment. However, there is a risk of reinfusing tumor cells. Allogeneic bone marrow transplantation is available only to younger patients who have an HLA matched sibling. This treatment is complicated by graft-versus-host disease in a significant fraction of patients. However, there is no risk of reinfusing tumor cells and there is some possibility that the graft might have an immunologic effect against the original tumor. Allogeneic bone marrow transplantation has only been performed rarely in patients with Hodgkin disease. The reported cases are listed in Table 1.

As can be seen, there was a high treatment related death rate. However, the number of patients alive and well after allogeneic transplantation is not different from that reported for autologous transplantation.

Table 1. Allogenic bone marrow transplantation in Hodgkin disease

Reference	Number of patients	Currently in initial CR	Treatment related deaths
Appelbaum, 1985	8	2	5
Phillips, 1986	3	2	1
Mascret, 1980	2	0	1

Autologous bone marrow transplantation or autologous peripheral stem cell transplantation has been the most frequently utilized high dose treatment approach in Hodgkin disease. Table 2 lists the largest reported series of patients undergoing autologous bone marrow transplantation for Hodgkin disease. As can be seen, although the treatment related death rate was lower than with allogeneic transplantation, the disease-free survival is approximately the same. The complete response rate has varied but has averaged 50% with approximately 30% of patients being long-term, disease-free survivors. However, the results have been superior for patients treated earlier in the course of their disease.

Table 2. Autologous bone marrow transplantation Hodgkin disease

Reference	Number of patients	Currently in initial CR	Treatment related deaths
Bierman, 1988	128	41 (32%)	11 (9%)
Goldstone, 1988	56	12 (21%)	5 (9%)
Carella, 1988	50	12 (24%)	2 (4%)
Phillips, 1989	26	7 (27%)	6 (23%)

The use of autologous peripheral stem cells to reestablish hematopoiesis after high dose therapy has been documented to be practical (Kessinger et al., 1988; Korbling et al., 1986). The results in patients treated with Hodgkin disease have been similar when peripheral stem cells or bone marrow stem cells are used for hematopoietic rescue (Kessinger et al., in press).

Results with bone marrow transplantation in Hodgkin disease

Bone marrow transplantation has not been used as a primary treatment in patients with Hodgkin disease. This treatment approach has been rarely utilized in non-Hodgkin lymphomas (Tura et al., 1986). Because of the high cure rate with primary chemotherapy regimens in Hodgkin Disease, it is unlikely that bone marrow transplantation will find a place in the initial management of this disease.

The prognostic factors reported in various series for bone marrow transplantation in Hodgkin disease are listed in Table 3. In one large series, the predominant prognostic factors identified were the performance status of the patients being treated and the extent of previous therapy (Jagannath et al., 1989). Healthy patients who had no more than two previous chemotherapy regimens had a disease-free survival of approximately 50% while patients with a poor performance status or multiple preceding chemotherapies had a disease-free survival of only approximately 10%. This outcome is similar to that reported in other illnesses when bone marrow transplantation has been utilized. In general, healthy patients with less disease, tumors that are still chemotherapy sensitive, and who do not have large amounts of disease have the best outlook.

Table 3. Reported important prognostic factors after autologous bone marrow transplantation in Hodgkin's disease

> Performance status
> Extent of preceding therapy
> Bulk
> Response to preceding therapy

The place of radiotherapy in the treatment of patients undergoing bone marrow transplantation is unclear. We have utilized radiotherapy to sites of previous bulk disease following bone marrow transplantation. In a group of 14 patients who received radiotherapy to sites of previously bulky disease after achieving a complete or partial remission with bone marrow transplantation, only 21% have subsequently progressed with follow up as long as four years. The results in patients achieving a complete or partial remission after autologous bone marrow transplantation at our institution but who did not receive radiotherapy revealed a relapse rate of approximately 40%. However, this was not a randomized controlled clinical trial and further reports will be necessary to document the efficacy of localized radiotherapy following autologous bone marrow transplantation. The place of radiotherapy to the chest preceding bone marrow transplantation, or the use of total body radiotherapy in Hodgkin disease is uncertain. Only a few patients will be able to receive total body radiotherapy because most will have had thoracic radiation therapy before coming to bone marrow transplantation. There is at least one report suggesting that chest radiotherapy preceding high dose therapy associated with an exessive incidence of interstitial pneumonitis (Phillips et al., 1989). At present, most investigators studying the treatment of Hodgkin disease with bone marrow transplantation use preparative regimens that contain only high dose chemotherapeutic agents.

Conclusions

Bone marrow transplantation has been demonstrated to be able to produce long-term, disease-free survival in some patients with relapsed Hodgkin disease. Although most patients have received autologous hematopoietic stem cells as their source of hematopoietic rescue, the ultimate survival rate seems comparable in the few cases of allogeneic bone marrow transplantation that have been reported. It is clear that patients who are treated soon after relapse from their initial combination chemotherapy regimen have a far better outlook than patients who are treated with end stage, resistant disease. At the present time, patients with Hodgkin disease who do not have other clinical problems such as major organ disfunction that would disqualify them from undergoing bone marrow transplantation should be offered this treatment immediately after failing regimens equivalent to MOPP and ABVD. To find the optimal application of high dose therapy and bone marrow transplantation in the treatment of Dpatients with Hodgkin disease will require prospective clinical trials. These trials will not be possible unless multiple institutions participate.

References

Armitage, J.O., et al. (1986): Bone Marrow Autotransplantation in Man. Report of an International Cooperative Study. *The Lancet* 2, 960-962.

Appelbaum, F.R., et al. (1985): Allogeneic marrow transplantation in the treatment of MOPP-resistant Hodgkin's disease. *J. Clin. Oncol.* 3, 1490-1494.

Bierman, P.J., et al. (1988): High dose cyclophosphamide, carmustine, etoposide (CBV) in 128 patients (Pts) with Hodgkin's disease. *Blood* 72, 239a.

Carella, A.M., et al. (1988): High-dose chemotherapy with autologous bone marrow transplantation in 50 advanced resistant Hodgkin's disease patients: An Italian study group report. *J. Clin. Oncol.* 6, 1411-1416.

Clamon, G.H., et al. (1978): ABVD treatment of MOPP failures in Hodgkin's disease: A re-examination of goals of salvage therapy. *Cancer Treat. Rep.* 62, 363-367.

DeVita, V.T., et al. (1980): Curability of advance Hodgkin's disease with chemotherapy. Long-term follow-up of MOPP-treated patients at the National Cancer Institute. *Ann. Intern. Med.* 92, 587-595.

Fisher, R.I., et al. (1979): Prolonged disease-free survival in Hodgkin's disease with MOPP reinduction after first relapse. *Ann. Intern. Med.* 90, 761-763.

Fox, K.A., et al. (1987): Radiation therapy salvage of Hodgkin's disease following chemotherapy failure. *J. Clin. Oncol.* 5, 38-45.

Goldstone, A.H., et al. (1988): Experience of autologous bone marrow transplantation in the first 100 lymphomas. *Bone Marrow Transplant* 3 (1), 65-66.

Gorin, N.C., et al. (1989): Autologous Bone Marrow Transplants. Different Indications in Europe and North America. *The Lancet* 2, 1273-1275.

Jagannath, S., et al. (1989): Prognostic factors for response and survival after high dose cyclophosphamide, carmustine, and etoposide with autologous bone marrow transplantation for relapsed Hodgkin's disease. *J. Clin. Oncol.* 7, 179-185.

Kessinger, A., et al. (1988): Autologous peripheral hematopoietic stem cell transplantation restores hematopoietic function following marrow ablative therapy. *Blood* 71, 723-727.

Kessinger, A., et al. (1989): High-dose therapy and autologous peripheral blood stem cell transplantation for patients with lymphoma. *Blood* 74, 1260-1265.

Korbling, M., et al. (1986): Autologous transplantation of blood-derived hematopoietic stem cells after myeloablative therapy in a patient with Burkitt's lymphoma. *Blood* 67, 529-532.

Krikorian, J.G., et al. (1978): Treatment of advanced Hodgkin's disease with adriamycin, bleomycin, vinblastine, and imidazole carboxamide (ABVD) after failure of MOPP therapy. *Cancer* 41, 2107-2111.

Mascret, B., et al. (1980): Treatment of malignant lymphoma with high dose chemo or chemoradiotherapy and bone marrow transplantation. *Eur. J. Cancer Clin. Oncol.* 22, 461-471.

Mauch, P., et al. (1987): Wide-field radiation therapy alone or with chemotherapy for Hodgkin's disease in relapsed from combination chemotherapy. *J. Clin. Oncol.* 5, 544-549.

Phillips, G.L., et al. (1986): High-dose chemotherapy, fractionated total-body irradiation, and allogeneic marrow transplantation for malignant lymphoma. *J. Clin. Oncol.* 4, 480-488.

Phillips, G.L., et al. (1989): Treatment of progressive Hodgkin's disease with intensive chemoradiotherapy and autologous bone marrow transplantation. *Blood* 73, 2086-2092.

Roach, M., et al. (1987): Radiotherapy with curative intent: An option in selected patients relapsing after chemotherapy for advanced Hodgkin's disease. *J. Clin. Oncol.* 5, 550-555.

Santoro, A., et al. (1982): Salvage chemotherapy with ABVD in MOPP-resistant Hodgkin's disease. *Ann. Intern. Med.* 96, 139-143.

Sutcliffe, S.B., et al. (1979): Adriamycin, bleomycin, vinblastine and imidazole carboxamide (ABVD) therapy for advanced Hodgkin's disease resistant to mustine, vinblastine, procarbazine and prednisolone (MVPP). *Cancer Chemother. Pharmacol.* 2, 209-213.

Tura, S., et al. (1986): High dose therapy followed by autologous bone marrow transplantation (ABMT) in previously untreated non-Hodgkin lymphoma. *Scand. J. Haematol.* 37, 374-382.

LONG TERM SURVIVAL AND SIDE-EFFECTS OF TREATMENT

SURVIE A LONG TERME ET MORBIDITE THERAPEUTIQUE

Second Malignancies following Hodgkin's disease

J.M. Kaldor[1], C. Lasset[2]

[1] International Agency for Research on Cancer, 150 Cours Albert Thomas, 69372 Lyon Cedex 08, France
[2] Centre Léon Bérard, 28 rue Laënnec, 69800 Lyon, France

Summary

Second cancer following Hodgkin's disease have been studied extensively from an epidemiological point of view. Some 18 major clinical series have reported on 662 second cancers arising in more than 14,000 patients. Several population-based cancer registries have compared cancer incidence following Hodgkin's disease to general population rates for over 30,000 patients. Case-control studies have permitted more detailed evaluation of the role of therapy for the first cancer in the etiology of selected types of second cancer. Acute leukaemia emerges as the cancer type for which relative risk is most elevated, and its association with chemotherapy is far stronger than its association with radiotherapy. Hodgkin's disease patients are also at a substancially increased risk of lung cancer, non-Hodgkin's lymphoma, and other cancers, but apart from leukaemia, none appear to be clearly associated with therapy.

Résumé

L'incidence des secondes tumeurs malignes survenant après maladie de Hodgkin a été étudiée de façon approfondie d'un point de vue épidémiologique. Six cent soixante-deux deuxièmes tumeurs ont été identifiées parmi plus de 14 000 malades issus de 18 cohortes hospitalières. L'incidence relative de ces secondes tumeurs par rapport aux taux observés dans la population générale a été analysée grace aux données de certains registres d'incidence regroupant plus de 30 000 cas de maladie de Hodgkin. Enfin des études cas-témoins ont permis des analyses plus détaillées en particulier en ce qui concerne le rôle étiologique des traitements reçus sur l'apparition de certains types de seconds cancers. Le risque relatif le plus important concerne les leucémies aiguës, et une association très étroite est retrouvée avec la chimiothérapie, loin devant celle que l'on a pu observer avec la radiothérapie. Les malades atteints d'une maladie de Hodgkin présentent aussi un risque non négligeable de cancer bronchique, lymphome non-Hodgkinien, et autres localisations. Toutefois, mise à part la leucémie, aucune de ces localisations n'apparait liée de façon évidente avec l'une ou l'autre des thérapeutiques étudiées.

Table 1. The major clinical series of Hodgkin's disease patients studied for second cancer occurrence

First author and publication year	Inclusion period	Total number of HD patients	PY of FU (median if unavailable)	Total number of second cancers	Subtypes of Second Cancers			Comments
					Leukemia	NHL	Solid Tumours	
Baccarani 1980	1969-1976	613	median: 3.5 yrs	12	7	0	5	
Blayney 1987	1964-1975	192	1606	29	12 ANLL		17	
Boivin 1984	1940-1975	2591	11446	74*	21 ANLL	3	50	Patients with incomplete information about treatment excluded
Colman 1988	1963-1978	583	3667	37	8 AML 1 CLL	2	26	Non-U.K. resident excluded
Coltman 1982	1971-1978	659	unknown	32	21		11	
Glicksman 1982	1966-1974	798	median: 4 yrs	27	10 ANLL	1	16	Stage III only. Patients who did not achieve CR excluded
Henry-Amar 1984	1964-1976	669 (in 2 groups)	medians: 10 and 8 yrs	36 (21+15)	6 ANLL (4+2)	5 (3+2)	25 (14+11)	Study of 2 successive cohorts. Stages I and II only
Henry-Amar 1989	1960-1984	871	5778	-	19 (9 MDS)	-	-	Leukemia studied only
Jacquillat 1983	1963-1976	1094	unknown	65	28	37		
Koletsky 1986	1969-1982	162	median: 8.3 yrs	14	5	3	6	Stages III and IV only. Patients who did not achieve CR excluded
List 1985	1970-1982	260	1423	-	-	-	4	Lung cancer study only
Meadows 1989	1955-1979	979	median: 7 yrs	38	17 1 CML	3	18	Children only
Nelson 1981	1960-1977	248	median: 5.7 yrs	10*	1	0	9	
Pedersen-Bjergaard 1987	1970-1981	391	2732	34	20 ANLL	0	14	
Tester 1984	1964-1981	473	median: 12 yrs	34*	8 ANLL 1 CML	3	22	Patients with unknown treatment excluded
Tucker 1988	1968-1985	1505	9239	83*	27 ANLL 1 other type	9	46	
Valagussa 1986	1965-1982	1392	median: 9.5 yrs	68 (6 children)	19 ANLL	6	43	Children included (207)
Van Leeuwen 1989	1966-1983	744	median: 6.4 yrs	69*	16 ANLL	9	32	

* Non melanoma skin cancers excluded
Abbreviations used in Table : ANLL: acute non-lymphocytic leukemia; CLL: chronic lymphocytic leukemia; CML: chronic myelonic leukemia; MDS: myelodysplastic syndrome; NHL: non Hodgkin's lymphoma; CR: complete remission; PY : person-years at risk; FU : follow up.

Introduction

Even before chemotherapy began to greatly improve the outcome of advanced stage Hodgkin's disease, cases of acute leukemia had been reported in survivors (Gill & McCall, 1943; Cohen et al., 1958). Several years later, careful clinical studies showed that there was indeed a substantial excess risk of leukemia following Hodgkin's disease, but that the excess was largely confined to patients who had been treated with chemotherapy (Arseneau et al., 1972).

Subsequently, it was established that other malignant diseases, including non-Hodgkin's lymphoma (Krikorian et al., 1979) and lung cancer (List et al., 1985) also occurred at an increased frequency in Hodgkin's disease survivors, when comparisons were made with rates among the general population of the same age and sex. Furthermore, it now appears that patients who were treated only with radiotherapy are at an increased risk for several types of second cancer.

In this chapter, we first review the principal published sources of information on second malignancies following Hodgkin's disease. We then return to discuss a number of specific issues, including the types of tumours observed in excess, the relative risk of second cancer for different types of therapy, the time pattern of the risk, and the role of splenectomy.

The major clinical series

The centralization of Hodgkin's disease treatment has lent itself to the establishment of patient registries and long-term follow-up in a number of larger treatment centres. Clinical trials groups have also been an important source of information on the long-term outcome of therapy. Table 1 summarizes the characteristics of the major clinical series which have been studied for the occurrence of second cancers. In each case, the reference cited is the most recent one for the series concerned. A series was included in the table if second cancers had been investigated, and if information was provided on the population of patients who were at risk for developing second cancers. All the studies referred to in the Table 1 give the total number of patients followed up, but relatively few give the total number of person-years for which they were followed.

Taken together, these studies evaluated second cancer occurrence in a total of over 14,000 patients initially diagnosed with Hodgkin's disease. There have been 662 second cancers reported among these patients, of which 249 were leukemias (mostly of the acute non-lymphocytic type) and 44 were non Hodgkin's lymphomas.

In order to evaluate the role of the therapy in the aetiology of second cancers, a variety of different statistical procedures have been adopted. Some studies calculated the actuarial rate of second cancer according to treatment category, as well as the corresponding standard error. The actuarial rate is useful as a means of correcting for competing causes of mortality and other forms of censoring among survivors. However, in its usual form it does not take into account possible differences among the treatment groups in age and sex, both of which could be strongly related to the risk of second cancer incidence. An alternative means of comparing treatment categories is to calculate the standardized incidence ratio or SIR, which, for each category, is the ratio of the number of observed second cancers of a particular type to the number expected on the basis of incidence rates in the general population among individuals of the same age and sex as the cancer survivors. Comparison can be made of SIR's among treatment groups, provided that the categories are comparable for age and sex. The calculation of the SIR requires that age- and sex-specific incidence rates be available from the appropriate reference population. Harris and Coleman discuss the relative merits of the various statistical procedures which have been used to study second cancer risk (Harris & Coleman, 1989).

Table 2 summarizes some of the actuarial estimates of leukemia incidence by treatment category obtained from those studies in Table 1 which clearly indicated a suitable categorization. There is clearly a wide range in the estimates, even within a single category of treatment. For example, Coltman and Dixon reported an actuarial rate of 6.2% after 7 years following chemotherapy only, while the rate calculated by Blayney et al. was only 1% (Coltman & Dixon, 1982; Blayney et al., 1987). Discrepancies of this kind can be attributed to a number of factors, including the above mentioned differences in the composition of the patient groups, variation in the types of therapy used within each broad category, and the small numbers of patients used in the calculations for each category. The main conclusion that can be drawn from the table is that the risk of leukemia is generally confined to patients who received chemotherapy. There is some suggestion that the combination of radiotherapy and chemotherapy leads to a higher actuarial risk.

Table 2. Actuarial rate of leukemia following Hodgkin's disease at 10 years (% +/- s.e.) by treatment category

First author and publication year	Chemotherapy only	Radiotherapy only	Chemotherapy and radiotherapy
Blayney et al. 1987	1.0 +/- 1	No patients	18 +/- 5
Valagussa et al.[1] 1986	1.4 +/- 2.3	0	3 chemotherapy categories: ABVD only 0 Alkylating agents 10.2 +/- 5.2 MOPP only 4.8 +/- 1.6
Tester et al. 1984	2 +/- 2	0	2 chemotherapy categories: initial 6 +/- 2.1 salvage 7.7 +/- 2.9
Coltman et al.[2] 1982	6.2 +/- 3.4	0	2 chemotherapy categories: initial 6.4 +/- 2.1 salvage 7.7 +/- 2.9
Henry-Amar et al. 1989	No patients	2 categories: limited RT 0 Extended RT 2.4 + 1.4	2 categories: no nitrogen mustard 0 nitrogen mustard 12.4 +/- 3.5

1. *Rates are at 12 years*
2. *Rates are at 7 years*

Abbreviations in Table : RT = Radiotherapy, ABVD = Adriamycin, Bleomycin, Vinblastine and Dacarbazine, MOPP = Nitrogen Mustard, Vincristine, Procarbazine, and Prednisone.

Table 3 summarizes the SIR for leukemia and solid tumours by category of treatment, relative to the risk in the general population. The results are somewhat more consistent across studies than they were for the actuarial analyses. Overall, it appears that the relative risk of leukemia is well over 100 for patients who had received chemotherapy, but that the addition of radiotherapy does not substantially modify this risk. Although only 5 cases have been reported altogether, there does appear to be an elevated risk of leukemia (5.0) associated with

Table 3A. Relative risk (SIR) of leukemia following Hodgkin's disease compared to the general population, by treatment category

First author and publication year	Chemotherapy alone			Radiotherapy alone			Radiotherapy & chemotherapy initial or at relapse		
	O	E	O/E	O	E	O/E	O	E	O/E
Van Leeuwen 1989	3	0.02	192	1	0.18	5.5	12	0.16	75
Boivin 1984	6	0.06	100	2	0.59	3.4	13	0.08	162.5
Tucker 1987	3	0.023	130	2	0.182	10.9	23	0.2	115
Colman 1988	2	0.01	200	0	0.044	0	6	0.039	158.8
TOTAL	14	0.113	123.9	5	0.996	5	54	0.479	112.7

Table 3B. Relative risk (SIR) of solid tumours following Hodgkin's disease compared to the general population, by treatment category

First author and publication year	Chemotherapy alone			Radiotherapy alone			Radiotherapy & chemotherapy initial or at relapse		
	O	E	O/E	O	E	O/E	O	E	O/E
Tucker 1987	1	0.91	1.1	16	5.7	2.8	25	4.94	5.06
Boivin[1] 1984	5	2.8	1.8	12	5.8	2.1	2	0.6	3.3
TOTAL	6	5.91	1.01	28	11.5	2.43	27	5.54	4.87

[1] Includes non-Hodgkin lymphoma.
Abbreviations used in Table: 0 = observed number of cases; E = expected number of cases.

Table 4. Observed numbers of second cancers and relative risk at least one year after Hodgkin's disease *(From Kaldor et al., 1987)*

Second cancer (ICD7)	Males Obs	Males RR	Females Obs	Females RR
Lip (140)	3	1.0	1	5.6
Tongue (141)	2	2.2	1	2.8
Salivary glands (142)	5	8.5**	3	6.5*
Mouth (143-4)	2	1.6	1	1.9
Other Pharynx (146,8-9)	2	1.5	1	3.2
Nasopharynx (147)	3	7.9*	1	9.1
Oesophagus (150)	5	1.6	2	1.8
Stomach (151)	28	1.5	4	0.5
Small intestine (152)	0	0.0	0	0.0
Colon (153)	23	1.3	16	1.1
Rectum (154)	14	1.1	7	1.0
Liver (155.0)	3	.17	0	0.0
Gall-bladder (155.1)	1	0.7	1	0.5
Pancreas (157)	10	1.2	5	1.1
Nasal sinuses (160)	2	3.4	1	4.2
Larynx (161)	3	0.8	3	9.1*
Trachea, bronchus (162-3)	89	1.9**	17	2.2**
Breast (170)	-	-	62	1.4**
Cervix (171)	-	-	23	2.1**
Corpus (172)	-	-	14	1.5
Other uterus (173-4)	-	-	0	0.0
Ovary (175)	-	-	7	0.7
Other females genital (176)	-	-	2	1.2
prostate (177)	43	1.3	-	-
Testis (178)	3	0.9	-	-
Other male genital (179)	3	4.5	-	-
Kidney (180)	12	1.8	7	2.3
Bladder (181)	19	1.2	8	2.2
Melanoma (190)	9	2.4*	5	1.3
Other skin (191)	37	2.3*	19	2.1**
Eye (192)	2	3.7	0	0.0
Brain, nervous system (193)	6	1.0	4	1.1
Thyroid (194)	3	2.8	5	2.2
Endocrine (195)	1	1.3	0	0.0
Bone (196)	1	1.3	4	10.6**
Connective tissue (197)		10.7	3	3.6
Non-Hodgkin's lymphoma (200, 202)	15	3.0**	9	3.1
Hodgkin's disease (201)	-	-	-	-
Multiple myeloma (203)	4	1.4	5	2.9
Other leukemia (204.0)	7	.26*	2	1.9
Acute leukemia (204.1-9)	53	17.5**	27	15.8**
All leukemia (204)	69	10.3**	37	10.9
TOTAL	430	1.8**	281	1.7**

* $p < 0.05$ (2-sided); ** $p < 0.01$ (2-sided)

radiotherapy alone. The picture for solid tumours is somewhat different. Based on 6 cases, there is no increase in risk for patients treated by chemotherapy alone (relative risk = 1.0), but there is for patients who had received radiotherapy, and the risk is about twice as high for patients treated with both modalities than those who only received radiotherapy.

No study has reported a sufficient number of cases of any particular type of solid tumour to permit a clear evaluation of differences in risk among treatment categories. In a review of lung cancer following Hodgkin's disease List et al. noted the high frequency of supradiaphragmatic irradiation and in-field tumours among reported lung cancer cases, but was unable to conclusively implicate radiotherapy as the causative factor in the increased incidence of lung cancer among Hodgkin's disease survivors (List et al., 1985). Non-Hodgkin's lymphoma incidence was identical between groups of patients treated by radiotherapy and chemotherapy (Tucker et al., 1987).

Cancer registry incidence studies

The principal strength of the clinical series is that they provide information on second cancer risk in a way which can be clearly related to oncological practice. However, even the largest studies are of limited size, and cannot provide information on the risk for rarer tumour types, or detect small increases in the risk of more common tumour types. For this purpose, descriptive studies of second cancer incidence carried out by cancer registries which have a large population base can be of considerable value. Registry studies have the further attraction that they generally include all patients in their region of coverage, rather than the selected groups seen in individual hospitals or entered into clinical trials and therefore give a broader picture of the incidence of second cancer. The cancer registries of Denmark, Finland and Connecticut have reported on the incidence of second cancer following Hodgkin's disease, and made comparisons of the numbers expected on the basis of rates among the general population (Storm et al., 1985; Teppo et al., 1985; Curtis et al., 1985). The largest descriptive study to date was a collaboration among 11 registries, including those of Denmark and Finland, and tabulated second primary cancers occurring at least one year after the diagnosis of Hodgkin's disease (Kaldor et al., 1987). The results are summarized in Table 4. Overall, 711 cases were reported as having occurred among over 28,000 patients initially diagnosed with Hodgkin's disease. In comparison with the general population, there was a substantially increased (17-fold) SIR of acute leukemia, as expected, and also of lung cancer (about 2-fold) and non-Hodgkin's lymphoma (about 3-fold). There were also significantly elevated risks for other cancer types which had not previously been thought to occur in excess following Hodgkin's disease. Among common malignancies the incidence of cancers of the breast, cervix, and skin (non-melanocytic) was increased. Based on much fewer cases, there were also substantially increases for cancers of the salivary glands and nasopharynx, the larynx and bone in women, and moderate increase in risk for cancers of the thyroid and melanoma. These increases cannot be attributed with any degree of certainty to Hodgkin's disease or its therapy. However, apart from non-melanoma skin cancer, they are unlikely to be artefactual consequences of increased medical surveillance following Hodgkin's disease.

The one apparent excess which may be due to difficulties of histological typing is non-Hodgkin's lymphoma. Consider a hypothetical situation in which 1%, or 280 of the original diagnoses of Hodgkin's disease were in fact misdiagnosed non-Hodgkin's lymphoma. If only 5% of these patients in turn relapsed following Hodgkin's disease therapy and were rediagnosed, this time correctly, as having non-Hodgkin's lymphoma, the apparent excess would be 14 cases, very close to the 18 observed in the study. Thus even a very low rate of misdiagnosis could produce a substantial apparent excess in the risk of non-Hodgkin's lymphoma.

Case-control studies

Another limitation of the clinical series is that the readily accessible information on therapy is frequently not as detailed as would be required for a full investigation of second cancer risk by treatment category. Rather than returning to the medical records of all available Hodgkin's disease patients, a more efficient strategy is to adopt the case-control design, under which the details of Hodgkin's disease therapy are only abstracted for patients who are diagnosed with second cancer, and suitable matched controls who were not. The first case-control study of second cancer in Hodgkin's survivors investigated the role of therapy in secondary acute leukemia (Van der Velden et al., 1988).

The principal drawback of the case-control approach is that it does not readily yield absolute estimates of second cancer risk. Its usual end-products are estimates of relative risk, comparing the risk associated with one or more treatment categories with the risk in a category which is arbitrarily chosen as the reference. In studies of Hodgkin's disease, the reference category depends to a large extent on which second cancer is being investigated. Since patients are generally treated by radiotherapy, chemotherapy or both, there is no group which could be designated as unexposed to carcinogenic or mutagenic agents.

Table 5. Acute or non-lymphocytic leukemia only. Relative risk[1] (95 percent confidence limits in brackets) by total radiation dose to the bone marrow and chemotherapy received *(From Kaldor et al., 1990)*

Chemotherapy	Bone marrow radiation dose (Gy)				
	0	<10	10-20	>20	Unknow
None	-	1.0	1.6 [0.26-10.0]	8.2** [1.7-39.0]	4 -
MP[2] only < 6 cycles	9.1* [1.6-53]	8.6** [1.9-39]	22*** [5.1-99]	9.4** [2.0-45]	19 [0.95-370]
> 6 cycles	50*** [8.1-310]	26*** [4.4-150]	63*** [9.6-410]	22*** [3.7-130]	4 -
Other chemotherapy[3]	17*** [4.4-68]	19*** [4.9-75]	25*** [6.1-99]	25*** [6.3-99]	18** [2.7-120

* $p < 0.05$; ** $p < 0.01$; *** $p < 0.001$

[1] *Relative to patients treated with radiotherapy only, who received less than 10 Gy to the bone marrow.*
[2] *MP: Combinations including nitrogen mustard and procarbazine, and no other alkylating agent.*
[3] *Includes 3 controls who received neither radiotherapy nor chemotherapy*
[4] *No cases in the category.*

In studies of leukemia, the reference category would most likely be patients who were treatment by radiotherapy only; in a case-control study of lung cancer, the reference category may well be patients who had not received radiation exposure to the lung, regardless of whether or not they had been treated with chemotherapy.

Although few case-control studies of second cancer following Hodgkin's disease have so far been published, they should in the future provide substantial information on the role of chemotherapy, radiotherapy and other factors. By far the largest investigation to date of leukemia in Hodgkin's disease survivors is a recently completed case-control study (Kaldor et al., 1990). A collaborative group, consisting of the cancer registries who had carried out the earlier linkage study as well as several large treatment centres, identified 163 cases of leukemia following Hodgkin's disease, and for each case, chose 3 controls matched by participating registry or centre, age, sex, and date of Hodgkin's disease diagnosis, who had survived free of a second cancer at least as long as the case (Kaldor et al., 1987). For all cases and controls, full details of Hodgkin's disease therapy were abstracted, and the relative risk associated with different categories of therapy was estimated.

The study confirmed that the addition of radiotherapy does not increase the risk conveyed by chemotherapy alone, and detected a clear increase in risk with the number of cycles of MOPP-type combination chemotherapy. This increase was shown to hold regardless of the total radiation exposure to the bone marrow, as shown in Table 5. The study also reproduced the earlier observation that splenectomy seems to be an independent risk factor for leukemia following Hodgkin's disease (Van Leeuwen et al., 1987). Other statistical analyses considered the relative leukemogenicity of different types of combination chemotherapy, and the evolution of the leukemia risk as a function of time since the first and last chemotherapy.

International Workshop, 1989

The recent initiative to combine the original records on Hodgkin's disease survivors from major clinical centres and cooperative groups has produced a data-base which potentially combines the strengths of the clinical series, the descriptive studies, and the case-control studies for investigating second cancer following Hodgkin's disease [*Statistical Report, part IX*]. Information on diagnosis, treatment and prognosis has been obtained for over 12,000 patients from 19 collaborating institutions and groups from Europe and North America. Among those patients, 631 second cancers, including 158 cases of leukemia, 106 cases of non-Hodgkin's lymphoma and 95 cases of lung cancer were recorded.

Evaluations of SIR were made using figures from the general population incidence rates matched for country, age, sex, and calendar year, as reference. There was a substantial consistency between this study and the registry-based study in the types of cancer which appeared in excess (Kaldor et al., 1987).

Detailed analyses of risk were carried out for all tumour types combined, leukemia, non-Hodgkin's lymphoma and all solid tumours combined. Of considerable interest were statistical analyses restricted to patients who achieved a complete remission after their first course of treatment. Concentrating on these patients was to a certain extent obliged by the lack of detail requested in the study on second and further courses, but it also produced estimates of second cancer risk which could be interpreted very readily. The principal findings for leukemia were a strongly increasing risk of leukemia with MOPP-like chemotherapy given alone or in association with radiation therapy (any type) and an increased risk associated with splenectomy [*Statistical Report, Table IX-12*]. For solid tumours, chemotherapy had no effect on risk, and total nodal irradiation increased risk by 80%, but for non-Hodgkin's lymphoma, no association could be detected with any treatment category [*Statistical Report, Tables IX-13 and IX-14*].

Discussion

As we have indicated, each approach described above for studying second cancers after Hodgkin's disease has contributed information of a somewhat different nature. Taken together, they provide a picture which is rather clear in several areas, although further work is required to resolve a number of questions.

Tumour types observed in excess

In terms of relative risk, leukemia is by far the most significant cancer occurring in excess following Hodgkin's disease, but as measured by the excess number of cases, lung cancer is almost of equal importance. The risk of non-Hodgkin lymphoma and several rarer types of cancer (salivary gland, thyroid, bone) is also substantially increased. Hodgkin's disease survivors may also be more susceptible than the general population to cancers of the colon, breast, cervix and skin. Only leukemia, and solid tumours as a group have been clearly demonstrated to be related to the type of therapy received.

The risk for the different types of therapy

Leukemia risk is clearly related to chemotherapy. Although the disease occurs more frequently among patients treated with radiotherapy alone than it does in the general population, chemotherapy increases the risk another 10-20 fold. It appears that the new type of combination chemotherapy known as ABVD is substantially less leukemogenic than the MOPP-type combinations but it is too early to state whether the combination is non-leukemogenic (Valagussa et al., 1986). Other combinations such as COPP (in which the nitrogen mustard of MOPP is replaced by cyclophosphamide) may be as leukemogenic as MOPP, but the number of patients so far studied is small (Kaldor et al., 1989). There is no evidence that radiotherapy enhances the leukemogenic effect of chemotherapy.

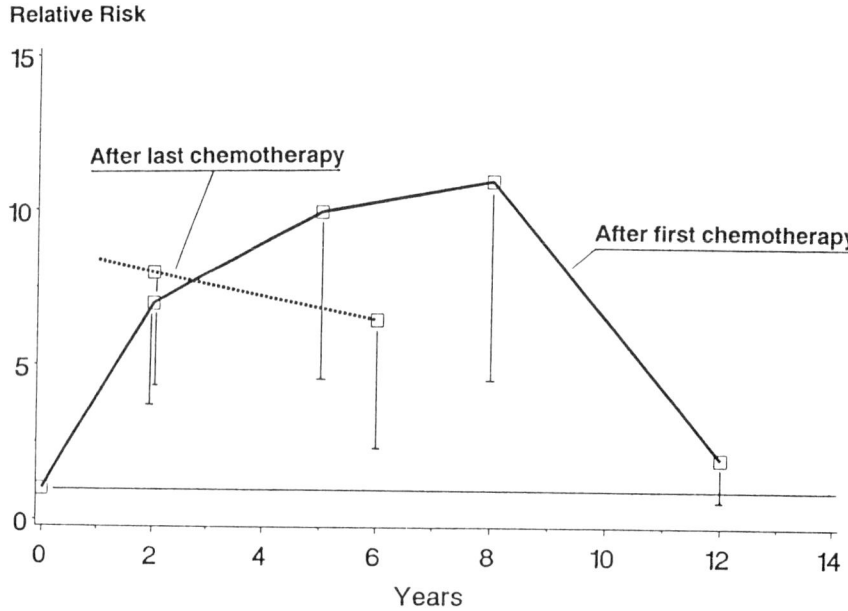

Figure 1. *Relative risk of leukemia in relation to chemotherapy as a function of time since first chemotherapy and time since last chemotherapy.*

Solid tumours so far appear to be related as a group to radiotherapy, rather than chemotherapy. Certainly ionizing radiation is well established as a multi-organ carcinogen, but studies of individual sites have not yet confirmed the role of radiotherapy in the induction of solid tumours after Hodgkin's disease.

Time patterns of risk

The risk of leukemia appears to be maximal 4-8 years after the diagnosis of Hodgkin's disease but, as Figure 1 shows, an increase in risk may persist for over a decade after treatment (Blayney et al., 1987; Kaldor et al., 1990). There is so far insufficient elapsed follow-up time to determine whether the risk ever returns to the level in patients treated by radiotherapy alone, or indeed to the level in the general population.

For solid tumours, the risk increase steadily, both in absolute and relative terms, for over 15 years, particularly among patients who were treated with total nodal irradiation [*Statistical Report, Table IX-3*]. An exception may be the risk of lung cancer, which seems to reach a peak within the first ten years (Kaldor et al., 1987).

The role of Hodgkin's disease

An important but unresolved question is whether Hodgkin's disease itself, rather than or in addition to its therapy, is a factor in increasing the risk of second cancer in surviving patients. Because virtually all patients receive potentially carcinogenic therapy, comparison cannot be made with the general population. If it were possible to control for the type of therapy, comparisons would be made with survivors of other forms of cancer, but they have so far not been attempted. Stage, which may be viewed as a marker of disease severity, has so far not been clearly identified or excluded as a risk factor for second cancer although it appears related to an increase in risk of secondary leukemia, and, to a lesser extent, of secondary non-Hodgkin lymphoma [*Statistical Report, Tables IX-12 and IX-13*].

Splenectomy

Several recent studies have shown that splenectomy is associated with an increased risk of leukemia following Hodgkin's disease (Van Leeuwen et al., 1987; Van der Velden et al., 1988; Kaldor et al., 1990). This observation was confirmed in the Workshop database analysis [*Statistical Report, Table IX-12*].

Conclusion

Hodgkin's disease survival has improved dramatically in the past two decades, to the extent that long-term side effects have become an important clinical issue. By studying second cancers in detail, it should be possible to reduce the long-term risk, and add to the already impressive gains which have been made in the number of patients who are truly cured of Hodgkin's disease.

References

Arsenau, J.C., et al. (1972): Non-lymphomatous malignant tumors complicating Hodgkin's disease. *N. Engl. J. Med.* 287, 119-1122.
Baccarani, M., et al. (1980): Second malignancy in patients treated for Hodgkin's disease. *Cancer* 46, 1735-1740.
Blayney, D.W., et al. (1987): Decreasing risk of leukemia with prolonged follow-up after chemotherapy and radiotherapy for Hodgkin's disease. *N. Engl. J. Med.* 318, 76-81.
Boivin, J.F., et al. (1984): Second primary cancers following treatment of Hodgkin's disease. *J. Nat. Cancer Inst.* 72, 233-241.
Cohen, M., et al. (1958): Hodgkin's disease (familial) associated with multiple malignant neoplasms. *Cancer* 11, 1267-1274.

Colman, M., et al. (1988): Second malignancies and Hodgkin's disease - The Royal Marsden Hospital experience. *Radiotherapy Oncol.* 11, 229-238.

Coltman, C.A., Jr & Dixon, D.O. (1982): Second malignancies complicating Hodgkin's disease: A Southwest Oncology Group 10-year follow-up. *Cancer Treat. Rep.* 66, 1023-1033.

Curtis, R.E., et al. (1985): Multiple primary cancers in Connecticut, 1935-82. *NCI Monogr.* 68, 219-242.

Gill, A.W. & Mc Call, A.J. (1943): Lymphoadenoma and leukemia. *Br. Med. J.* 1, 284-286.

Glicksman, A.S., et al. (1982): Second malignant neoplams in patients successfully treated for Hodgkin's diseases: A Cancer And Leukemia Group B study. *Cancer Treat. Rep.* 66.

Harris, T.R., & Coleman, C.N. (1989): Estimating the Risk of second primary tumours following cancer treatment. *J. Clin. Onc.* 7, 5-6.

Henry-Amar, M. (1985): Second cancers after treatment in two successive cohorts of patients with early stages of Hodgkin's disease. In *Malignant lymphomas and Hodgkin's disease : Experimental and therapeutic advances*, ed. F. Cavalli, G. Bonadonna, & M. Rozencweig, pp. 417-428. Boston: Martinus Nijhoff.

Henry-Amar, M., et al. (1989): Risk of secondary acute leukemia and preleukemia after Hodgkin's disease: The Institute Gustave-Roussy Experience. In *New aspects in the diagnosis and treatment of Hodgkin's disease*, ed. V. Diehl, M. Pfreundschuh, & M. Löffler, pp. 270-283. Recent results in Cancer Research 117. Berlin: Springer-Verlag..

Jacquillat, C., et al. (1983): Leucémies aiguës et tumeurs solides dans l'évolution de la maladie de Hodgkin. *Bull. Cancer (Paris)* 70, 61-66.

Kaldor, J.M., et al. (1987): Second malignancies following testicular cancer, ovarian cancer and Hodgkin's disease: An International collaborative study among cancer registries. *Int. J. Cancer* 39, 571-585.

Kaldor, J.M., et al. (1990): Leukemia following Hodgkin's disease. *N. Engl. J. Med.* 322, 7-13.

Krikorian, J.G., et al. (1979): Occurrence of non-Hodgkin's lymphoma after therapy for Hodgkin's disease. *N. Engl. J. Med.* 300, 452-458.

Koletsky, A.J., et al. (1986): Second neoplasms in patients with Hodgkin's disease following combined modality therapy - The Yale Experience. *J. Clin. Oncol* 4, 311-317.

List, A.F., et al. (1985): Lung cancer in Hodgkin's disease: association with previous radiation therapy. *J. Clin. Oncol.* 3, 215-221.

Meadows, A.T., et al. (1989): Second malignant neoplasms following childhood Hodgkin's disease: Treatment and splenectomy as risk factors. *Med. Ped. Oncol.* (in press).

Nelson, D.F., et al. (1981): Second malignant neoplasm in patients treated for Hodgkin's disease with radiotherapy or radiotherapy and chemotherapy. *Cancer* 48, 2386-2393.

Pedersen-Bjergaard, J., et al. (1987): Risk of therapy-related leukaemia and preleukaemia after Hodgkin's disease. *Lancet* ii, 83-88.

Storm, H.H., et al. (1985): Multiple primary cancers in Denmark, 1943-80. *NCI Monogr.* 68, 411-430.

Tester, W.J., et al. (1984): Second malignant neoplasms complicating Hodgkin's disease: The National Cancer Institute experience. *J. Clin. Oncol.* 2, 762-769.

Teppo, L., et al. (1985): Multiple cancer - an epidemiologic exercise in Finland. *J. Nat. Cancer Inst.* 75, 207-217.

Tucker, M.A., et al. (1987): Risk of second cancers after treatment for Hodgkin's disease. *N. Engl. J. Med.* 318, 76-81.

Valagussa, P., et al. (1986): Second acute leukemia and other malignancies following treatment for Hodgkin's disease. *J. Clin. Oncol.* 4, 83-837.

Van Leeuwen, F.E., et al. (1987): Splenectomy in Hodgkin's disease and second leukaemias (letter). *Lancet* ii, 210-211.

Van Leeuwen, F.E., et al. (1989): Increased risk of lung cancer, non-Hodgkin's lymphoma, and leukemia following Hodgkin's Disease. *J. Clin. Oncol.* 7, 1046-1059.

Van der Velden, J.W., et al. (1988): Subsequent development of acute non-lymphocytic leukemia in patients treated for Hodgkin's disease. *Int. J. Cancer* 42, 252-255.

Long term survival in early stages Hodgkin's disease : the EORTC experience

M. Henry-Amar[1], R. Somers[2],
for the EORTC Lymphoma Cooperative Group[3]

1 Institut Gustave-Roussy, 94805 Villejuif, France
2 Antoni van Leeuwenhoek Huis, 1066 CX Amsterdam, The Netherlands
3 EORTC members are listed in appendix

Summary

From 1963 to 1988, 1,660 early stage Hodgkin disease patients were treated on four successive clinical trials conducted by the European Organization for Research and Treatment of Cancer (EORTC) Lymphoma Cooperative Group. Treatments used were radiation therapy alone (56%), radiation therapy followed by adjuvant chemotherapy (14%), or combined modality treatments including MOPP (20%) or ABVD (10%) for 6 courses in association with mantle field irradiation. Overall, 320 deaths were observed (O) compared to 40.14 expected (E) from general population (SMR (ie, O/E) = 7.97; $p<0.001$). Causes of death were disease progression in 169 cases, toxic deaths in 26 cases, second cancer in 46 cases (SMR = 3.84; $p<0.001$), cardiac failure in 24 cases (SMR = 8.63; $p<0.001$). The remaining 55 deaths were from intercurrent disease (32 cases) or unspecified cause (23 cases). Overall, intercurrent deaths were responsible for a difference in the 20-year survival rate of 15% compared to the general population and an excess mortality of 3.11 ($p<0.001$). The evolution of SMR by 3-year interval was : 0-2 years, 1.91 ($p<0.01$); 3-5 years, 3.43 ($p<0.001$); 6-8 years, 2.89 ($p<0.001$); 9-11 years, 5.79 ($p<0.001$); 12-14 years, 3.73 ($p<0.001$); 15-17 years, 3.85 ($p<0.001$); and 0.89 ($p>0.20$) 18 years or more after Hodgkin disease diagnosis. The 9-11 year and the 12-14 year excess mortality were mostly related to an excess in second cancer and cardiac failure deaths. While toxic deaths or deaths from disease progression were rather uncommon 10 years or more after initial treatment, those from intercurrent diseases, especially second cancer and cardiac failure, appeared to increase regularly in all age groups, an observation that should encourage investigators to continue long-term follow-up in successfully treated Hodgkin disease patients.

Résumé

Entre 1963 et 1988, le Groupe Coopérateur Lymphome de l'Organisation Européenne de Recherche et de Traitement des Cancer (OERTC) a successivement conduit 4 essais thérapeutiques comparatifs dans lesquels ont été inclus 1 660 malades atteints d'une maladie de Hodgkin au stade localisé. Les traitements administrés étaient soit une radiothérapie exclusive (56% des cas), une association radiothérapie et chimiothérapie adjuvante (14% des cas), ou une association radiothérapie-chimiothérapie utilisant 6 cycles de MOPP (20% des cas) ou d'ABVD (10% des cas). Globalement, 320 décès ont été observés (O) alors que 40,14 étaient attendus (E) (SMR (ie, O/E) = 7,97; $p<0,001$). La cause du décès était la progression de la maladie dans 169 cas, une complication thérapeutique dans 26 cas, la survenue d'une seconde tumeur maligne dans 46 cas (SMR = 3,84; p<0,001), une cardiopathie ischémique dans 24 cas (SMR = 8,63; p<0,001). Les autres causes de décès se répartissaient entre autre maladie intercurrente que second cancer ou cardiopathie ischémique (32 cas) et cause non spécifiée (23 cas). Par rapport à la survie attendue, les décès de cause intercurrente (second cancer, cardiopathie ischémique, autres causes intercurrentes) étaient responsables d'une diminution de 15% du taux de survie attendu à 20 ans. La surmortalité qui peut leur être attribuée est égale à 3,11 (p<0,001). L'évolution du SMR par intervalle de 3 ans était le suivant : 0-2 ans, 1,91 (p<0,01); 3-5 ans, 3,43 (p<0,001); 6-8 ans, 2,89 (p<0,001); 9-11 ans, 5,79 (p<0,001); 12-14 ans, 3,73 (p<0,001); 15-17 ans, 3,85 (p<0,001); et 0,89 (p>0,20) 18 ans ou plus après le diagnostic de maladie de Hodgkin. L'excès de risque de décès observé pendant les intervalles 9-11 ans et 12-14 ans était en grande partie du à un excès de décès lié aux secondes tumeurs malignes et aux décès par cardiopathie ischémique. Alors que les décès liés à la progression de la maladie ou aux complications thérapeutiques étaient peu fréquents parmi les malades ayant un recul dépassant 10 ans, ceux liés à d'autres causes, en particulier les seconds cancers et les cardiopathies ischémiques, augmentaient régulièrement avec le temps, et ce quel que soit l'âge. Une constatation qui devrait inciter les médecins à continuer de suivre attentivement tout malade même "guéri" d'une maladie de Hodgkin.

Introduction

The use of modern therapies, such as a combination of radiotherapy and chemotherapy, or a better adaptation of these therapies to the *a priori* patient's prognosis have led to very high survival rates, particularly for early stages of the disease. There is now evidence that a patient with early stage I-II disease can be cured with a probability as high as 90 %, perhaps higher. However, cure rate estimates refer to tumour mortality, including disease progression and treatment-related deaths. Besides patients who die from treatment failure or toxic death are patients who after a period of complete remission die from intercurrent diseases. These particularly include second cancers and cardiac failure. The distinction between Hodgkin disease-related deaths and intercurrent deaths is of great interest, especially in a disease that has a long expected survival after treatment, and occurs mostly in young populations.

The risk of dying from specific causes after Hodgkin disease has rarely been reported. In 1986, Rubin et al. reported no significant difference between overall survival and survival corrected for second cancer mortality in a series of 320 clinical stage I-IV patients while the European Organization for Research and Treatment of Cancer (EORTC) and the Groupe Pierre et Marie Curie (GPMC) reported a 5 % difference in the 15-year survival rates between crude and corrected survival in a series of 1,501 clinical stage I-II patients (Rubin et al., 1986; Henry-Amar, 1988). Similar findings were reported by the Stanford University group (Hancock et al., 1988).

The risk of dying from cardiac failure was investigated in three retrospective series. In a cohort of 957 patients diagnosed with Hodgkin disease between 1942-1975, 25 coronary heart disease deaths were observed giving a death rate relative to the general population rate of 0.91 not statistically significant from 1 (Boivin & Hutchison, 1982). Similary, Hancock et al. reported no increase in the death rate from acute myocardial infarction (Hancock et al., 1988). In this last series, the comparison of observed deaths from intercurrent disease with the general population rates indicated a relative risk of 1.25 (p=0,07) while in a series of 340 clinical stage I-IV patients treated in the Netherlands, successfully treated patients were still at an increased risk of dying (Relative risk = 1.97, p<0.001) (van Rijswijk et al., 1987).

This study examines the overall risks and specific causes of death unrelated to active Hodgkin disease in a series of clinical stage I-II patients enrolled in four successive randomized clinical trials that were conducted by the EORTC Lymphoma Cooperative Group over 25 years.

Patients and methods

From 1963 to 1988, 1,660 adult patients with early stage Hodgkin disease were treated on four successive prospective clinical trials (Hayat, 1972; Tubiana et al., 1981; Carde et al., 1988; Carde et al., 1990). Initial patients characteristics are listed in Table 1.

Table 1. Initial patients characteristics and treatment

Age in years	mean (SD)	31.3 (11.8)		
15-19 years		225		14 %
20-29		600		36 %
30-39		466		28 %
40-49		218		13 %
50 +		141		9 %
Sex-ratio		1.35		
Clinical stage	I	610		37 %
	II	1040		63 %
Laparotomy & splenectomy		514		31 %
Radiation therapy alone		925		56 %
Mantle field			347	21 %
STNI [a]			426	26 %
TNI [a]			152	9 %
Combined treatment :		725		44 %
Mantle field + VLB [b]			136	8 %
STNI + VLB w/wo PCZ [c]			98	6 %
MOPP x 3 - mantle field - MOPP x 3 [d]			325	20 %
ABVD x 3 - mantle field - ABVD x 3 [e]			166	10 %
Initial complete response		1624		98 %

(a) Subtotal (STNI) or total (TNI) nodal + spleen irradiation
(b) Vinblastine
(c) Procarbazine
(d) Mechlorethamine hydrochloride, vincristine, procarbazine and prednisone
(e) Doxorubicin, bleomycin, vinblastine and dacarbazine

The first trial H1 (1963-1971; N=288) compared regional radiotherapy alone with a combination of the same irradiation followed by vinblastine for 2 years. No laparotomy was performed, and no prophylactic irradiation was given to the other side of the diaphragm.

The second trial H2 (1972-1976; N=300) compared staging laparotomy and splenectomy with spleen irradiation. All patients received subtotal nodal irradiation (mantle-field and paraaortic lymph node irradiation). Moreover, patients with mixed cellularity or lymphocytic depletion histological subtypes subsequently were administered adjuvant chemotherapy with vinblastine or vinblastine and procarbazine for 2 years.

In the third trial H5 (1977-1981; N=494) patients were subgrouped into two subsets according to their initial characteristics. Those with favourable prognostic features were submitted to staging laparotomy and splenectomy and were randomized, in case of pathological stage I-II, to either mantle-field irradiation alone or subtotal nodal irradiation. Patients with unfavourable indicators at onset or those with pathological stage III-IV were randomized between total nodal irradiation (including spleen irradiation) and combined modality treatment, i.e. 3 courses of MOPP (mechlorethamine, vincristine, procarbazine, prednisone) - Mantle-field irradiation - 3 courses of MOPP.

The last trial H6 (1981-1988; N=578) also considered two groups of patients according to initial characteristics. In patients with favourable prognostic indicators, the protocol compared subtotal nodal irradiation (including spleen irradiation) to staging laparotomy and splenectomy followed by an adapted treatment according to laparotomy findings. Pathological stage I-II patients were administered mantle-field irradiation alone (or mantle-field + paraaortic irradiation in patients with unfavourable histological subtypes), while pathological stage III-IV patients received combined modality treatment identical to that given in the unfavourable group. Patients with unfavourable pronostic indicators were randomly assigned to receive either 3 courses of MOPP - mantle-field irradiation - 3 courses of MOPP or 3 courses of ABVD (adriamycin, bleomycin, vinblastine, dacarbazine) - mantle-field irradiation - 3 courses of ABVD.

Overall, 31 % of the patients underwent a staging laparotomy and splenectomy; 56 % were treated with irradiation alone, 14 % with irradiation followed by adjuvant chemotherapy, and 30 % with combined modality treatments (Table 1).

Initial complete remission was achieved in 98 % of the patients. Results expressed as disease-free survival and overall survival according to trials and treatment groups were recently published (Tubiana et al., 1989). Overall, survival curves by trial are plotted on Figure 1.

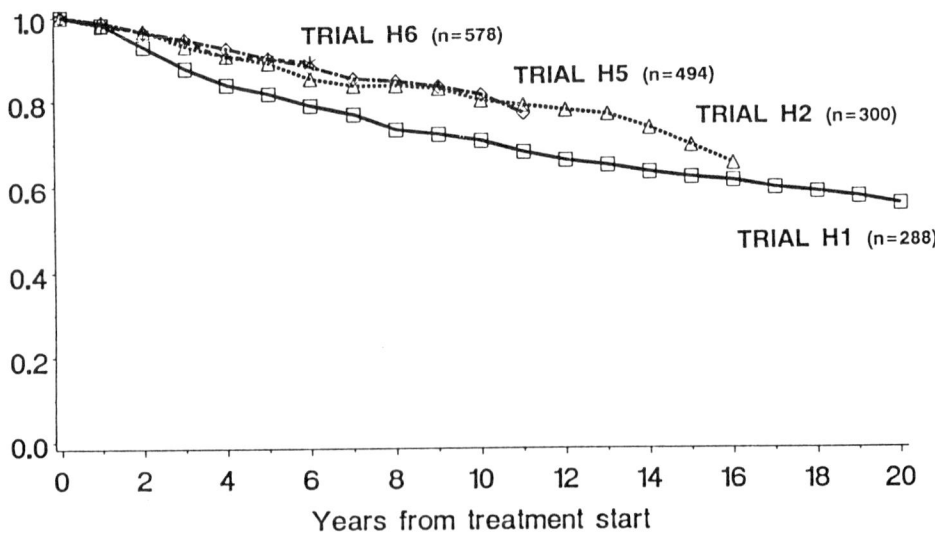

Figure 1. *Overall survival for patients included in the 4 successive EORTC clinical trials on early stage Hodgkin disease.*

All patients were prospectively followed and detailed causes of death were reported as follows: *1)* Hodgkin disease progression, *2)* treatment-related death without evidence of active disease, *3)* second cancer, *4)* cardiac failure, *5)* other intercurrent deaths, and *6)* deaths from cause unspecified. Data were updated January 1, 1990. A death was considered as cardiac failure if history of cardiac disease has previously been reported, or if the cause of death was specified, possibly after an autopsy was performed. Sudden death from cause unspecified were classified in the sixth group.

The time at risk for death was computed from the start of initial treatment, and the date of death, date of last known vital status, or January 1, 1990, whichever came first. Mortality rates were compared between the population of patients with Hodgkin disease and the general population. The exposure to the risk was based on the accumulation of person-years (PY) of observation. The excess of deaths was computed as the difference between the observed number of deaths (O) and the expected number (E) divided by PY and multiplied by 100. Expected numbers were calculated with the use of mortality rates, for Belgium, France, and the Netherlands, specific for age, sex, and calendar year that have been published by the World Health Organization (World Health Statistics Annual, 1965-1988). The expected numbers were then pooled and compared with the observed ones giving an estimation of the standardized mortality ratio (SMR). SMR was defined as the ratio of O to E. Although biased, SMR is an easy parameter to use in estimating the excess mortality of a particular cohort (Hakulinen, 1982). In diseases like Hodgkin disease where deaths occur early in the follow-up, i.e. after progression or early relapse, the SMR is obviously over estimated. Nevertheless, the SMR was used since it easily permits comparisons between expected and observed survival curves. Confidence limits (CL) of SMRs and excess of death were calculated using exact Poisson probabilities (Berry, 1983; Breslow & Day, 1987). Expected and observed survival were calculated by the life-table method from the date of first therapy. Excess mortality was also estimated as the difference between expected and observed rates at 10 years and 15 years after first treatment start. Cumulative death rate was calculated as 1-S(t), where S(t) is the proportion of cases surviving at time t.

Results

The population study is composed of 1,650 patients, survival data being not available in 10 cases (0.6 %). The mean follow-up was 7.8 years (range 1-23 years) giving 12,863 person-years at risk (Table 2).

Three hundred twenty (19 %) deaths were observed, 1 to 22 years after the start of treatment. There were 169 (53 %) deaths related to disease progression, 26 (8 %) deaths related to treatment adverse effect without evidence of active Hodgkin disease, 46 (14 %) deaths related to second cancer, 56 (18 %) deaths due to intercurrent disease including 24 (8 %) cardiac failures, and 23 (7 %) deaths from unspecified causes. Early deaths, within 5 years since treatment start, occurred in 74 %, 73 %, 66 % and 61 % of those due to disease progression, treatment adverse effect, intercurrent disease (cardiac failure excluded) and cause unspecified, respectively. By contrast, second cancer deaths and cardiac failures occurred mostly (63% and 50%, respectively) in the 6-14 year interval after the start of treatment.

Toxic deaths occurred in 26 (1.6 %) patients, 12 being in first complete remission after extended field irradiation (6 cases) or combined modality treatment with MOPP (4 cases) or ABVD (2 cases). In addition, 3 patients died from acute or late complication after staging laparotomy. The other 11 patients died after having developed a relapse. Overall, toxic deaths were radiationy-related in 14 deaths (including 2 cases where patients were given ABVD) and chemotherapy in 9 cases. The other causes of death such as second cancer, cardiac failure and intercurrent deaths became more and more important as follow-up time increased. The 20-year specific survival rate was only 79 % compared to 94 % expected from the general population.

Table 2. Study population characteristics by sex

		Patients at risk	Person-years at risk
Overall population			
Males		949	7 272
Females		701	5 591
Total		1 650	12 863
Time since initial treatment start			
0-2 years	males	198	2 600
	females	137	1 948
3-5 years	males	245	1 858
	females	175	1 422
6-8 years	males	172	1 219
	females	143	927
9-11 years	males	136	782
	females	87	608
12-14 years	males	85	458
	females	72	366
15-17 years	males	57	244
	females	34	208
18+ years	males	56	111
	females	53	112

Second cancers were the main cause of intercurrent death with a 20-year cumulative rate of 9.3 %. Of the 46 second cancer deaths observed, 13 were from acute non-lymphocytic leukemia or myelodysplastic syndrome. Two of them occurred in patients in first complete remission initially treated by mantle-field irradiation (1 case) or total nodal irradiation (1 case). The other 11 cases were all previously treated with MOPP either as first line treatment (2 cases) or on the occasion of a relapse (7 cases). These 13 patients died 18 to 151 months after Hodgkin disease diagnosis (median 76 months) and 12 to 121 months post first course of MOPP (median 60 months). Non-Hodgkin lymphoma was the cause of death for 9 patients. They occurred 22 to 163 months after Hodgkin disease diagnosis (median 99 months) and in 6 cases, 22 to 161 months after a first course of MOPP chemotherapy was administered (median 64 months). Solid tumour deaths were observed in 24 patients of whom 8 were bronchus carcinomas, and 6 were localized in the digestive tract. All but one developed within a previous irradiated area as it was the case for an additional breast carcinoma. These 15 cases can be considered as radiation-related. Overall, solid tumour deaths occurred 18 to 184 months after Hodgkin disease diagnosis (median 112 months), mostly in patients in first complete remission (18 out of 24). Compared to expected survival, second cancer was responsible for a 7.3 % difference in the 20-year survival rate.

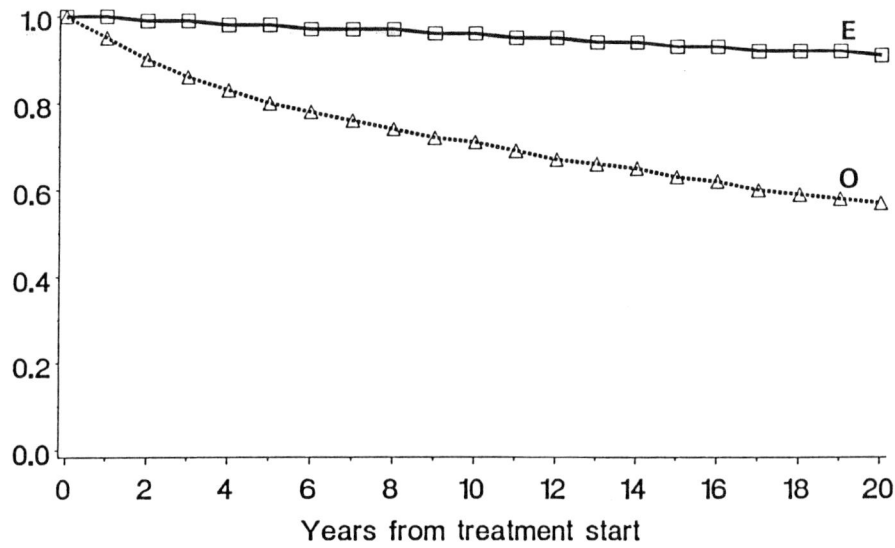

Figure 2. *Expected (solid line) and observed (dash line) survival for the cohort of EORTC patients overall (1964 - 1988; N = 1,650).*

Overall, the 10-year survival rate was 79 % and the 15-year survival rate was 69 %. Compared to the general population, the difference is equal to -18 % at 10 years and -26 % at 15 years (Figure 2) giving a SMR of 7.97 (95% CL 7.12-8.90, $p<0.001$) (Table 3). Deaths were more frequently observed in males than in females with a difference of -22 % and -13 % between expected and observed survival rates at 10 years, respectively. Overall the SMR was 7.31 (95% CL 6.38-8.33, $p<0.001$) in males and was 10.05 (95% CL 8.16-12.25, $p<0.001$) in females. Deaths were also more frequently observed in patients aged 40 years or more at Hodgkin disease diagnosis than in younger age groups. At 10 years, the differences between expected and observed survival rates were -29 % (SMR = 5.22, 95% CL 4.33-6.25; $p<0.001$) and -15% (SMR = 11.59, 95% CL 10.04-13.30; $p<0.001$) respectively.

The cumulative death rate (all causes) steadily increased with time. SMR by 3-year interval showed a significant increase in all the interval studied, even in the latest one (Table 4). These findings were also true whether survival was analyzed by sex or age.

The distribution of the deaths by cause shows that death related to Hodgkin disease or treatment-related occurred earlier (Figure 3). Annual mortality decreased with time from 2.5% during years 1 to 8 to less than 1% in year 9 and after. On the other hand there was a small increase in rate for death from other causes (from 0.5% in year 1 to 1.5% in year 15 and after) with a peak as high as 2.5% annually during years 8 to 12. This peak was clearly explained by an increase in mortality from second cancer or intercurrent disease during this interval (Figure 4). After 20 years, the main intercurrent causes of death were second cancer (cumulative death rate 9.3 %), followed by intercurrent death (cumulative death rate 7.6 %) and death from cardiac failure (cumulative death rate 5.7 %).

Cause-specific survival analysis was then performed under the following assumption. In the general population the annual risk of death from Hodgkin disease is very low compared to overall risk. For example, in 1979 in France, the risk of dying from Hodgkin disease for a male aged 35-44 years was 3.3/100.000 while it was 223.6/100,000 overall (World Health Statistics Annual, 1979). Consequently, the risk of dying from Hodgkin disease can be neglected, the excess of death being then estimated as the ratio of the observed number of deaths from other causes than disease progression and treatment-related to the expected number. In this procedure patients who died from disease progression or treatment-related death are censored at the time they died. Such an approach permits to estimate the excess mortality that can be related to Hodgkin disease itself and/or late treatment sequellae.

Table 3. Observed (O) and expected (E) deaths by cause for the entire cohort

	O	E	Excess of deaths	SMR	95 % C.L
All deaths	320	40.14	2.18	7.97 ***	7.12, 8.90
Deaths from Hodgkin disease	169				
Treatment-related deaths	26				
Deaths from second cancer	46	11.98	0.26	3.84 ***	2.81, 5.12
ANLL or MDS	13	0.49	0.10	26.53 ***	14.12, 45.37
NHL	9	0.41	0.07	21.95 ***	10.04, 41.66
ST	24	11.07	0.10	2.17 ***	1.39, 3.23
Intercurrent deaths	56				
Cardiac failure	24	2.78	0.17	8.63 ***	5.53, 12.85
Cause unspecified	23				
Intercurrent deaths + cause unspecified	79	28.16	0.40	2.81 ***	2.22, 3.50
Intercurrent deaths + cause unspecified + second cancer	125	40.14	0.66	3.11 ***	2.59, 3.71

SMR : ratio of O to E
ANLL : acute non-lymphocytic leukemia; MDP : myelodysplastic syndrome; NHL : non-Hodgkin lymphoma;
ST : solid tumours
Excess of deaths : (O-E) x 100/person-years at risk; p value : * < 0.05; ** < 0.01; *** < 0.001 (two-sided test)
95 % CL : 95 % confidence limits assuming a Poisson distribution for O

Overall, patients "cured" from Hodgkin disease had a relative risk of dying multiplied by 3.11 (95% CL 2.59-3.71; $p<0.001$) compared to the general population (Table 3). This risk differed whether specific causes were considered. It was 8.63 (95% CL 5.53-12.85; $p<0.001$) for cardiac failure, and was 3.84 (95% CL 2.81-5.12; $p<0.001$) for second cancer. The SMR also differed with sex, being higher in males (SMR = 3.06, 95% CL 2.47-3.75; $p<0.001$) than in females (SMR = 3.28, 95% CL 2.25-4.63; $p<0.001$). It also differed with age at diagnosis (SMR = 3.46, 95% CL 2.64-4.45, $p<0.001$, in patients younger than 40; SMR = 2.85, 95% CL 95% CL 2.20-3.64, $p<0.001$, in patients age 40 or more). Cardiac failures were observed in males only with an associated SMR of 10.17 (95% CL 6.52-15.13; $p<0.001$). Age was also a major risk for dying from cardiac failure but an excess in risk was observed both in patients younger than 40 (SMR = 15.38, 95% CL 7.38-28.29; $p<0.001$) and in older patients (SMR = 8.24, 95% CL 4.50-13.82; $p<0.001$). Overall, deaths from second cancer were more frequently

Table 4. Observed (O) and expected (E) deaths as a function of time since initial treatment start. **All causes of death.**

Time in years		0-2	3-5	6-8	9-11	12-14	15-17	18+
All patients	O	110	92	42	38	21	11	6
	E	12.59	9.90	6.91	4.84	2.95	1.82	1.12
	SMR	8.74***	9.29***	6.08***	7.85***	7.12***	6.04***	5.36**
	95% CL	7.18, 10.53	7.49, 11.40	4.38, 8.22	5.56, 10.78	4.41, 10.88	3.02, 10.81	1.96, 11.66
Males	O	69	70	30	29	12	9	3
	E	9.96	7.61	5.17	3.51	2.08	1.27	0.78
	SMR	6.93***	9.20***	5.80***	8.26***	5.77***	7.09***	3.85
	95% CL	5.39, 8.77	7.17, 11.62	3.91, 8.28	5.53, 11.87	2.98, 10.08	3.24, 13.45	0.79, 11.24
Females	O	41	22	12	9	9	2	3
	E	2.63	2.29	1.74	1.33	0.87	0.55	0.34
	SMR	15.59***	9.61***	6.90***	6.77***	10.34***	3.64	8.82**
	95% CL	11.19, 21.15	6.02, 14.55	3.56, 12.05	3.09, 12.84	4.73, 19.63	0.44, 13.13	1.82, 25.79
Age[a] <40 yrs	O	69	57	25	22	15	9	4
	E	4.61	3.84	3.03	2.36	1.66	1.12	0.73
	SMR	14.97***	14.84***	8.25***	9.32***	9.04***	8.04***	5.48*
	95% CL	11.64, 18.94	11.24, 19.23	5.34, 12.18	5.84, 14.11	5.06, 14.90	3.67, 15.25	1.51, 14.03
Age >40 yrs	O	41	35	17	16	6	2	2
	E	7.98	6.06	3.88	2.48	1.29	0.70	0.35
	SMR	5.14***	5.78***	4.38***	6.45***	4.65**	2.86	5.71
	95% CL	3.69, 6.97	4.02, 8.03	2.55, 7.02	3.69, 10.48	1.71, 10.12	0.35, 10.31	0.69, 20.63

SMR : ratio of O to E; 95 % CL : 95 % confidence limits assuming a Poisson distribution for O
(a) Age at Hodgkin's disease diagnosis; p value: * < 0.05; ** < 0.01; *** < 0.001 (two-sided test)

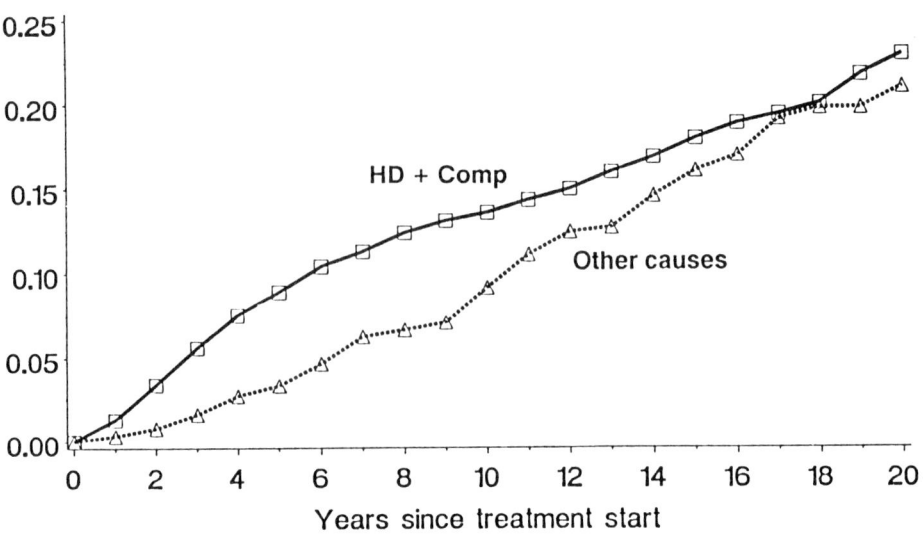

Figure 3. *Cumulative death rate by cause for the cohort of EORTC patients overall (1964 - 1988, N=1,650) (HD+Comp: disease progression or toxic death).*

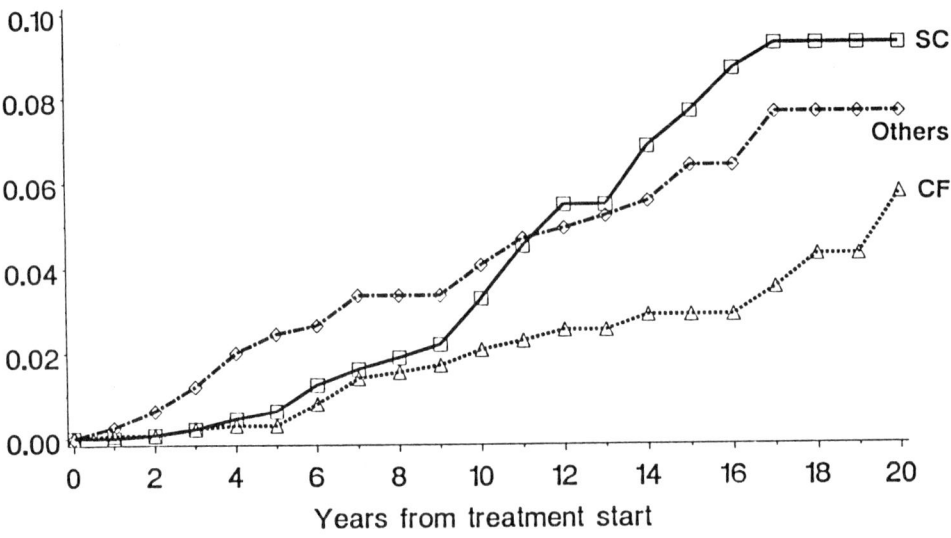

Figure 4. *Cumulative death rate by cause for the cohort of EORTC patients overall (1964 - 1988, N=1,650) (SC: second cancer; CF: cardiac failure; Others: other causes of death, Hodgkin-related death and toxic death excluded).*

Table 5. Observed (O) and expected (E) deaths as a function of time since initial treatment start. Deaths from intercurrent disease, cause unspecified and second cancer

Time in years		0-2	3-5	6-8	9-11	12-14	15-17	18+
All patients	O E SMR 95% CL	24 12.59 1.91** 1.22, 2.84	34 9.90 3.43*** 2.38, 4.80	20 6.91 2.89*** 1.77, 4.47	28 4.84 5.79*** 3.85, 8.36	11 2.95 3.73*** 1.86, 6.67	7 1.82 3.85** 1.54, 7.92	1 1.12 0.89 0.02, 4.97
Males	O E SMR 95% CL	15 9.96 1.51 0.84, 2.48	27 7.61 3.55*** 2.34, 5.16	15 5.17 2.90*** 1.82, 4.79	22 3.51 6.27*** 3.93, 9.49	7 2.08 3.37** 1.35, 6.93	6 1.27 4.72** 1.73, 10.28	1 0.78 1.28 0.03, 7.14
Females	O E SMR 95% CL	9 2.63 3.42** 1.57, 6.49	7 2.29 3.06** 1.23, 6.30	5 1.74 2.87 0.93, 6.71	6 1.33 4.51** 1.65, 9.82	4 0.87 4.60* 1.25, 11.77	1 0.55 1.82 0.05, 10.13	0 0.34 0 0, 10.85
Age[a] <40 yrs	O E SMR 95% CL	10 4.61 2.17* 1.04, 3.99	15 3.84 3.91*** 2.19, 6.44	9 3.03 2.97** 1.36, 5.64	14 2.36 5.93*** 3.24, 9.95	6 1.66 3.61* 1.33, 7.87	5 1.12 4.46* 1.45, 10.42	1 0.73 1.37 0.03, 7.63
Age>40 yrs	O E SMR 95% CL	14 7.98 1.75 0.96, 2.94	19 6.06 3.14*** 1.89, 4.90	11 3.88 2.84** 1.41, 5.07	14 2.48 5.65*** 3.08, 9.47	5 1.29 3.88* 1.26, 9.05	2 0.70 2.86 0.35, 10.31	0 0.35 0 0, 10.54

SMR: ratio of O to E; 95% CL: 95% confidence limits assuming a Poisson distribution for O
(a) Age at Hodgkin's disease diagnosis; p value: * < 0.05; ** < 0.01; *** < 0.001 (two-sided test)

observed in males than in females, the SMR being 4.17 (95% CL 2.92-5.77; p<0.001) and 3.00 (95% CL 1.44-5.52; p<0.001), respectively. While SMRs for acute leukaemia (SMR = 25.0, 95% CL 10.04-51.50, p<0.001; and SMR = 28.57, 95% CL 10.49-62.19, p<0.001; in younger and older patients, respectivelly) or non-Hodgkin lymphoma (SMR = 19.05, 95% CL 5.19-48.76, p<0.001; and SMR = 25.0, 95% CL 8.12-58.35, p<0.001; respectivelly) were similar in both age groups, the risk for dying from solid tumour was increased in the youngest only (SMR = 3.02, 95% CL 1.45-5.56; p<0.01).

SMRs by time intervals are given in Table 5 for all deaths not related to Hodgkin disease and in Table 6 for death from cardiac failure. When all intercurrent deaths were considered, a peak was observed during the 9-11 year interval, the SMR still being significantly increased after 15 years of follow-up (Table 5). Similar findings were observed when the analysis was made by sex or by age, although males and patients younger than 40 were at greater risk to die than females and older patients.

SMRs for second cancer increased with time, mostly in males, but independently with age at diagnosis. The evolution of the SMR by 3-year interval was : 0-2 years, 0.88 (95% CL 0.18-2.59, ns); 3-5 years, 3.93 (95% CL 1.96-7.03, p<0.001); 6-8 years, 3.40 (95% CL 1.36-7.0, p<0.01); 9-11 years, 10.13 (95% CL 5.78-16.44, p<0.001); 12-14 years, 6.12 (95% CL 2.24-13.33, p<0.001); 15-17 years, 4.69 (95% CL 0.97-13.70, ns). No second cancer were observed 18 years or more after Hodgkin disease diagnosis.

SMRs for intercurrent death other than second cancer and cardiac failure were significantly increased but at a constant level until year 11. The evolution of the SMR by 3-year interval was : 0-2 years, 2.28 (95% CL 1.41-3.49, p<0.001); 3-5 years, 3.24 (95% CL 2.05-4.86, p<0.001); 6-8 years, 2.68 (95% CL 1.43-4.58, p<0.01); 9-11 years, 3.68 (95% CL 1.90-6.43, p<0.001); 12-14 years, 2.54 (95% CL 0.82-5.92, ns); 15-17 years, 3.39 (95% CL 0.92-8.69, ns); and 18 years or more, 1.47 (95% CL 0.04-8.19, ns).It was more important in males than in females, while age did not appear to play a major role.

At last, fatal cardiac failures were observed in males only. They occurred mostly from year 3 to year 11 post treatment start with a peak during the 6-8 year interval. When analysing by age, the SMRs were two-times higher in younger than in older patients (Table 6). Cause-specific survival for cardiac failure death shows that the difference in the 20-year survival rate was 5.7 % compared to the general population, a figure that is certainly underestimated since patients who died from "sudden death of unspecified cause" were not considered in the analysis.

Discussion

During the last three decades, survival after Hodgkin disease diagnosis has dramatically improved. It was generally the consequence of a better use of the radiation therapy technique, the description and use of new chemotherapy regimen like MOPP and the use of combined modality treatments. The recognition of adverse treatment side-effects also encouraged investigators to better adapt the treatment strategy to the *a priori* patients prognosis using pronostic factors. This was the attitude of the EORTC Lymphoma Group which always favoured radiation therapy as first line treatment, reserving aggressive chemotherapy for patients with unfavourable initial prognostic features or for relapsing patients (Tubiana et al., 1989). The hope was then that more patients will be cured from Hodgkin disease and that long-term survival will not very much differ from that of the general population. Obviously this goal was not reached, although better overall long-term survival is observed in trials H2, H5 and H6 compared to H1 trial (Figure 1). Nevertheless, the long-term overall mortality observed in these series is still much higher than that expected from the general population matched for age, sex, calendar period and country (Figure 2).

Table 6. Observed (O) and expected (E) deaths as a function of time since initial treatment start. Deaths from cardiac failure

Time in years		0-2	3-5	6-8	9-11	12-14	15-17	18+
All patients	O E SMR 95% CL	3 0.78 3.85 0.79, 11.24	6 0.68 8.82*** 3.24, 19.21	7 0.48 14.58*** 5.85, 30.04	4 0.37 10.81*** 2.95, 27.68	1 0.22 4.55 0.12, 25.32	2 0.13 15.38* 1.86, 55.57	1 0.10 10.0 0.25, 55.70
Males	O E SMR 95% CL	3 0.70 4.29 0.88, 12.52	6 0.58 10.34*** 3.79, 22.52	7 0.40 17.50*** 7.03, 36.05	4 0.30 13.33*** 3.63, 34.13	1 0.18 5.56 0.14, 30.94	2 0.12 16.67* 2.02, 69.21	1 0.08 12.50 0.32, 69.63
Age[a] <40 yrs	O E SMR 95% CL	0 0.10 0 0, 36.90	2 0.12 16.67* 2.02, 60.21	3 0.12 25.0*** 5.16, 73.06	2 0.12 16.67* 2.02, 60.21	0 0.08 0 0, 46.13	2 0.06 33.33** 4.04, 120	1 0.04 25.0 0.63, 139
Age >40 yrs	O E SMR 95% CL	3 0.60 5.0* 1.03, 14.61	4 0.46 8.70** 2.37, 22.26	4 0.28 14.29*** 3.89, 36.57	2 0.18 11.11* 1.35, 40.14	1 0.10 10.0 0.25, 55.70	0 0.06 0 0, 61.50	0 0.04 0 0, 92.25

SMR : ratio of O to E; 95 % CL : 95 % confidence limits assuming a Poisson distribution for O
(a) Age at Hodgkin's disease diagnosis; p value: * < 0.05; ** < 0.01; *** < 0.001 (two-sided test)

Irradiation technique as well as chemotherapies and combined modality treatments have changed since the first trial H1 was initiated. These changes involved the machines, the energy and the fractionation in radiation therapy, as radiations fields were better delimited. On the other hand the total dose delivered in radiation fields was kept constant to 40 Gy. Aggressive therapies, such as combination of radiotherapy and MOPP or ABVD, have first been used as second line treatment in the early seventies, or as part of initial treatment thereafter. This attitude resulted in a large decrease in the proportion of deaths from Hodgkin disease progression and in an increase in death from other causes. Among the latter, the SMR corresponding to cardiac failure and second cancer remained approximately constant over years. Thus the ratio of the number of deaths from disease progression or treatment related to that of other causes was 3.41 in the H1 trial, 0.88 in the H2 trial, 0.82 in the H5 trial, and 2.5 in the H6 trial but, in this last series, the mean follow-up is only 3.6 years.

Deaths not related to Hodgkin disease became more and more frequent as follow-up time increased. In the EORTC series the SMR was significantly increased (Table 3). This is to be compared to what was observed in the database [*Workshop Statistical Report, Table X-8a*] where the relative risk of death was only 2.07 ($p<0.001$). Although a large proportion of the patients from the EORTC series were included in the database, the results are not completely superimposable demonstrating the superiority of collecting information prospectively.

In the EORTC series, none of the patients treated with vinblastine and procarbazine or vinblastine alone as adjuvant chemotherapy (N=234) or with combined modality treatment included ABVD (N=166) developped an acute leukemia which confirm previous studies (Amadori et al.,1983; Valagussa et al., 1988). Overall, the excess mortality from non-Hodgkin lymphoma was similar to that observed from acute leukemia suggesting a direct relationship to treatment. Solid tumour deaths occurred mostly after 10 years post treatment initiation, which is in accordance with a longer delay before development of second solid tumour compared to that for acute leukemia or non-Hodgkin lymphoma as it was previously stated (Nelson et al., 1981; Boivin et al., 1984; Schull, 1984; Green & Wilson, 1985; Storm & Prener, 1985; Rubin et al., 1986; Tucker et al., 1988).

Although numerously limited second cancer deaths have a great impact on physicians psyche. Second cancer patients had a very poor outcome. Overall 15 acute leukemias or myelodysplastic syndromes were observed, and 13 patients died mostly within few months after the diagnosis was made; thirteen non-Hodgkin lymphomas were observed, 9 patients died from their second cancer and one patient died from cardiac failure; fifty-six patients developed a second solid tumour of whom 24 died from second cancer progression and 6 died from intercurrent disease. Thus in the EORTC series, cause specific survival for second cancer is likely to reflect at least two-thirds of the second cancer incidence in the outcome of Hodgkin disease patients.

The last cause of death that was analyzed concerns cardiac failures. Twenty-four cardiac failure deaths were observed in male patients with a SMR of 10.17 ($p<0.001$). Cardiac failure death, i.e. ischaemic heart disease (ICD-9 270 and 279) is very unexpected in a population in which the mean age is 31 years. For example, the annual death rate was, in 1979 in France, 67.0/100,000 in males aged 45-54 years (World Health Statistics Annual, 1979). In the present series, significant increases in relative risk were observed in patients younger and older than 40 years of age at Hodgkin disease diagnosis. These findings, although they appear contradictory to previously published data, are not surprising (Van Rijswijk et al., 1987; Hancock et al., 1988). There is little evidence in the literature that irradiation induces cardiac dysfunction. Most series studied were small in numbers or in follow-up time, presented only case-reports, or were conducted in retrospect.

In a retrospective study on 957 patients, Boivin and Hutchison reported a SMR of death from coronary heart disease to 2.1 (95% CL 1.0-3.9, $p<0.05$) in heart irradiated patients while the risk was not increased in patients who were not irradiated (SMR = 1.5, 95% CL 0.6-3.1) (Boivin & Hutchison, 1982). Similarly Cosset and coworkers reported a 3.9 % 10-year cumulative incidence of acute myocardial infarction in 499 patients treated by mantle irradiation at the Institut Gustave-Roussy while no cases of acute myocardial infarction were observed among 138 patients who were not irradiated (Cosset et al., 1990). In the EORTC series, the 24 patients who died from cardiac failure were heart irradiated as part of the mantle-field technique. Since the series comprises upper-diaphragmatic early stage Hodgkin disease patients for whom initial therapy involved systematic mediastinal irradiation, no comparison can be made with unirradiated patients. Total dose delivered to the mediastinum and upper part of the heart was 40 Gy with very few exceptions. In addition, 21 patients were in first complete remission at the time the cardiac failure occurred. Also the radiation dose was delivered in most cases using 5 fractions a week or more (16 cases out of 24). These findings confirm that of the Institut Gustave Roussy where the myocardial infarction risk was not found to be related to dose nor to fraction size (Cosset et al., 1990).

Although the risk for first recurrence and death from Hodgkin disease appears very small 10 years or more after initial therapy (only 6 patients relapsed in the EORTC series and 19 patients died from disease progression or treatment-related death), risks for intercurrent death are not negligible. The observation that deaths from second cancer, cardiac failure, and other intercurrent diseases are still increasing 10 years after first therapy clearly shows that patients, even "cured" from Hodgkin disease, are at higher risk for death than expected from the general population. This finding should encourage carefull evaluation of patients at regular intervals even a long time after the patients have been successfully treated for Hodgkin disease.

References

Amadori, S., et al. (1983): Acute promyelocytic leukemia following ABVD (doxorubicin, bleomycin, vinblastine and dacarbazine) and radiotherapy for Hodgkin's disease. *Cancer Treat. Rep.* 67, 603-604.

Berry, G. (1983): The analysis of mortality by the subject-years method. *Biometrics* 39, 173-184.

Boivin, J.F. & Hutchison, G.B. (1982): Coronary heart mortality after irradiation for Hodgkin's disease. *Cancer* 49, 2470-2475.

Boivin, J.F., et al. (1984): Second primary cancers following treatment of Hodgkin's disease. *JNCI* 72, 233-241.

Breslow, N.E. & Day, N.E. (1987): *Statistical methods in cancer research*. Vol. 2. The design and analysis of cohort studies. IARC scientific publication n° 82. Lyon: International Agency for Research on Cancer.

Carde, P., et al. (1988): Clinical stages I and II Hodgkin's disease : A specifically tailored therapy according to prognostic factors. *J. Clin. Oncol.* 6, 239-252.

Carde, P., et al. (1990): H6 EORTC controlled trials in clinical stage I-II Hodgkin's disease. First report on the results of a randomized staging laparotomy in favorable cases and of a randomized MOPP versus ABVD combined radiotherapy modality in unfavorable cases. *Proc. Am. Soc. Clin. Oncol.* (in press).

Cosset, J.M., et al. (1990): Pericarditis and myocardial infarctions after Hodgkin disease therapy at the Institut Gustave Roussy. *Int. J. Radiat. Oncol. Biol. Phys.* (in press).

Greene, M.H. & Wilson, J. (1985): Second cancer following lymphatic and hematopoietic cancers in Connecticut, 1935-1982. *NCI Monogr.* 68, 191-217.

Hakulinen, T. (1982): Cancer survival corrected for heterogeneity in patient withdrawal. *Biometrics* 38, 933-942.

Hancock, S.L., et al. (1988): Intercurrent death after Hodgkin disease Therapy in radiotherapy and adjuvant MOPP trials. *Ann. Int. Med.* 109, 183-189.

Hayat, M. (1972): A randomized study of irradiation and vinblastine in clinical stages I and II of Hodgkin's disease. Preliminary results. *Eur. J. Cancer* 8, 353-362.

Henry-Amar, M. (1988): Quantitative risk of seconf cancer in patients in first complete remission from early stages of Hodgkin's disease. *NCI Monogr.* 6, 65-72.

Nelson, D.F., et al. (1981): Second malignant neoplasms and solid tumors in patients treated for Hodgkin's disease with radiotherapy and chemotherapy. *Cancer* 48, 2386-2393.
Rubin, Ph., et al. (1986): Hodgkin's disease : Is there a price for successful treatment? A 25-year experience. *Int. J. Radiat. Oncol. Biol. Phys.* 12, 153-166.
Schull, W.J. (1984): Atomic bomb survivors : Pattern of cancer risk. In *Radiation carcinogenesis : Epidemiology and biological significance*, ed. J.D. Boice, Jr. & J.F. Fraumeni, Jr., pp. 21-36. New-York: Raven Press.
Storm, H.H. & Prener, A. (1985): Second cancer following lymphatic and hematopoietic cancers in Denmark, 1943-1980. *NCI Monogr.* 68, 389-409.
Tubiana, M., et al. (1981): Five-year results of the EORTC randomized study of splenectomy and spleen irradiation in clinical stages I and II of Hodgkin's disease. *Eur. J. Cancer* 17, 355-363.
Tubiana, M., et al. (1989): Toward comprehensive management tailored to prognostic factors of patients with clinical stages I and II in Hodgkin's disease. The EORTC Lymphoma Group controlled clinical trials : 1964-1987. *Blood* 73, 47-56.
Tucker, M.A., et al. (1988): Risk of second cancers after treatment for Hodgkin's disease. *N. Engl. J. Med.* 318, 76-81.
Valagussa, P., et al. (1988): Hodgkin's disease and second malignancies. *Proc. Am. Assoc. Clin. Oncol.* 7, 227.
Van Rijswijk, R.E.N., et al. (1987): Major complications and causes of death in patients treated for Hodgkin's disease. *J. Clin. Oncol.* 5, 1624-1633.
World Health Statistics Annual (1965 to 1988). Ed. World Health Organization. Geneva: World Health Organization.

Appendix

Chairmen of the EORTC Lymphoma Cooperative group : M. Tubiana (1964-1967), K. Breur (1967-1969), B. van der Werf-Messing (1969-1972), J. Henry (1973-1975), J. Abbatucci (1975-1977), J.M.V. Burgers (1977-1980), M. Hayat (1980-1982), R. Somers (1983-1987), and J.H. Meerwaldt (1987-present). *Statistician :* M. Henry-Amar. *Data manager :* N. Dupouy. *Scientific secretaries :* A. Laugier (1964-1972), M. Hayat (1972-1975), M. Urbajtel (1975-1977), E. van der Schueren (1977-1980), P. Carde (1980-1985), J.H. Meerwaldt (1985-1987), and J. Thomas (1987-present). *Committee of pathologists :* M.J.J.T. Bogman, J. Bosq, B. Caillou, N. Duplay, R. Gérard-Marchant, E. Halkin, P. van Heerde, R. Heiman, P.M. Kluin, A.M. Mandard, R. Menon, M.F. Prins, J.A.M. van Unnik, L. Vrints, and C. de Wolf-Peeters. *Committee of radiologists :* C. Bergiron, J.L. Chassard, W. Feremans, R.W. Kropholler, J. Masselot, and P. Markovits.

Cooperating centers in The Netherlands : Antoni van Leeuwenhoek Ziekenhuis, Amsterdam *(J.M.V. Burgers and R. Somers)*; University Hospital, Leiden *(E.M. Noordijk)*; St. Radboud Academic Hospital, Nijmegen *(C. Haanen, B.E. de Pauw, and D. Wagener)*; Rotterdamsch-Radiotherapeutisch Instituut, Rotterdam *(J.H. Meerwaldt, M. Qasim, W. Sizoo, and B. van der Werf-Messing)*; Ziekenhuis Leyenburg, The Hague *(H. Kerkhofs)*; University Hospital, Utrecht *(J.G. Nyssen, H. van Peperzeel, and L. Verdonck)*; Stichting Ignatius-Ziekenhuis, Breda *(A.C.J.M. Holdrinet)*; Catharina Ziekenhuis, Eindhoven *(W.P.M. Breed)*; and Acad. Ziekenhuis, Rotterdam *(J. Michiels)*. *Cooperating centers in Belgium :* Institut Jules Bordet, Brussels *(D. Bron, J. Henry, J. Lustmann-Maréchal, R. Reinier)*; Centre René Goffin, La Louvière *(J.C. Goffin)*; Hôpital de Bavière, Liège *(R. Lemaire)*; Acad. Ziekenhuis St. Rafaël, Leuven *(J. Thomas and E. van der Schueren)*; and Ziekenhuis St Jan, Brugge *(A. Van Hoof and A. Louwagie)*. *Cooperating centers in Italy :* Instituto di Radiologia, Universita di Firenze *(L. Cionini and G. De Giuli)*; and Ospedale San Giovanni, Torino *(R. Musella)*. *Cooperating centers in France :* Fondation Bergonié, Bordeaux *(B. Hoerni and C. Lagarde)*; Centre François-Baclesse, Caen *(J.S. Abbatucci and A. Tanguy)*; Centre G.F. Leclerc, Dijon *(P. Fargeot and J.C. Horiot)*; Centre Léon-Bérard, Lyon *(J. Papillon and L. Revol)*; Centre Antoine-Lacassagne, Nice *(C. Lalanne, M. Schneider, and A. Thyss)*; Hôtel-Dieu, Paris *(M.C. Blanc and R. Zittoun)*; Institut Jean-Godinot, Reims *(A. Cattan)*; Centre Henri-Becquerel, Rouen *(R. Le Fur, M. Monconduit, and H. Piguet)*; Centre Cl. Regaud, Toulouse *(F. Rigal-Huguet)*; Institut Gustave-Roussy, Villejuif *(J.L. Amiel, P. Carde, J.M. Cosset, M. Hayat, and M. Tubiana)*; and Institut de Cancérologie et d'Immunogénétique, Hôpital Paul Brousse, Villejuif *(G. Mathé and J.L. Misset)*. *Cooperating center in West Germany :* Universitat zu Köln *(H. Sack)*.

WORKSHOP STATISTICAL REPORT

RAPPORT STATISTIQUE

Treatment strategy in Hodgkin's disease. Eds R. Somers, M. Henry-Amar, J.H. Meerwaldt, P. Carde. Colloque INSERM/John Libbey Eurotext Ltd. © 1990, Vol. 196, pp. 169-418.

Workshop statistical report

M. Henry-Amar[1], in collaboration with D.M. Aeppli[2], J. Anderson[3], S. Ashley[4], F. Bonichon[5], R.S. Cox[6], S.J. Dahlberg[7], G. DeBoer[8], D.O. Dixon[9], P.G. Gobbi[10], W. Gregory[11], D. Hasenclever[12], M. Löffler[12], V. Pompe Kirn[13], M.T. Santarelli[14], L. Specht[15], R. Swindell[16], B. Vaughan Hudson[17]

1 *Institut Gustave-Roussy, 94805 Villejuif, France;* 2 *University of Minnesota Hospital and Clinic, Minneapolis MN 55455, USA;* 3 *Harvard School of Public Health, Boston MA 02115, USA;* 4 *The Royal Marsden Hospital, Sutton, Surrey SM2 5PT, England;* 5 *Fondation Bergonié, 33076 Bordeaux, France;* 6 *Stanford University Medical Center, Stanford CA 94305, USA;* 7 *Fred Hutchinson Cancer Research Center, Seattle WA 98104-2092, USA;* 8 *The Princess Margaret Hospital, Toronto, Canada M4X 1K9;* 9 *University of Texas, M.D. Anderson Cancer Center, Houston TX 77030, USA;* 10 *Università di Pavia, Clinica Medica II, 27100 Pavia, Italy;* 11 *Guy's Hospital, London SE1 9RT, England;* 12 *Medizinische Universitätsklinik 1, 5000 Köln, Federal Republic of Germany;* 13 *Cancer Registry of Slovenia, 61000 Ljubljana, Yougoslavia;* 14 *Pacheco de Melo 3081, (1425) Capital Federal, Buenos Aires, Argentina;* 15 *Rigshospitalet, 2100 Copenhagen, Denmark;* 16 *Christie Hospital & Holt Radium Institute, Manchester M20 9BX, England;* 17 *The Middlesex Hospital, London W1N 8AA, England*

Foreword

This present report has been achieved with the help of most of the Workshop participants, clinicians and biostatisticians, who provided data. Prior to the Workshop, three meetings were organized in order to *i)* define a common data collection form (July 1988 Paris meeting), and *ii)* to review the first draft of the statistical report (May 1989 Paris and San Francisco meetings). The Paris meetings involved European biostatisticians and clinicians who reported from the Workshop during the Friday Symposium. At the San Francisco meeting there were American biostatisticians and clinicians from various countries. During these two 1989 meetings the first draft of the statistical report was extensively discussed and suggestions for additional analyses made. Moreover some other participants have sent comments and suggestions which were taken into consideration whenever possible.

Nevertheless this report does not include some relevant information. The main reason is the lack of time for statistical analysis before the Workshop held. To remedy that, an international association involving most of the contributors was founded in January 1990 and named "International Database on Hodgkin's Disease" (IDHD). Its aim is to *i)* study data already collected; *ii)* provide information to design future collaborative studies; and *iii)* to collect data from other sources. There is no doubt that the tremendous effort made for the first time in collecting such an amount of data will be rewarded by results from future studies.

Avant-propos

Le rapport qui suit a été élaboré avec l'aide de la plupart des participants à la réunion de travail, cliniciens et bio-statisticiens ayant collaboré à la base de données. Avant la réunion de Juin, trois réunions ont été organisées afin i) de rédiger le questionnaire de recueil des données (Paris, Juillet 1988), et ii) de relire le premier rapport statistique (Paris, Mai 1989, et San Francisco, Mai 1989). Les bio-statisticiens européens ainsi que les cliniciens rapporteurs de la réunion de travail au cours du Symposium ont participé à la réunion organisée à Paris. La réunion de San Francisco a réuni des cliniciens et des bio-statisticiens de plusieurs pays. Au cours de ces deux réunions, le premier rapport statistique a été entièrement revu et critiqué, et des analyses complémentaires ont été suggérées. En outre, plusieurs participants avaient adressé des commentaires détaillés. Ainsi la plupart des suggestions ont pu être prises en considération dans l'analyse finale.

Néanmoins certaines informations qui pourraient sembler pertinentes à certains ne sont pas incluses dans ce rapport. La raison principale en est le manque de temps nécessaire à l'analyse. Afin de combler cette lacune, une association internationale à laquelle a adhéré la grande majorité des participants a été créée en Janvier 1990. Cette association, intitulée "International Database on Hodgkin's Disease" (IDHD), s'est donnée pour but i) d'analyser en détails les données recueillies; ii) de fournir des informations susceptibles de servir à l'élaboration de nouvelles études; et iii) de rassembler des données en provenance d'autres équipes. Il ne fait aucun doute que l'effort très important qui a été déployé pour réaliser, pour la première fois, une telle base de données sera récompensé par les résultats qu'on en pourra tirer dans le future.

Part I - *Première partie*

INTRODUCTION AND STATISTICAL CONSIDERATIONS

INTRODUCTION ET CONSIDERATIONS STATISTIQUES

Introduction

The aim of this study was to assess the relevance of parameters commonly used in the management of Hodgkin disease patients with respect to treatment response and prognosis. Since the use of such parameters differs from one country to another, and, within one country, from one institution or cooperative group to another, it appeared at the time the study was initiated that the greater the recruitment was, the more general the conclusions could be assessed.

Most of the largest institutions or cooperative groups in the western world with extensive experience in the management of Hodgkin disease were approached in 1988. Of them 20 agreed to participate in sending data to be analyzed in a common statistical design. Baseline data collected were intentionally restricted to those that had previously been reported to be of prognostic importance. Also data concerning treatment were simplified. Radiation therapy was categorized into three groups, i.e. localized radiotherapy, regional radiotherapy, or extended radiotherapy. Although the type of chemotherapy administered (drugs used, single or in association like MOPP, ABVD, etc.) and the number of cycles given were recorded, it was necessary that patients be subgrouped into several broad categories. In particular, no attempt was made to analyze the influence of treatment intensity (i.e. number of cycles given) on response, relapse-free survival, survival, or second cancer risk. It must be stated that treatment recorded was most often the treatment *given*. Consequently a patient who progressed during first line therapy appears to be under treated. It must also be emphasized that data collected do not always come from randomized clinical trials, although most of the cases were treated according to protocols. The date of initiation of therapy was recorded (in particular, staging laparotomy and splenectomy were considered as treatment) but not the date on which the patient was considered in complete remission. Consequently, in all cases time at risk started from the date of start of initial therapy. Data concerning relapses were also restricted to the date of relapse occurrence, and the type of relapse (i.e. nodal or extranodal, within a previous irradiated field or not, previously involved (true relapse) or not (extension). Detailed relapse therapy was not recorded. For survival analysis, the following items were recorded: date of last known vital status, vital status (dead or alive), cause of death in 5 broad categories (related to Hodgkin disease, treatment related without evidence of Hodgkin disease, second malignancy, intercurrent, or cause unspecified), and clinical status if the patient was alive (in complete remission, or with active disease). Finally, information collected on second cancer was the date of diagnosis, the type of second cancer (acute leukemia or myelodysplastic syndrome, non-Hodgkin lymphoma, and solid tumor), and, in case of solid tumor, the site where it developed, its localization in relation to previously irradiated fields, and the tumor type using the ICD-O code published by the World Health Organization (World Health Organization, 1976).

Overall, 14,702 cases of Hodgkin disease patients treated from the early sixties to 1987 have been enrolled in the study. After checking the data, 387 cases (2.6%) had to be excluded for the following reasons:
- The protocol design clearly stated that only patients 15 years of age and older could be included. Thus cases aged 14 or younger were excluded.
- Also cases for whom discrepancies were noticed between date of initial start of therapy and that of possible events were excluded when they could not be corrected in time.

After these exclusions, the series was composed of 14,315 cases, 20.9% of clinical stage (CS) I, 42.6% of CS II, 23.4% of CS III, and 13.1% of CS IV (Table I). Previous publications in which patient characteristics, treatments, and results were described are listed after the present report.

Description

The present report consists of ten parts, namely:
- Part I: Introduction and statistical considerations;
- Part II: Description of pretreatment patient characteristics;
- Part III: Description of initial treatment types;
- Part IV: Relationships between pretreatment clinical and biological parameters;
- Part V: Prognostic study of laparotomy findings;
- Part VI: Analysis of response to initial therapy;
- Part VII: Prognostic study of relapse-free survival;
- Part VIII: Prognostic study of overall survival;
- Part IX: Study of second cancer risk;
- Part X: Long term survival and study of causes of death.

Each chapter is composed of a limited text describing the results, tables, and figures.

Statistical considerations

Data were analysed on a 785 VAX/VMS computer with the use of a specific database management program (PIGAS) developed at the Institut Gustave-Roussy Department of Medical Statistics (Wartelle et al., 1983). For analysis, the programs 3S, LR, 1L and 2L of BMDP Statistical Software were used (Dixon et al., 1987a). Curves were plotted using the actuarial method.

No statistical test was applied when comparing the distributions since the large amount of cases would always induce a statistical significance. Correlations between biological parameters were assessed using nonparametric models: the Kruskal-Wallis one-way analysis of variance and the Spearman rank correlation test, as appropriate.

A stepwise multiple logistic regression model was applied when studying the relationships between initial characteristics and laparotomy findings, or between initial characteristics and response to initial treatment. In the latter, the type of initial treatment was not taken into consideration in the analysis since the purpose of the study was only the assessment of prognostic parameters on several endpoints. The logistic regression model is a multiplicative regression model for analysis of data predicting for a success E, expressed as Prob.(E). The regression model has the following form:

$$\text{Prob.}(E) = \exp(a + b_1 z_1 + ... + b_i z_i + ... + b_n z_n)/[1 + \exp(a + b_1 z_1 + ... + b_i z_i + ... + b_n z_n)]$$

where α is the intercept (constant) and z_i the patient baseline characteristics. Thus the success of an event is being predicted by the predictor variables z_1 to z_i, each variable z_i being multiplied by a corresponding regression coefficient b_i (Kleinbaum et al., 1982).

Relapse-free survival analysis was restricted to cases who achieved a complete remission following initial therapy. Time at risk for relapse was defined as time from date of start of initial therapy to date of first relapse, date of last known vital status, or January 1, 1989, whichever came first. Date of first treatment was chosen instead of that at which the patients were considered in complete remission since this last information was not available. Patients who died from other causes than Hodgkin's disease were considered as censored data (Dixon et al., 1987b). In a first step, the influence of each variable considered separately on relapse-free survival was analyzed with the use of the logrank test (for heterogeneity) stratified on treatment period (i.e. 1960s, 1970s, and 1980s), initial treatment type (i.e. radiation therapy alone, chemotherapy alone, or combined modalities) and staging laparotomy (i.e. performed or not performed). Then the stepwise proportional hazards model (Cox model) was used to assess the independent prognostic value of each variable included in the model (Cox, 1972).

The regression model proposed by Cox is a multiplicative regression model for analysis of censored survival data. The regression model has the following form:

$$\lambda(t,z) = \lambda_0(t) \exp(b_1 z_1 + ... + b_i z_i + ... + b_n z_n)$$

where $\lambda(t,z)$ is the hazard at time t after a defined starting point (date of first treatment) for an individual with variables (characteristics) $z = (z_1 ... z_i ... z_n)$. Thus $\lambda(t,z)$ is being dependent on or explained or predicted by $\lambda_0(t)$, the so-called underlying hazard at time t, and the predictor variables z_1 to z_n (recorded at time zero), each variable z_i being multiplied by a corresponding regression coefficient b_i (Christensen, 1987; see also *Introduction* by Gregory & Löffler, present issue).

Each analysis was performed with stratification on the three variables mentioned above. When biological factors were studied, they were only considered one at the time otherwise the numbers of patients for whom all data were available decreased in such a proportion that no conclusion could reasonably be considered. When categorical ordered variables were analyzed, an overall chi-square was used.

The same approach was used in the overall survival analysis. All cases with data available were used. Time at risk for survival was defined as time from date of start of initial therapy to date of last known vital status, or January 1, 1989, whichever came first. The Cox model with a stepwise approach was used in which only initial patient characteristics were included in the model. Again, each analysis was performed with stratification on type of initial therapy given, period of treatment, and staging laparotomy. In both analyses three end points were used in succession. The first one was "death from any causes"; the second was "death from Hodgkin disease" where patients who died from other causes than Hodgkin disease were censored; and the third one was "death from other causes than Hodgkin disease" where patients who died from Hodgkin disease or treatment side-effects were censored.

In the analyses mentioned above, biological parameters were never included at the first step in the model since data were missing in so many cases that it would have restricted the analysis to less than one-half of the patients. Therefore, these variables were included in the models one at a time and their influence on the results previously obtained carefully analysed (see below).

The second cancer risk was estimated using two different approaches. The first one compares observed (0) numbers of second cancers to those expected (E) from the general population. Expected numbers were calculated, country by country, with the use of cancer incidence specific for age, sex, and calendar year that have been published by the International Agency for Research on Cancer (Waterhouse et al., 1982). The expected numbers were then pooled and compared with the observed ones. The equality of O and E was tested by assuming the Poisson distribution for O. A two-sided test was used. In the second approach, the quantification of the relationship between the time of occurrence of second cancer and concomitant variables was calculated using the Cox model.

For long term survival analysis and that of causes of death, the same approach as that described above was used. Expected numbers were calculated, country by country, with the use of mortality rates specific for age, sex, and calendar year that have been published by the World Health Organization (World Health Statistics Annual, 1965 to 1985). The expected numbers were then pooled and compared with the observed ones giving an estimation of the standardized mortality ratio (SMR). Although biased the SMR is an easy parameter to be used in estimating the excess mortality of a particular cohort. In diseases like Hodgkin disease where deaths occur early in the follow-up, i.e. after progression or early relapse in patients with advanced stages, the SMR is obviously overestimated. Nevertheless the SMR was used since it easily permits comparisons between expected and observed survival curves.

In all stepwise regressions a significance level of 0.01 was used.

Curves, all crude, were plotted using the actuarial method. Cumulative incidence was calculated as 1-S(t), where S(t) is the proportion of cases surviving, or free of relapse, or free of second cancer, at time t. The instantaneous death rate, or cancer incidence rate, was estimated at the midpoint of each interval using the BMDP program 1L (Dixon et al., 1987a).

Table I. Distribution of patients included by center and clinical stage

	I	II	III	IV	Total
B.N.L.I. (UK)	623	837	615	463	2,538
EORTC Lymphoma Group	593	987	110	111	1,801
Stanford Univ Med Center (USA)	186	886	481	110	1,663
Princess Margaret Hospital (CDN)	228	430	229	160	1,047
Southwest Oncology Group (USA)	72	274	334	255	935
MD Anderson Cancer Center (USA)	190	422	157	101	872*
Royal Marsden Hosp, London (UK)	214	357	159	0	730
St Bartholomew's Hosp, London (UK)	129	231	146	104	610
G.A.T.L.A. (ARG)	64	163	250	114	591
Universita di Pavia (I)	41	180	222	86	532*
Joint Center for Radiat Therap (USA)	133	303	83	3	522
Finsen Institute (DK)	122	182	88	86	478
Fondation Bergonié, Bordeaux (F)	117	179	116	29	441
German Hodgkin Study Group (FRG)	29	140	144	87	400
Groupe Pierre et Marie Curie (F)	105	204	26	0	335
Christie Hosp, Manchester (UK)	38	76	58	127	301*
The Institute of Oncology Ljubljana (YU)	47	64	71	18	200
Univ Minnesota Health Sc Center (USA)	39	135	7	0	181
University of Nebraska (USA)	10	32	28	8	78
Yale University (USA)	6	23	23	8	60
TOTAL :	2,986	6,105	3,347	1,870	14,315

* *including patients for whom stage is not available (n = 7)*

Part II - *Deuxième partie*

PRETREATMENT PATIENT CHARACTERISTICS
DESCRIPTION BY CLINICAL AND PATHOLOGICAL STAGE

Caractéristiques pré-cliniques
Description en fonction du stade clinique et du stade pathologique

Pretreatment patient characteristics

In this chapter, the distribution of each characteristic is given first by clinical stage (Table II-1), and second by pathological stage for those patients who underwent a staging laparotomy (Table II-2). The distribution of missing data varies somewhat from one characteristic to another. Number of major lymph node areas involved is missing in 11.7% of cases. When there was mediastinum involvement, information on bulky disease was missing in 56% of cases.

Biological parameters were very often unreported: 39.4% for erythrocyte sedimentation rate (ESR), 87.2% for serum LDH, 46.3% for alkaline phosphatase, 62.7% for serum albumin, and 26.6% for hemoglobin.

Distributions of ESR and hemoglobin were similar when compared between centres. They could therefore be used as quantitative data in the following analyses. The distribution of the other three biological parameters were so different between centres that it appeared necessary to use surrogate variables defined as quartiles calculated within each centre.

Table II-1. Initial patient characteristics by clinical stage

	CS I (n=2,986)	CS II (n=6,105)	CS III (n=3,347)	CS IV (n=1,870)
SEX M/F (sex ratio)	2,014/972 (2.07)	3,213/2,891 (1.11)	2,239/1,108 (2.02)	1,201/669 (1.80)
AGE at diagnosis Mean (SD)	36.6 (15.1)	31.4 (12.9)	35.7 (15.1)	39.1 (16.3)
15-19 (%)	273 (9.2)	879 (14.4)	356 (10.7)	176 (9.4)
20-29	952 (32.0)	2,460 (40.4)	1,110 (33.2)	503 (26.9)
30-39	675 (22.7)	1,465 (24.0)	732 (21.9)	381 (20.4)
40-49	441 (14.0)	654 (10.7)	460 (13.8)	280 (15.0)
50-59	328 (11.0)	355 (5.8)	357 (10.7)	252 (13.5)
60-69	218 (7.3)	201 (3.3)	239 (7.2)	197 (10.5)
70-79	77 (2.6)	63 (1.0)	82 (2.5)	71 (3.8)
80 +	12 (0.4)	20 (0.3)	6 (0.2)	9 (0.5)
unspecified	10	8	5	1
range	15-88	15-93	15-87	15-85
SEX and AGE Mean (SD)				
Males	36.7 (14.6)	32.4 (12.8)	36.1 (14.7)	39.9 (15.5)
Females	36.4 (16.1)	30.4 (12.9)	34.9 (15.7)	37.8 (17.6)
PRESENTATION				
above diaphragm (%)	2,789 (95.0)	5,532 (93.4)	–	265 (14.2)
below	147 (5.0)	394 (6.6)	–	47 (2.5)
above and below	–	–	3,114 (100)	1,554 (83.3)
unspecified	50	179	233	4

Table II-1. Initial patient characteristics by clinical stage (continued)

		CS I (n=2,986)	CS II (n=6,105)	CS III (n=3,347)	CS IV (n=1,870)
NUMBER OF MAJOR LYMPH NODE AREAS INVOLVED	(%)				
0		—	—	—	212 (11.4)
1		2,639 (100)	—	—	324 (17.4)
2		—	2,657 (49.0)	461 (17.0)	299 (16.1)
3		—	1,653 (30.5)	598 (22.1)	283 (15.2)
4		—	712 (13.1)	548 (20.2)	228 (12.3)
5		—	328 (6.1)	412 (15.2)	173 (9.3)
6		—	50 (0.9)	295 (10.9)	142 (7.6)
7		—	17 (0.3)	173 (6.4)	98 (5.3)
8		—	2	126 (4.6)	46 (2.5)
9		—	—	69 (2.5)	34 (1.8)
10+		—	—	28 (1.0)	22 (1.2)
unspecified		345	686	637	9
MEDIASTINAL INVOLVEMENT	(%)	334 (11.2)	4,207 (69.1)	1,848 (55.7)	1,094 (59.2)
bulky mediastinum	(%)	59/186 (31.7)	717/2,092 (34.3)	188/677 (27.8)	124/339 (36.6)
LOCALIZED EXTRANODAL INVOLVEMENT	(%)	251 (8.4)	748 (12.3)	238 (7.1)	350 (18.7)
BONE MARROW INVOLVEMENT *	(%)	4 (0.1)	21 (0.3)	66 (2.0)	432 (23.1)
PRESENCE OF SYSTEMIC SYMPTOMS	(%)	277 (9.3)	1,697 (27.8)	1,779 (53.3)	1,449 (77.9)

* PS IV after laparotomy (CS I to III)

Table II-1. Initial patient characteristics by clinical stage (continued)

	CS I (n=2,986)	CS II (n=6,105)	CS III (n=3,347)	CS IV (n=1,870)
ERYTHROCYTE SEDIMENTATION RATE (mm/1st hour)				
Mean (SD)	22.1 (24.6)	41.5 (32.1)	51.6 (37.4)	65.6 (38.1)
(%)				
1 - 9	818 (40.6)	572 (16.1)	237 (12.5)	82 (6.9)
10-19	444 (22.0)	537 (15.1)	222 (11.7)	73 (6.1)
20-29	240 (11.9)	416 (11.7)	182 (9.6)	94 (7.9)
30-39	142 (7.0)	441 (12.4)	194 (10.2)	96 (8.0)
40-49	110 (5.5)	355 (10.0)	174 (9.2)	92 (7.7)
50-59	87 (4.3)	297 (8.4)	168 (8.9)	108 (9.0)
60-69	48 (2.4)	243 (6.8)	159 (8.4)	109 (9.1)
70-79	30 (1.5)	181 (5.1)	106 (5.6)	112 (9.4)
80-89	39 (1.9)	149 (4.2)	103 (5.4)	86 (7.2)
90-99	21 (1.0)	107 (3.0)	99 (5.2)	74 (6.2)
100 +	38 (1.9)	254 (7.2)	255 (13.4)	271 (22.6)
unspecified	969	2,552	1,448	673
range	1-170	1-163	1-185	1-161
SERUM L.D.H.				
< 25th percentile (%)	75 (34.3)	148 (21.6)	102 (30.0)	81 (18.6)
25 - 75th	134 (61.2)	427 (62.4)	268 (55.1)	212 (48.6)
> 75th	10 (4.5)	109 (16.0)	116 (23.9)	143 (32.8)
unspecified	2,767	5,421	2,861	1,434

Table II-1. Initial patient characteristics by clinical stage (continued)

	CS I (n=2,986)	CS II (n=6,105)	CS III (n=3,347)	CS IV (n=1,870)
ALKALINE PHOSPHATASE				
< 25th percentile (%)	460 (30.2)	679 (21.0)	364 (20.7)	149 (12.8)
25 - 75th	852 (55.8)	1,868 (57.9)	961 (54.0)	435 (37.4)
< 75th	213 (14.0)	680 (21.1)	446 (25.3)	580 (49.8)
unspecified	1,461	2,878	1,586	706
SERUM ALBUMIN				
< 25th percentile (%)	56 (5.2)	289 (14.7)	310 (23.0)	431 (46.4)
25 - 75th	523 (48.1)	1,049 (43.3)	738 (54.7)	402 (43.3)
> 75th	508 (46.7)	631 (32.0)	300 (22.3)	96 (10.3)
unspecified	1,899	4,136	1,999	941
HEMOGLOBIN ($mmol.L^{-1}$)				
Mean (SD)	8.7 (1.0)	8.1 (1.1)	7.8 (1.2)	7.1 (1.3)
(%)				
< 4.0	2 (0.1)	8 (0.2)	6 (0.2)	19 (1.2)
4.0- 4.9	7 (0.3)	20 (0.5)	24 (1.0)	71 (4.3)
5.0- 5.9	15 (0.7)	87 (2.1)	148 (5.8)	182 (11.0)
6.0- 6.9	87 (4.0)	432 (10.5)	455 (18.0)	462 (28.0)
7.0- 7.9	333 (15.2)	1,138 (27.6)	677 (26.7)	449 (27.2)
8.0- 8.9	779 (35.5)	1,473 (35.8)	744 (29.4)	335 (20.3)
9.0- 9.9	777 (35.4)	800 (19.4)	405 (16.0)	113 (6.9)
10.0-10.9	185 (8.4)	142 (3.5)	69 (2.7)	14 (0.9)
>11.0	12 (0.6)	15 (0.4)	6 (0.2)	4 (0.2)
unspecified	789	1,989	813	221
range	3.2-12.5	3.2-12.4	2.3-11.7	2.9-13.0

Table II-1. Initial patient characteristics by clinical stage (continued)

	CS I (n=2,986)	CS II (n=6,105)	CS III (n=3,347)	CS IV (n=1,870)
DATE OF INITIATION OF THERAPY				
1960 - 1969 (%)	260 (8.7)	546 (8.9)	246 (7.4)	62 (3.3)
1970 - 1979	1,681 (56.3)	3,413 (55.9)	1,950 (58.3)	1,054 (56.4)
1980 - 1988	1,045 (35.0)	2,145 (35.1)	1,151 (34.3)	754 (40.3)
HISTOLOGICAL TYPE LP (%)*	455 (15.4)	299 (4.9)	193 (5.8)	64 (3.4)
NS	1,400 (42.2)	4,424 (72.8)	1,841 (55.0)	1,017 (54.5)
MC	1,021 (34.4)	1,137 (18.7)	1,079 (32.3)	538 (28.8)
LD	30 (1.0)	114 (1.9)	124 (3.7)	160 (8.6)
unclassified	59 (2.0)	103 (1.7)	109 (3.3)	87 (4.7)
unspecified	21	28	1	4

* LP = *lymphocytic predominance*
NS = *nodular sclerosing*
MC = *mixed cellularity*
LD = *lymphocytic depleted*

Table II-1. Initial patient characteristics by clinical stage (continued)

			CS I (n=2,986)	CS II (n=6,105)	CS III (n=3,347)	CS IV (n=1,870)
HISTOLOGICAL TYPE						
LP	1960 - 1969	(%)	41 (16.9)	38 (7.3)	21 (8.5)	2 (3.2)
	1970 - 1979		245 (14.6)	178 (5.2)	121 (6.2)	42 (4.0)
	1980 - 1988		169 (16.2)	83 (3.9)	51 (4.4)	20 (2.7)
NS	1960 - 1969	(%)	110 (45.3)	323 (61.8)	115 (46.8)	21 (33.9)
	1970 - 1979		800 (47.7)	2,473 (72.3)	1,055 (54.1)	536 (50.9)
	1980 - 1988		490 (47.0)	1,628 (76.0)	671 (58.4)	460 (61.3)
MC	1960 - 1969	(%)	79 (32.5)	123 (23.5)	86 (35.0)	25 (40.3)
	1970 - 1979		588 (35.0)	654 (19.2)	644 (33.0)	326 (30.9)
	1980 - 1988		354 (33.9)	360 (16.8)	349 (30.4)	187 (24.9)
LD	1960 - 1969	(%)	6 (2.5)	19 (3.6)	9 (3.7)	10 (16.1)
	1970 - 1979		21 (1.3)	72 (2.1)	83 (4.3)	109 (10.3)
	1980 - 1988		3 (0.3)	23 (1.1)	32 (2.8)	41 (5.5)
Unclassified	1960 - 1969	(%)	7 (2.9)	20 (3.8)	15 (6.1)	4 (6.5)
	1970 - 1979		25 (1.5)	34 (1.0)	47 (2.4)	41 (3.9)
	1980 - 1988		27 (2.6)	49 (2.3)	47 (4.1)	42 (5.6)

LP = lymphocytic predominance
NS = nodular sclerosing
MC = mixed cellularity
LD = lymphocytic depleted

Table II-2. Initial patient characteristics by pathological stage

	PS I (n=1,071)	PS II (n=2,362)	PS III (n=2,164)	PS IV (n= 496)
SEX M/F (sex ratio)	700/371 (1.89)	1,197/1,165 (1.03)	1,456/708 (2.06)	358/138 (2.59)
AGE at diagnosis Mean (SD)	33.2 (12.3)	29.2 (10.7)	31.0 (12.4)	38.0 (14.8)
15-19 (%)	109 (10.3)	366 (15.5)	305 (14.1)	49 (9.9)
20-29	380 (35.8)	1,079 (45.6)	931 (43.1)	131 (26.4)
30-39	289 (27.2)	564 (23.9)	457 (21.1)	108 (21.8)
40-49	148 (13.9)	207 (8.8)	241 (11.1)	76 (15.3)
50-59	96 (9.0)	99 (4.2)	153 (7.1)	82 (16.5)
60-69	37 (3.5)	46 (1.9)	67 (3.1)	44 (8.9)
70-79	3 (0.3)	1 (0.1)	7 (0.3)	6 (1.2)
80 +	0	0	1 (<0.1)	0
unspecified	9	–	2	–
range	15-74	15-76	15-91	15-78
SEX and AGE Mean (SD)				
Males	33.3 (12.3)	30.2 (10.9)	31.5 (12.3)	38.8 (14.4)
Females	32.8 (12.3)	28.1 (10.3)	30.1 (12.4)	35.9 (15.8)
PRESENTATION				
above diaphragm (%)	952 (89.5)	1,989 (84.2)	1,218 (56.3)	104 (21.0)
below	59 (5.5)	155 (6.6)	4 (0.2)	22 (4.4)
above and below	53 (5.0)	218 (9.2)	942 (43.5)	369 (74.6)
unspecified	7	–	–	1

Table II-2. Initial patient characteristics by pathological stage (continued)

	PS I (n=1,071)	PS II (n=2,362)	PS III (n=2,164)	PS IV (n= 496)
NUMBER OF MAJOR LYMPH NODE AREAS INVOLVED (%)				
0	1 (0.1)	1 (<0.1)	7 (0.3)	42 (8.8)
1	999 (93.6)	21 (0.9)	347 (16.1)	93 (18.8)
2	57 (5.3)	1,200 (50.8)	728 (33.8)	128 (25.9)
3	4 (0.4)	636 (26.9)	401 (18.6)	72 (14.6)
4	4 (0.4)	313 (13.3)	287 (13.3)	49 (9.9)
5+	2 (0.2)	191 (8.1)	385 (17.9)	110 (22.3)
unspecified	4	—	9	2
MEDIASTINAL INVOLVEMENT (%)	120 (11.3)	1,741 (73.8)	1,115 (51.8)	225 (45.7)
bulky mediastinum (%)	22/63 (34.0)	257/728 (35.3)	101/367 (27.5)	5/ 28 (20.0)
LOCALIZED EXTRANODAL INVOLVEMENT (%)	92 (8.6)	297 (12.6)	161 (7.4)	133 (26.7)
BONE MARROW * INVOLVEMENT (%)	88 (10.8)	211 (10.7)	155 (8.7)	106 (28.2)
PRESENCE OF SYSTEMIC SYMPTOMS (%)	73 (6.8)	554 (23.5)	713 (33.0)	320 (64.5)

* PS IV after laparotomy (CS I to III)

Table II-2. Initial patient characteristics by pathological stage (continued)

	PS I (n=1,071)	PS II (n=2,362)	PS III (n=2,164)	PS IV (n= 496)
ERYTHROCYTE SEDIMENTATION RATE (mm/1st hour)				
Mean (SD)	17.7 (19.8)	36.1 (29.2)	38.9 (33.2)	49.7 (37.5)
(%)				
1- 9	277 (47.1)	180 (19.1)	211 (22.0)	33 (15.0)
10-19	125 (21.3)	150 (16.0)	150 (15.7)	25 (11.0)
20-29	76 (12.9)	125 (13.3)	103 (10.8)	23 (11.0)
30-39	36 (6.1)	128 (13.6)	97 (10.1)	15 (7.0)
40-49	25 (4.3)	106 (11.3)	88 (9.2)	24 (11.0)
50-59	22 (3.7)	75 (8.0)	71 (7.4)	23 (11.0)
60-69	10 (1.7)	52 (5.5)	52 (5.4)	14 (6.0)
70-79	3 (0.5)	36 (3.8)	38 (4.0)	15 (7.0)
80-89	6 (1.0)	26 (2.8)	48 (5.0)	10 (5.0)
90-99	4 (0.7)	19 (2.0)	31 (3.2)	9 (4.0)
100 +	4 (0.7)	43 (4.6)	69 (7.2)	27 (12.0)
unspecified	483	1,422	1,206	278
SERUM L.D.H.				
< 25th percentile (%)	43 (34.0)	74 (20.0)	99 (27.0)	17 (18.0)
25 - 75th	73 (58.0)	235 (63.0)	203 (55.0)	47 (50.0)
> 75th	9 (8.0)	62 (17.0)	65 (18.0)	30 (32.0)
unspecified	946	1,991	1,797	402

Table II-2. Initial patient characteristics by pathological stage (continued)

	PS I (n=1,071)	PS II (n=2,362)	PS III (n=2,164)	PS IV (n= 496)
ALKALINE PHOSPHATASE				
< 25th percentile (%)	188 (37.5)	259 (26.2)	278 (27.5)	40 (17.0)
25 - 75th	259 (51.6)	555 (56.2)	533 (53.0)	108 (45.0)
< 75th	55 (10.9)	173 (17.6)	196 (19.5)	92 (38.0)
unspecified	569	1,375	1,159	256
SERUM ALBUMIN				
<25th percentile (%)	19 (5.1)	97 (13.9)	82 (13.1)	57 (31.0)
25 - 75th	148 (39.9)	380 (54.4)	341 (54.3)	90 (50.0)
> 75th	204 (55.0)	221 (31.7)	205 (32.6)	35 (19.0)
unspecified	700	1,664	1,536	314
HEMOGLOBIN $(mmol.L^{-1})$				
Mean (SD)	8.7 (1.0)	8.1 (1.1)	8.2 (1.2)	7.6 (1.3)
(%)				
< 4.0	1 (0.1)	2 (0.1)	4 (0.3)	39 (0.8)
4.0- 4.9	4 (0.5)	6 (0.4)	7 (0.5)	6 (1.6)
5.0- 5.9	7 (0.9)	31 (2.2)	53 (3.6)	26 (7.0)
6.0- 6.9	24 (3.2)	148 (10.6)	176 (11.8)	80 (21.7)
7.0- 7.9	115 (15.2)	467 (33.4)	349 (23.4)	101 (27.4)
8.0- 8.9	279 (36.9)	418 (29.9)	476 (31.9)	96 (26.0)
9.0- 9.9	259 (34.3)	287 (20.5)	349 (23.4)	49 (13.3)
10.0-10.9	63 (8.3)	40 (2.9)	71 (4.8)	7 (1.9)
>11.0	4 (0.5)	1 (0.1)	5 (0.3)	1 (0.3)
unspecified	315	962	674	127

Table II-2. Initial patient characteristics by pathological stage (continued)

	PS I (n=1,071)	PS II (n=2,362)	PS III (n=2,164)	PS IV (n= 496)
DATE OF INITIATION OF THERAPY				
1960 - 1969 (%)	9 (0.8)	64 (2.7)	45 (2.0)	11 (2.2)
1970 - 1979	765 (71.4)	1,683 (71.3)	1,570 (72.6)	379 (76.4)
1980 - 1988	297 (27.8)	615 (26.0)	549 (25.4)	106 (21.4)
HISTOLOGICAL TYPE LP (%)*	185 (17.3)	105 (4.4)	116 (5.4)	15 (3.0)
NS	547 (51.3)	1,901 (80.5)	1,348 (62.3)	262 (52.9)
MC	314 (29.4)	307 (13.0)	602 (27.8)	172 (34.7)
LD	4 (0.4)	20 (0.8)	38 (1.8)	26 (5.2)
unclassified	17 (1.6)	29 (1.2)	60 (2.8)	21 (4.2)
unspecified	4	-	-	-

* *LP* = *lymphocytic predominance*
NS = *nodular sclerosing*
MC = *mixed cellularity*
LD = *lymphocytic depleted*

Part III - *Troisième partie*

INITIAL TREATMENT TYPES
DESCRIPTION BY CLINICAL STAGE

TRAITEMENTS INITIAUX
DESCRIPTION EN FONCTION DU STADE CLINIQUE

Initial treatments given

Overall initial treatment was not specified in only 21 cases (0.1%). In addition, 77 patients (0.5%) were not treated (58 cases) or treated with surgery alone (19 cases) (Table III-1).

Initial treatments by pathological stage are listed in Table III-2.

A summary is also given by clinical stage in tables III-3 to III-6.

Types of chemotherapy used are given in Table III-7. Single (or bi-)agent chemotherapies and combination chemotherapies were then grouped into three categories each. When combination chemotherapy was used, MOPP-like regimens were given in more than 80% of the cases, including in most cases 4 to 6 cycles.

Table III-1. Description of initial therapy given by clinical stage

	CS I (n=2,986)	CS II (n=6,105)	CS III (n=3,347)	CS IV (n=1,870)
LAPAROTOMY and SPLENECTOMY (%)	1,386 (46.4)	3,077 (50.4)	1,318 (39.4)	327 (17.5)
Pathological stage I (%)	1,017 (73.4)	—	53 (4.0)	1 (4.9)
II	—	2,124 (69.0)	221 (16.8)	16 (4.9)
III	340 (24.6)	877 (28.6)	899 (68.2)	45 (13.8)
IV	27 (1.9)	72 (2.3)	139 (10.5)	262 (80.1)
unspecified	2	4	6	3
RADIOTHERAPY (%)	2,819 (94.4)	5,489 (89.9)	1,985 (59.3)	513 (27.4)
IF irradiation *	737 (26.1)	812 (16.3)	542 (27.3)	227 (44.2)
Mantle or inverted Y RT	1,153 (40.9)	2,236 (40.7)	223 (11.2)	97 (18.9)
STNI or TNI **	876 (31.1)	2,301 (41.9)	1,188 (59.8)	135 (26.3)
Unspecified	53	60	32	54
CHEMOTHERAPY (%)	1,015 (34.0)	2,995 (54.6)	2,694 (80.5)	1,816 (97.1)
Single or bi-agent CT (%)	122 (12.0)	170 (5.7)	57 (2.1)	30 (1.7)
Combination CT ***	891 (87.8)	2,825 (94.3)	2,637 (97.9)	1,786 (98.3)
- MOPP-like	792	2,435	2,290	1,470
- ADM containing	65	181	29	10
- Alternated	27	186	299	267
- Others	7	23	19	39
Unspecified	2	—	—	—

* involved field irradiation
** subtotal or total nodal irradiation
*** including patients with both single or bi-agent and combination CT (ie CS II, 10 patients; CS III, 19 patients; CS IV, 13 patients)

Table III-1. Description of initial therapy given by clinical stage (continued)

	CS I (n=2,986)	CS II (n=6,105)	CS III (n=3,347)	CS IV (n=1,870)
OVERALL TREATMENT				
no Lap (*), RT (%)	989 (33.1)	1,252 (20.5)	214 (6.4)	24 (1.3)
Lap + RT	960 (32.2)	1,831 (30.0)	427 (12.8)	13 (0.7)
no Lap + RT + single or bi-agent CT	96 (3.2)	139 (2.3)	49 (1.5)	15 (0.8)
no Lap + RT + combination CT	450 (15.1) **	1,282 (21.0)	732 (21.9)	391 (20.9)
Lap + RT + single or bi-agent CT	25 (0.8)	27 (0.4)	3	–
Lap + RT + Combination CT	299 (10.0)	958 (15.7)	560 (16.7)	70 (3.7)
no Lap, single or bi-agent CT	1	4	5	15 (0.8)
no Lap, combination CT	51 (1.7)	326 (5.3)	1,013 (30.3)	1,075 (57.5)
Lap + single or bi-agent CT	–	–		
Lap + combination CT	92 (3.1)	253 (4.1)	327 (9.8)	242 (12.9)
no treatment/surgery alone	13/9	18/8	12/0	15/2
unspecified	1	7	5	8

* Lap = staging laparotomy and splenectomy
** including 2 patients with type of CT unspecified

Table III-2. Description of initial therapy given by pathological stage

	PS I (n=1,071)	PS II (n=2,362)	PS III (n=2,164)	PS IV (n=496)
RADIOTHERAPY (%)	1,059 (98.9)	2,303 (97.5)	1,663 (76.8)	138 (27.8)
IF irradiation	194 (18.3)	310 (13.5)	234 (14.1)	34 (25.0)
Mantle or inverted Y RT	427 (40.3)	728 (31.6)	185 (11.1)	26 (19.0)
STNI or TNI	432 (40.8)	1,254 (54.5)	1,188 (71.4)	71 (51.0)
Unspecified	6	11	56	7
CHEMOTHERAPY (%)	146 (13.8)	633 (26.8)	1,591 (73.5)	484 (97.4)
Single or bi-agent CT (%)	20 (14.0)	17 (2.7)	17 (1.1)	1 (0.2)
Combination CT*	126 (86.0)	616 (97.3)	1,574 (98.9)	483 (99.8)
OVERALL TREATMENT				
RT alone (%)	915 (85.4)	1,727 (73.1)	573 (26.5)	11 (2.2)
. IF irradiation	130	148	2	1
. M or inverted Y RT	374	501	10	2
. STNI or TNI	405	1,069	557	8
Single or bi-agent CT	–	–	–	–
Combination CT	2 (0.2)	57 (2.4)	501 (23.2)	357 (72.0)
RT + single or bi-agent CT	20 (1.9)	17 (0.7)	17 (0.8)	1 (0.2)
RT + Combination CT	124 (11.6)	559 (23.7)	1,073 (49.6)	126 (25.4)
. MOPP-like	123	528	990	100
. ADM Containing	0	1	16	1
. Alternated	1	26	63	20
Others	10 (0.9)	2 (0.1)	–	1 (0.2)

* including 2 patients with type of CT unspecified

Table III-3. Description of initial therapy given in clinical stage I by time period

	1960-69 (n=260)	1970-79 (n=1,681)	1980+ (n=1,045)
LAPAROTOMY and SPLENECTOMY (%)	9 (4.0)	965 (57.4)	412 (39.4)
Pathological stage I (%)	7	721 (74.7)	289 (70.1)
III	1	228 (23.6)	112 (27.2)
IV	0	16 (1.7)	10 (2.4)
unspecified	1	0	1
RADIOTHERAPY (%)	256 (98.0)	1,599 (95.1)	964 (92.2)
IF irradiation	47 (18.0)	388 (24.3)	302 (31.3)
Mantle or inverted Y RT	194 (76.0)	585 (36.6)	374 (38.8)
STNI or TNI	14 (5.0)	591 (37.0)	271 (28.1)
Unspecified	1	35	17
CHEMOTHERAPY (%)	62 (24.0)	540 (32.1)	413 (39.5)
Single or bi-agent CT (%)	58 (94.0)	61 (11.3)	3 (0.7)
Combination CT*	3 (5.0)	478 (88.5)	410 (99.3)
Unspecified	1 (1.0)	1	0
OVERALL TREATMENT			
no Lap, RT (%)	185 (71.0)	456 (27.1)	348 (33.3)
Lap + RT	9 (4.0)	672 (40.0)	279 (26.7)
no Lap+RT+single/bi-agent CT	58 (22.0)	35 (2.1)	3
no Lap + RT + combination CT	3	204 (12.1)	243 (23.3)
Lap + RT + single/bi-agent CT	0	25 (1.5)	0
Lap + RT + combination CT	0	208 (12.4)	91 (8.7)
no Lap, single or bi-agent CT	0	1	0
no Lap, combination CT	0	15 (0.9)	36 (3.4)
Lap + single or bi-agent CT	0	0	0
Lap + combination CT	0	52 (3.1)	40 (3.8)
no treatment/surgery alone	4/0	6/7	3/2
unspecified	1	0	0

* including patients with both single or bi-agent and combination CT

Table III-4. Description of initial therapy given in clinical stage II by time period

	1960-69 (n=546)	1970-79 (n=3,413)	1980+ (n=2,145)
LAPAROTOMY and SPLENECTOMY (%)	78 (14.3)	2,141 (62.7)	858 (40.0)
Pathological stage			
II (%)	58 (74.0)	1,493 (69.7)	574 (66.9)
III	18 (23.0)	600 (28.0)	261 (30.4)
IV	2	46 (2.1)	21 (2.4)
unspecified	0	2	2
RADIOTHERAPY (%)	533 (97.6)	3,145 (92.1)	1,811 (84.4)
IF irradiation	83 (15.6)	517 (16.4)	292 (16.1)
Mantle or inverted Y RT	303 (56.8)	1,055 (33.5)	878 (48.5)
STNI or TNI	147 (27.6)	1,545 (49.1)	609 (33.6)
Unspecified	0	28	32
CHEMOTHERAPY (%)	111 (20.3)	1,539 (45.1)	1,345 (62.7)
Single or bi-agent CT (%)	76 (68.0)	88 (5.7)	6
Combination CT*	35 (32.0)	1,451 (94.3)	1,339 (99.6)
Unspecified	0	0	0
OVERALL TREATMENT			
no Lap, RT (%)	365 (66.8)	580 (17.0)	307 (12.7)
Lap + RT	58 (10.6)	1,287 (37.7)	486 (20.1)
no Lap+RT+single/bi-agent CT	75 (13.7)	58 (1.7)	6
no Lap + RT + combination CT	17 (3.1)	528 (15.5)	737 (30.5)
Lap + RT + single/bi-agent CT	1	26 (0.8)	0
Lap + RT + combination CT	17 (3.1)	666 (19.5)	275 (11.4)
no Lap, single or bi-agent CT	0	4	0
no Lap, combination CT	0	101 (3.0)	225 (9.3)
Lap + single or bi-agent CT	0	0	0
Lap + combination CT	1	156 (4.6)	96 (4.0)
no treatment/surgery alone	11/1	1/6	6/1
unspecified	0	0	0

* *including patients with both single or bi-agent and combination CT*

Table III-5. Description of initial therapy given in clinical stage III by time period

	1960-69 (n=246)	1970-79 (n=1,950)	1980+ (n=1,151)
LAPAROTOMY and SPLENECTOMY (%)	37 (15.0)	1,029 (52.8)	252 (21.9)
Pathological stage I (%)	2	45 (4.4)	6
II	5	170 (16.5)	46 (18.0)
III	25 (68.0)	703 (68.3)	171 (68.0)
IV	4	108 (10.5)	27 (11.0)
unspecified	1	3	2
RADIOTHERAPY (%)	214 (87.0)	1,248 (64.0)	523 (45.4)
IF irradiation	26 (12.0)	287 (23.0)	229 (43.8)
Mantle or inverted Y RT	30 (14.0)	125 (10.0)	68 (13.0)
STNI or TNI	156 (73.0)	824 (66.0)	208 (39.8)
Unspecified	2	12	18
CHEMOTHERAPY (%)	86 (35.0)	1,529 (78.4)	1,079 (93.7)
Single or bi-agent CT (%)	17 (20.0)	38 (2.5)	2
Combination CT*	69 (80.0)	1,491 (97.5)	1,077 (99.8)
Unspecified	0	0	0
OVERALL TREATMENT			
no Lap, RT (%)	126 (51.0)	86 (4.4)	2
Lap + RT	26 (11.0)	333 (17.1)	68 (5.9)
no Lap+RT+single/bi-agent CT	13 (5.0)	34 (1.7)	2
no Lap + RT + combination CT	39 (16.0)	345 (17.7)	348 (30.2)
Lap + RT + single/bi-agent CT	1	2	0
Lap + RT + combination CT	9 (4.0)	448 (23.0)	103 (8.9)
no Lap, single or bi-agent CT	3	2	0
no Lap, combination CT	20 (8.0)	452 (23.2)	541 (47.0)
Lap + single or bi-agent CT	0	0	0
Lap + combination CT	1	246 (12.6)	80 (7.0)
no treatment/surgery alone	8/0	2/0	2/0
unspecified	0	0	5

* *including patients with both single or bi-agent and combination CT*

Table III-6. Description of initial therapy given in clinical stage IV by time period

	1960-69 (n=62)	1970-79 (n=1,054)	1980+ (n=754)
LAPAROTOMY and SPLENECTOMY (%)	7 (11.0)	259 (24.6)	61 (8.1)
Pathological stage I (%)	0	0	1
II	1	14 (6.0)	1
III	1	37 (14.0)	7
IV	5	208 (80.0)	49 (80.0)
unspecified	0	0	3
RADIOTHERAPY (%)	33 (53.0)	254 (24.1)	226 (30.0)
IF irradiation	12 (36.0)	93 (37.0)	122 (54.0)
Mantle or inverted Y RT	7	44 (17.0)	46 (20.0)
STNI or TNI	14 (42.0)	99 (39.0)	22 (10.0)
Unspecified	0	18	36
CHEMOTHERAPY (%)	43 (69.0)	1,029 (97.6)	744 (98.7)
Single or bi-agent CT (%)	7	21 (2.0)	2
Combination CT*	36 (84.0)	1,008 (98.0)	742 (99.7)
Unspecified	0	0	0
OVERALL TREATMENT			
no Lap, RT (%)	14 (23.0)	7	3
Lap + RT	2	10 (0.9)	1
no Lap+RT+single/bi-agent CT	5	10 (0.9)	0
no Lap + RT + combination CT	10 (16.0)	178 (16.9)	203 (26.9)
Lap + RT + single/bi-agent CT	0	0	0
Lap + RT + combination CT	2	49 (4.6)	19 (2.5)
no Lap, single or bi-agent CT	2	11 (1.0)	2
no Lap, combination CT	21 (34.0)	580 (55.0)	474 (62.9)
Lap + single or bi-agent CT	0	0	0
Lap + combination CT	3	200 (19.0)	39 (5.2)
no treatment/surgery alone	3/0	8/0	4/2
unspecified	1	1	7

* *including patients with both single or bi-agent and combination CT*

Table III-7. Description of initial chemotherapy administered by clinical stage (continued)

	CS I (n=2,986)	CS II (n=6,105)	CS III (n=3,347)	CS IV (n=1,870)
COMBINATION CHEMOTHERAPY *				
number of patients (%)	891 (29.8)	2,825 (46.3)	2,637 (78.8)	1,786 (95.5)
1. MOPP-like regimen				
MOPP	516 (57.9)	1,568 (55.5)	1,236 (46.9)	760 (42.6)
C-MOPP	8	37 (1.3)	75 (2.8)	40 (2.2)
Bleo-MOPP	4	6	18 (0.7)	71 (4.0)
PAVe	4	57 (2.0)	64 (2.4)	10
LOPP	33 (3.7)	132 (4.7)	278 (10.5)	197 (11.0)
BOPP	1	7	18 (0.7)	10
COPP	5	26 (0.9)	23 (0.9)	10
MVPP	64 (7.2)	207 (7.3)	188 (7.1)	194 (10.9)
CVPP	151 (16.9)	384 (13.6)	376 (14.3)	173 (9.7)
LVPP	6	6	4	2
2. Adriamycin containing regimen				
ABVD	42 (4.7)	156 (5.5)	16 (0.6)	5
EBVD	23 (2.6)	23 (0.8)	9	2
miscellaneous	–	2	4	3

* see glossary in appendix

Table III-7. Description of initial chemotherapy administered by clinical stage (continued)

	CS I (n=2,986)	CS II (n=6,105)	CS III (n=3,347)	CS IV (n=1,870)
COMBINATION CHEMOTHERAPY *				
3. Alternated regimen				
MOPP/ABVD or ABV or BAP or BCAVe or MCAVe-CEC	24 (2.7)	137 (4.8)	243 (9.2)	239 (13.4)
MVPP or CVPP/ABDIC or (B)EVA	3	47 (1.7)	31 (1.2)	10
PAVe/ABVD	–	2	16 (0.6)	6
miscellaneous	–	5	19 (0.7)	15 (0.8)
unspecified	7 (0.8)	23 (0.8)	19 (0.7)	39 (2.2)
Total subgroups :				
1. MOPP-like	792 (88.9)	2,430 (86.0)	2,280 (86.5)	1,467 (82.1)
2. Adriamycin containing	65 (7.3)	181 (6.4)	29 (1.1)	10 (0.6)
3. Alternated	27 (3.0)	191 (6.8)	309 (11.7)	270 (15.1)

see glossary in appendix

Part IV - *Quatrième partie*

RELATIONSHIP BETWEEN PRETREATMENT CLINICAL AND BIOLOGICAL PARAMETERS

LIAISONS STATISTIQUES DES CARACTERISTIQUES CLINIQUES ET BIOLOGIQUES INITIALES ENTRE ELLES

Relationships between pretreatment characteristics

Only associations that are generally published have been examined and are presented here.

Table IV-1 shows the relationship between biological parameters and the presence or absence of systemic symptoms. When B symptoms were present ESR was elevated above 50 mm in 62.5% of the cases, mean hemoglobin was lower, there was an increase in mean serum LDH and alkaline phosphatase, and a decrease in serum albumin level.

Distribution of hemoglobin according to sex and systemic symptoms is given in Table IV-2. In further analyses, hemoglobin was then considered as normal if above 7.0 mmol/l in females and above 8.0 mmol/l in males. Otherwise it was considered abnormal.

Mediastinal involvement was associated with female gender, as was nodular sclerosing histological type. The latter association still exists when adjustment for mediastinal involvement was made (Table IV-3).

Mediastinal involvement was also associated with clinical stage II and consequently with the number of major lymph node areas involved (Table IV-4). This latter association disappeared when considering only stage III and IV patients.

Pairwise associations berween biological parameters are examined in Table IV-5. Major relationships are observed between alkaline phosphatase and ESR, alkaline phosphatase and hemoglobin, serum albumin and ESR, and hemoglobin and ESR.

Pairwise correlations between biological parameters are given in Table IV-6. These correlations are to be compared with the distributions given in Table IV-5.

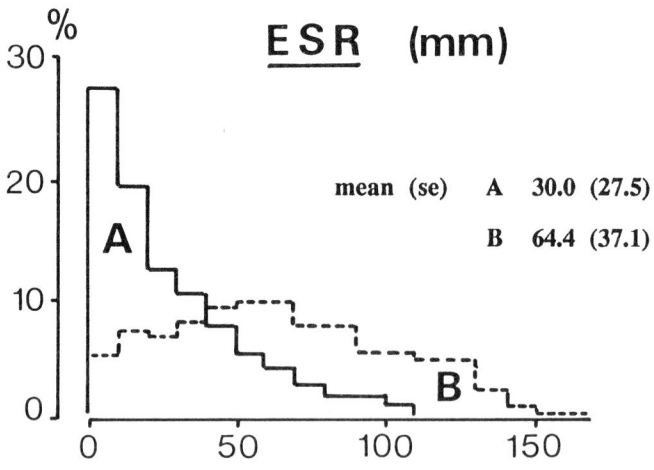

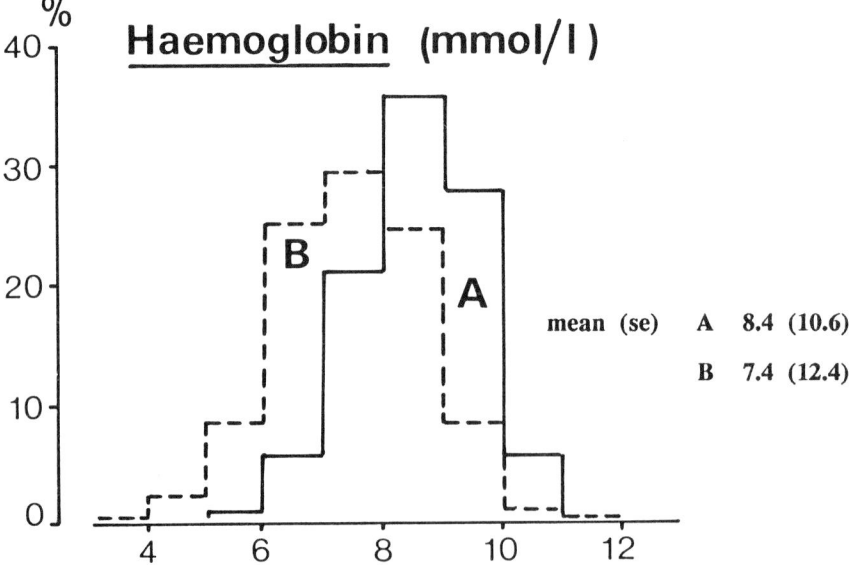

Table IV-1. Relationship between systemic symptoms and biological parameters

	Systemic Symptoms	
	absent	present

ERYTHROCYTE SEDIMENTATION RATE

	absent	present
< 9 mm/1st hour	27.8 %	5.7 %
10- 19	18.8	7.7
20- 29	13.1	6.8
30- 39	11.2	8.2
40- 49	8.1	9.1
50- 59	6.4	9.7
60- 69	4.4	10.0
70- 79	3.2	8.0
80- 89	2.3	7.9
90- 99	1.9	6.2
100-109	1.3	5.9
110-119	0.8	5.2
120-129	0.5	5.2
130-139	0.2	2.5
140-149	0.1	1.4
150-159	< 0.1	0.5
160-169	< 0.1	0.1
170-179	< 0.1	-
180 +	-	< 0.1
number of patients	5,501	3,168

HEMOGLOBIN

	absent	present
< 4.0 mmol/l	0.1 %	0.7 %
4.0- 4.9	0.3	2.6
5.0- 5.9	1.2	8.7
6.0- 6.9	6.6	24.9
7.0- 7.9	21.8	29.3
8.0- 8.9	36.3	24.6
9.0- 9.9	27.6	7.9
10.0-10.9	5.7	1.1
11.0 +	0.4	0.3
number of patients	6,412	4,072

Table IV-1. Relationship between systemic symptoms and biological parameters (continued)

	Systemic Symptoms	
	absent	present
L.D.H. IU/l		
< 25th percentile	25.0 %	19.2 %
25-75th percentile	61.1	52.4
> 75th percentile	13.9	28.4
number of patients	965	855
ALKALINE PHOSPHATASE IU/l		
< 25th percentile	24.8 %	16.5 %
25-75th percentile	58.1	46.6
> 75th percentile	17.1	36.9
number of patients	4,610	3,061
SERUM ALBUMIN micro mol/l		
< 25th percentile	8.6 %	38.3 %
25-75th percentile	52.9	47.7
> 75th percentile	38.5	14.0
number of patients	3,221	2,115

Table IV-2. Distribution of hemoglobin according to sex and
systemic symptoms

	Hemoglobin	Males	Females
All patients	< 4.0 mmol/l	0.4 %	0.2 %
	4.0- 4.9	1.0	1.4
	5.0- 5.9	3.6	5.0
	6.0- 6.9	10.3	19.0
	7.0- 7.9	17.8	35.7
	8.0- 8.9	31.4	32.2
	9.0- 9.9	28.9	5.9
	10.0-10.9	6.2	0.4
	11.0 +	0.4	0.2
	mean (SD)	8.3 (1.3)	7.6 (1.0)
	# of patients	6,414	4,088
B Symptoms		absent	present
Males	< 4.0 mmol/l	0.1 %	1.0 %
	4.0- 4.9	0.1	1.9
	5.0- 5.9	0.9	7.1
	6.0- 6.9	2.8	21.5
	7.0- 7.9	10.5	27.2
	8.0- 8.9	33.7	28.3
	9.0- 9.9	41.1	11.2
	10.0-10.9	10.1	1.6
	11.0 +	0.7	0.2
	mean (SD)	8.9 (1.0)	7.5 (1.3)
	# of patients	3,778	2,557
	p value *		<0.001
Females	< 4.0 mmol/l	0.1 %	0.4 %
	4.0- 4.9	0.4	2.4
	5.0- 5.9	1.6	10.3
	6.0- 6.9	11.0	31.2
	7.0- 7.9	36.7	31.9
	8.0- 8.9	41.4	20.9
	9.0- 9.9	8.4	2.3
	10.0-10.9	0.4	0.3
	11.0 +	0.1	0.4
	mean (SD)	7.8 (0.9)	7.1 (1.1)
	# of patients	2,590	1,461
	p value *		<0.001

* *Kruskal-Wallis one-way analysis of variance*

Table IV-3. Relationship between sex, mediastinal involvement and histological type

			Males	Females
MEDIASTINAL INVOLVEMENT	no (%)		4,737 (55.0)	2,013 (35.8)
	yes		3,872 (45.0)	3,611 (64.2)
HISTOLOGICAL TYPE	LP (%)		773 (8.9)	239 (4.3)
	NS		4,616 (53.4)	4,068 (72.5)
	MC		2,742 (31.7)	1,036 (18.5)
	LD		288 (3.3)	141 (2.5)
	unclassified		230 (2.7)	128 (2.2)
WITHOUT MEDIASTINAL INVOLVEMENT				
HISTOLOGICAL TYPE	LP (%)		659 (14.0)	183 (9.2)
	NS		1,848 (39.1)	1,127 (56.4)
	MC		1,946 (41.2)	582 (29.1)
	LD		153 (3.2)	60 (3.0)
	unclassified		119 (2.5)	47 (2.3)
WITH MEDIASTINAL INVOLVEMENT				
HISTOLOGICAL TYPE	LP (%)		113 (2.9)	56 (1.5)
	NS		2,729 (70.7)	2,925 (81.4)
	MC		779 (20.2)	450 (12.5)
	LD		130 (3.4)	81 (2.3)
	unclassified		111 (2.9)	81 (2.3)

Table IV-4. Relationship between clinical stage, mediastinal involvement, and number of lymph node areas involved

			mediastinal involvement	
			no	yes
CLINICAL STAGE (upper torso)				
	I	(%)	2,449 (88.2)	334 (11.8)
	II		1,419 (25.7)	4,207 (74.3)
Number of lymph node areas involved				
CS I	1	(%)	2,449 (88.2)	329 (11.8)
CS II	2		1,045 (35.1)	1,929 (64.9)
	3		212 (13.9)	1,310 (86.1)
	4		121 (18.8)	523 (81.2)
	5 +		17 (4.8)	335 (95.2)
CLINICAL STAGE	III	(%)	1,470 (44.3)	1,848 (55.7)
	IV		755 (40.8)	1,094 (59.2)
Number of lymph node areas involved				
	0	(%)	174 (100)	—
	1		106 (30.9)	237 (69.1)
	2		717 (53.3)	629 (46.7)
	3		332 (37.7)	549 (62.3)
	4		307 (39.6)	469 (60.4)
	5 +		561 (34.7)	1,057 (65.3)
CS III	2	(%)	601 (57.3)	448 (42.7)
	3		236 (39.5)	362 (60.5)
	4		223 (40.7)	325 (59.3)
	5 +		390 (35.4)	713 (64.6)
CS IV	0	(%)	174 (100)	—
	1		106 (30.9)	237 (69.1)
	2		116 (39.1)	181 (60.9)
	3		96 (33.9)	187 (66.1)
	4		84 (36.8)	144 (63.2)
	5 +		171 (33.2)	344 (66.8)

Table IV-5. Pairwise associations between biological parameters

	L.D.H. (percentile)		
	< 25th	25-75th	> 75th

ERYTHROCYTE SEDIMENTATION RATE mm/1st hour

number of patients		150	341	154
mean (SD)		54 (37)	51 (36)	64 (40)
0-19	(%)	28 (19)	85 (25)	23 (15)
20-39		31 (21)	59 (17)	24 (16)
40-59		32 (21)	65 (19)	27 (18)
60-79		26 (17)	54 (16)	23 (15)
80-99		8 (5)	40 (12)	21 (13)
100 +		25 (17)	38 (11)	36 (23)

ALKALINE PHOSPHATASE UI/l

< 25th percentile (%)	104 (26)	217 (21)	51 (14)
25 - 75th percentile	225 (57)	564 (56)	158 (44)
> 75th percentile	68 (17)	229 (23)	154 (42)

SERUM ALBUMIN micromol/l

< 25th percentile (%)	12 (14)	48 (19)	31 (34)
25 - 75th percentile	60 (67)	141 (55)	45 (50)
> 75th percentile	17 (19)	65 (26)	14 (16)

HEMOGLOBIN mmol/l

number of patients		398	1,016	370
mean (SD)		8.0 (1.3)	7.9 (1.3)	7.4 (1.3)
< 5.0	(%)	7 (2)	13 (1)	11 (3)
5.0- 6.9		80 (20)	213 (21)	131 (35)
7.0- 8.9		221 (56)	574 (57)	183 (49)
9.0-10.9		88 (22)	212 (21)	44 (12)
11.0 +		2 (<1)	4 (<1)	1 (<1)

Table IV-5. Pairwise associations between biological parameters (continued)

	ALKALINE PHOSPHATASE (percentile)		
	< 25th	25-75th	> 75th
ERYTHROCYTE SEDIMENTATION RATE mm/1st hour			
number of patients	1,150	3,013	1,317
mean (SD)	34 (31)	42 (33)	62 (40)
0-19 (%)	524 (45.6)	975 (32.4)	232 (17.6)
20-39	231 (20.1)	691 (22.9)	225 (17.1)
40-59	160 (13.9)	529 (17.6)	227 (17.2)
60-79	95 (8.3)	379 (12.6)	188 (14.3)
80-99	81 (7.0)	221 (7.3)	162 (12.3)
100 +	59 (5.1)	218 (7.2)	283 (21.5)
SERUM ALBUMIN micromol/l			
< 25th percentile (%)	100 (14.5)	258 (15.9)	295 (38.6)
25 - 75th percentile	339 (49.3)	892 (55.0)	326 (42.7)
> 75th percentile	249 (36.2)	472 (29.1)	143 (18.7)
HEMOGLOBIN mmol/l			
number of patients	1,562	3,808	1,776
mean (SD)	8.2 (1.2)	8.1 (1.2)	7.5 (1.4)
< 5.0 (%)	13 (0.8)	42 (1.1)	72 (4.1)
5.0- 6.9	216 (13.8)	570 (15.0)	534 (30.1)
7.0- 8.9	919 (58.8)	2,209 (58.0)	910 (51.2)
9.0-10.9	410 (26.3)	965 (25.3)	255 (14.4)
11.0 +	4 (0.3)	22 (0.6)	5 (0.2)

Table IV-5. Pairwise associations between biological parameters (continued)

		SERUM ALBUMIN (percentile)		
		< 25th	25 - 75th	> 75th

ERYTHROCYTE SEDIMENTATION RATE   mm/1st hour

number of patients		918	2,358	1,362
mean	(SD)	74 (37)	42 (32)	24 (26)
0-19	(%)	80 (8.7)	715 (30.3)	778 (57.1)
20-39		107 (11.7)	564 (23.9)	299 (21.9)
40-59		152 (16.6)	445 (18.9)	143 (10.5)
60-79		160 (17.4)	313 (13.3)	71 (5.2)
80-99		159 (17.3)	152 (6.4)	42 (3.1)
100 +		260 (28.3)	169 (7.2)	29 (2.2)

HEMOGLOBIN   mmol/l

number of patients		1,064	2,663	1,320
mean	(SD)	6.9 (1.2)	8.1 (1.1)	8.7 (1.0)
< 5.0	(%)	60 (5.6)	18 (0.7)	3 (0.2)
5.0- 6.9		491 (46.2)	377 (14.1)	60 (4.6)
7.0- 8.9		459 (43.1)	1,694 (63.6)	677 (51.3)
9.0-10.9		53 (5.0)	569 (21.4)	576 (43.6)
11.0 +		1 (0.1)	5 (0.2)	4 (0.3)

Table IV-5. Pairwise associations between biological parameters (continued)

			HEMOGLOBIN	mmol/l		
E.S.R. mm/1st hour	< 5.0	5.0-6.9	7.0-8.9	9.0-10.9	11.0+	Total
0- 19	12 (10.0)	100 (7.7)	1,152 (26.5)	1,325 (68.6)	19 (63)	2,608
20- 39	16 (13.0)	120 (9.1)	1,609 (24.6)	374 (19.4)	1	1,580
40- 59	16 (13.0)	181 (13.9)	903 (20.8)	159 (8.2)	3	1,262
60- 79	13 (11.0)	231 (17.7)	606 (13.9)	49 (2.5)	3	902
80- 99	10 (9.0)	246 (18.8)	345 (7.9)	16 (0.8)	1	618
100-119	18 (15.0)	206 (15.8)	197 (4.5)	6	1	428
120 +	34 (29.0)	222 (17.0)	73 (1.8)	2	2	333
Total	119	1,306	4,345	1,931	30	7,731

Overall group: mean E.S.R. (SD) = 43 (36) mm/1st hour
mean Hemoglobin (SD) = 8.1 (1.3) mmol/l

Table IV-6. Pairwise correlations between biological parameters

		ESR	LDH	AP	SA
ALL STAGES	LDH	**(+)			
	AP	***(+)	***(+)		
	SA	***(−)	* (−)	***(−)	
	Hb	***(−)	***(−)	***(−)	***(+)
CS I-II	LDH	n.s.			
	AP	***(+)	***(+)		
	SA	***(−)	n.s.	** (−)	
	Hb	***(−)	** (−)	***(−)	***(+)
CS III-IV	LDH	n.s.			
	AP	***(+)	***(+)		
	SA	***(−)	* (−)	***(−)	
	Hb	***(−)	***(−)	***(−)	***(+)

ESR : Erythrocyte sedimentation rate
LDH : Serum lacticodeshydrogenase
AP : Alkaline phosphatase
SA : Serum albumin
Hb : Hemoglobin

p value = * < 0.05; ** < 0.01; *** < 0.001
(-) negative or (+) positive correlation

Part V - *Cinquième partie*

PROGNOSTIC STUDY OF LAPAROTOMY FINDINGS BY CLINICAL STAGE

ANALYSE PRONOSTIQUE DES RESULTATS DE LA LAPAROTOMIE EXPLORATRICE EN FONCTION DU STADE CLINIQUE

Prognostic study of laparotomy findings

Overall a staging laparotomy was performed in 6,108 cases (42.7%) (Table III-1). Since staging laparotomy is rarely performed nowadays in clinical stage IV patients, the study was limited to stages I to III. Cases were subdivided into 5 subgroups, i.e. clinical stage IA, IIA, IB-IIB, IIIA, and IIIB.

In the analyses performed, only variables which have reached the 0.01 level of significance are presented in the Tables V-2, V-4, V-6, V-8, V-10, and V-11.

In clinical stage IA patients, only male gender, mixed cellularity (MC) and lymphocytic depleted (LD) histological types and age above 50 were significantly associated with a higher probability of positive laparotomy (Table V-2). Biological parameters had no independent influence when included in the model.

In clinical stage IIA patients, the absence of mediastinal involvement, a large number of lymph node areas involved, MC or LD histological types, and male gender were significantly associated with a higher probability of positive laparotomy (Table V-4). When ESR was added in the model, ESR above 60 mm reached the 0.01 significance level in third position after mediastinal involvement and histology, and before sex. None of the other biological parameters were significantly associated with a high probability of positive laparotomy.

In clinical stage IB-IIB patients three variables displayed significant association with positive laparotomy: male gender, absence of mediastinal involvement, and extra nodal localization (E+) (Table V-6). Biological parameters had no independent influence when included in the model.

In clinical stage IIIA patients, only age below 40 was significantly associated with an increased probability of pathological IV (Table V-8), while in clinical stage IIIB patients the three variables which were associated with a pathological stage IV were: MC or LD histological types, a few numbers of lymph node areas involved, and age above 30 (Table V-10). Here again biological parameters had no independent influence when included in the model.

False positivity of stage III (PS I-II patients) was associated with the absence of B symptoms, limited number of lymph node areas involved, mediastinal involvement, LP or NS histological types and age below 50 (Table V-11).

Table V-1. Prognostic factors of positive laparotomy findings in CS IA supradiaphragmatic patients (N=1,169)

Factors studied	SEX	males	800	68,4 %
		females	369	31.6 %
	AGE	15-19 years	122	10.4 %
		20-29	410	35.1 %
		30-39	309	26.4 %
		40-49	155	13.3 %
		50 +	173	14.8 %
	MEDIASTINUM	not involved	1,065	91.1 %
		not bulky	87	7.4 %
		bulky	17	1.5 %
	HISTOLOGY	LP	169	14.5 %
		NS	573	49.0 %
		MC	400	34.2 %
		LD	6	0.5 %
		unclassified	21	1.8 %
	EXTRA NODAL LOCALIZATION (E+)		94	8.0 %
Other factors	E.S.R.	available	690	59.0 %
		mean (SD)	18 (19)	
	SERUM L.D.H.	available	146	12.5 %
		< 25th percentile	50	
		25-75th	89	
		> 75th	7	
	ALKALINE PHOSPHATASE	available	576	49.3 %
		< 25th percentile	215	
		25-75th	296	
		> 75th	65	
	SERUM ALBUMIN	available	414	35.4 %
		< 25th percentile	14	
		25-75th	180	
		> 75th	220	
	HEMOGLOBIN	available	863	73.8 %
		mean (SD)	8.8 (1.0)	

Table V-2. Prognostic factors of positive laparotomy findings in CS IA
supradiaphragmatic patients (N=1,169)

Patients with positive laparotomy *(PS III - IV)*: n = 287 (24.6 %)

STEPWISE LOGISTIC REGRESSION

Parameters included in the model (number of dummy variables) =
sex, age (4), mediastinal involvement (2), histological
subtype (2), extra nodal localization.

Step	Variable (codes)	log. likelihood	Coeff/s.e.	p value
0		- 649.84		
1	SEX (M=-1, F=1)	- 635.03	- 0.396/0.084	< 0.001
2	HISTOLOGY (LP-NS=-1, MC-LD-uncl.=1)	- 625.90	+ 0.295/0.070	< 0.001
3	AGE (<50=-1, 50+=1)	- 622.50	+ 0.243/0.091	0.009
	CONSTANT		- 1.079/0.102	

Pattern	number of patients	observed proportion of LAP +	predicted probability of LAP +
Male, 50+ yrs, MC-LD	50	0.38	0.46
Female, 50+ yrs, MC-LD	22	0.36	0.28
Male, <50 yrs, MC-LD	276	0.36	0.35
Male, 50+ yrs, LP-NS	66	0.32	0.32
Female, 50+ yrs, LP-NS	35	0.26	0.18
Male, <50 yrs, LP-NS	402	0.23	0.23
Female, <50 yrs, MC-LD	76	0.17	0.19
Female, <50 yrs, LP-NS	236	0.11	0.12

Table V-3. Prognostic factors of positive laparotomy findings in CS IIA supradiaphragmatic patients (N=2,141)

Factors studied				
	SEX	males	1,069	49.9 %
		females	1,072	50.1 %
	AGE	15-19 years	371	17.3 %
		20-29	990	46.2 %
		30-39	510	23.8 %
		40-49	176	8.2 %
		50 +	94	5.5 %
	MEDIASTINUM	not involved	543	25.4 %
		not bulky	1,392	65.0 %
		bulky	206	9.6 %
	NUMBER OF NODAL AREAS INVOLVED			
		2	1,107	51.7 %
		3	574	26.8 %
		4	284	13.3 %
		5 +	176	8.2 %
	HISTOLOGY	LP	88	4.1 %
		NS	1,739	81.2 %
		MC	280	13.1 %
		LD	14	0.7 %
		unclassified	20	0.9 %
	EXTRA NODAL LOCALIZATION (E+)		248	11.6 %
Other factors	E.S.R.	available	924	43.2 %
		mean (SD)	32 (25)	
	SERUM L.D.H.	available	341	15.9 %
		< 25th percentile	76	
		25-75th	217	
		> 75th	48	
	ALKALINE PHOSPHATASE available		921	43.0 %
		< 25th percentile	244	
		25-75th	529	
		> 75th	148	
	SERUM ALBUMIN	available	588	27.5 %
		< 25th percentile	47	
		25-75th	317	
		> 75th	224	
	HEMOGLOBIN	available	1,301	60.8 %
		mean (SD)	8.3 (1.0)	

Table V-4. Prognostic factors of positive laparotomy findings in CS IIA
supradiaphragmatic patients (N=2,141)

Patients with positive laparotomy *(PS III - IV)*:   n = 600   (28.0 %)

STEPWISE LOGISTIC REGRESSION

Parameters included in the model (number of dummy variables) =
sex, age (4), mediastinal involvement (2), number of lymph
node areas involved (3), histological subtype (2), extra
nodal localization.

Step	Variable (codes)	log. likelihood	Coeff/s.e.	p value
0		- 1267.37		
1	**MEDIASTINUM** (not involved=-1, involved=1)	- 1252.37	- 0.250/0.057	< 0.001
2	**# OF LYMPH NODE AREAS** (2-3=-1, 4-5=1)	- 1242.99	+ 0.233/0.058	< 0.001
3	**HISTOLOGY** (LP-NS=-1, MC-LD-uncl.=1)	- 1235.06	+ 0.243/0.067	< 0.001
4	**SEX** (M=-1, F=1)	- 1230.84	- 0.147/0.051	0.004
	CONSTANT		- 0.541/0.075	

Table V-4. Prognostic factors of positive laparotomy findings in CS IIA supradiaphragmatic patients (N=2,141) (continued)

Pattern	number of patients	observed proportion of LAP +	predicted probability of LAP +
Female, LP-NS, 4-5 Areas, MED-	13	0.69	0.39
Male, MC-LD, 4-5 Areas, MED-	25	0.56	0.58
Male, MC-LD, 2-3 Areas, MED-	98	0.50	0.47
Female, MC-LD, 4-5 Areas, MED-	4	0.50	0.51
Male, MC-LD, 2-3 Areas, MED+	77	0.39	0.35
Male, LP-NS, 2-3 Areas, MED-	213	0.34	0.35
Female, LP-NS, 4-5 Areas, MED+	181	0.33	0.28
Male, LP-NS, 4-5 Areas, MED+	179	0.32	0.34
Male, LP-NS, 4-5 Areas, MED-	20	0.30	0.46
Female, MC-LD, 2-3 Areas, MED-	30	0.30	0.39
Female, MC-LD, 4-5 Areas, MED+	10	0.30	0.39
Male, MC-LD, 4-5 Areas, MED+	27	0.30	0.46
Female, MC-LD, 2-3 Areas, MED+	51	0.27	0.28
Female, LP-NS, 2-3 Areas, MED-	133	0.27	0.29
Male, LP-NS, 2-3 Areas, MED+	432	0.25	0.25
Female, LP-NS, 2-3 Areas, MED+	650	0.19	0.20

Table V-5. Prognostic factors of positive laparotomy findings in
CS IB - IIB supradiaphragmatic patients (N=739)

Factors studied				
	SEX	males	421	57.0 %
		females	318	43.0 %
	AGE	15-19 years	100	13.5 %
		20-29	338	45.7 %
		30-39	164	22.2 %
		40-49	76	10.3 %
		50 +	61	8.3 %
	MEDIASTINUM	not involved	195	26.4 %
		not bulky	422	57.1 %
		bulky	122	16.5 %
	NUMBER NODAL AREAS INVOLVED			
		1 CS I	112	15.2 %
		2 CS II	272	36.8 %
		3	171	23.1 %
		4	112	15.2 %
		5 +	72	9.7 %
	HISTOLOGY	LP	21	2.8 %
		NS	573	77.5 %
		MC	116	15.7 %
		LD	10	1.4 %
		unclassified	19	2.6 %
	EXTRA NODAL LOCALIZATION (E+)		92	12.4 %
Other factors	E.S.R.	available	307	41.5 %
		mean (SD)	54 (36)	
	SERUM L.D.H.	available	134	18.1 %
		< 25th percentile	26	
		25-75th	86	
		> 75th	22	
	ALKALINE PHOSPHATASE	available	330	44.7 %
		< 25th percentile	77	
		25-75th	172	
		> 75th	81	
	SERUM ALBUMIN	available	244	33.0 %
		< 25th percentile	61	
		25-75th	129	
		> 75th	54	
	HEMOGLOBIN	available	458	62.0 %
		mean (SD)	7.8 (1.1)	

Table V-6. Prognostic factors of positive laparotomy findings in CS IB - IIB supradiaphragmatic patients (N=739)

Patients with positive laparotomy *(PS III - IV)*: n = 242   (32.7 %)

STEPWISE LOGISTIC REGRESSION

Parameters included in the model (number of dummy variables) = sex, age (4), mediastinal involvement (2), number of lymph node areas involved (3), histological subtype (2), extra nodal localization.

Step	Variable (codes)	log. likelihood	Coeff/s.e.	p value
0		- 466.53		
1	SEX (M=-1, F=1)	- 452.45	- 0.382/0.086	< 0.001
2	MEDIASTINUM (not involved= -1, involved=1)	- 446.99	- 0.276/0.090	0.001
3	EXTRA LOCALIZATION (absent=-1, present=1)	- 441.92	- 0.435/0.146	0.001
	CONSTANT		- 1.023/0.155	

Pattern	number of patients	observed proportion of LAP +	predicted probability of LAP +
Male, MED-, E+ absent	134	0.51	0.52
Female, MED-, E+ absent	44	0.41	0.33
Male, MED+, E+ absent	238	0.39	0.38
Male, MED+, E+ present	39	0.21	0.21
Female, MED+, E+ absent	229	0.20	0.22
Female, MED+, E+ present	37	0.19	0.11
Male, MED-, E+ present	9	0.11	0.31
Female, MED-, E+ present	7	0	0.17

Table V-7. Prognostic factors of positive laparotomy findings
CS IIIA patients (N=756)

Factors studied	SEX	males	504	66.7 %
		females	252	33.3 %
	AGE	15-19 years	100	13.2 %
		20-29	309	40.9 %
		30-39	156	20.6 %
		40-49	99	13.1 %
		50 +	92	12.2 %
	MEDIASTINUM	not involved	381	50.9 %
		not bulky	349	46.6 %
		bulky	19	2.5 %
	NUMBER OF NODAL AREAS INVOLVED			
		2	342	45.5 %
		3	146	19.4 %
		4	108	14.4 %
		5 +	156	20.7 %
	HISTOLOGY	LP	58	7.7 %
		NS	450	59.6 %
		MC	219	28.9 %
		LD	9	1.2 %
		unclassified	20	2.6 %
	EXTRA NODAL LOCALIZATION (E+)		49	6.5 %
Other factors	E.S.R.	available	300	39.7 %
		mean (SD)	31 (28)	
	SERUM L.D.H.	available	89	11.8 %
		< 25th percentile	18	
		25-75th	51	
		> 75th	20	
	ALKALINE PHOSPHATASE	available	267	35.3 %
		< 25th percentile	78	
		25-75th	159	
		> 75th	30	
	SERUM ALBUMIN	available	233	30.8 %
		< 25th percentile	17	
		25-75th	135	
		> 75th	81	
	HEMOGLOBIN	available	453	59.9 %
		mean (SD)	8.3 (1.1)	

Table V-8. Prognostic factors of positive laparotomy findings in CS IIIA patients (N=756)

Patients with positive laparotomy *(PS IV)*: n = 59   (7.8 %)

STEPWISE LOGISTIC REGRESSION

Parameters included in the model (number of dummy variables) = sex, age (4), mediastinal involvement (2), number of lymph node areas involved (3), histological subtype (2), extra nodal localization.

Step	Variable (codes)	log. likelihood	Coeff/s.e.	p value
0		− 203.590		
1	AGE (<40=−1, 40+=1)	− 197.823	+ 0.486/0.140	< 0.001
	CONSTANT		− 2.310/0.140	

Pattern		Number of patients	Proportion of LAP +
AGE	40+ yrs	187	0.14
	<40 yrs	556	0.06

Table V-9. Prognostic factors of positive laparotomy findings in CS IIIB patients (N=554)

Factors studied				
	SEX	males	395	71.3 %
		females	159	28.7 %
	AGE	15-19 years	71	12.8 %
		20-29	227	41.0 %
		30-39	127	22.9 %
		40-49	62	11.2 %
		50 +	67	12.1 %
	MEDIASTINUM	not involved	206	37.6 %
		not bulky	329	60.0 %
		bulky	13	2.4 %
	NUMBER OF NODAL AREAS INVOLVED			
		2	164	29.9 %
		3	108	19.7 %
		4	83	15.2 %
		5 +	193	35.2 %
	HISTOLOGY	LP	7	1.3 %
		NS	370	66.8 %
		MC	138	24.9 %
		LD	17	3.0 %
		unclassified	22	4.0 %
	EXTRA NODAL LOCALIZATION (E+)		77	13.9 %
Other factors	E.S.R.	available	190	34.3 %
		mean (SD)	63 (38)	
	SERUM L.D.H.	available	79	14.3 %
		< 25th percentile	16	
		25-75th	38	
		> 75th	25	
	ALKALINE PHOSPHATASE available		237	42.8%
		< 25th percentile	61	
		25-75th	101	
		> 75th	75	
	SERUM ALBUMIN	available	143	25.8 %
		< 25th percentile	48	
		25-75th	71	
		> 75th	24	
	HEMOGLOBIN	available	352	63.5 %
		mean (SD)	7.4 (1.2)	

Table V-10. Prognostic factors of positive laparotomy findings in CS IIIB patients (N=554)

Patients with positive laparotomy *(PS IV)*:   n= 80   (14.7 %)

STEPWISE LOGISTIC REGRESSION

Parameters included in the model (number of dummy variables) =
sex, age (4), mediastinal involvement (2), number of lymph node areas involved (3), histological subtype (2), extra nodal localization.

Step	Variable (codes)	log. likelihood	Coeff/s.e.	p value
0		- 227.160		
1	HISTOLOGY (LP-NS=1 MC-LD-uncl.=-1)	- 216.460	- 0.569/0.128	< 0.001
2	# LYMPH NODES INVOLVED (<3=-1, 4+=1)	- 210.858	+ 0.429/0.132	0.001
3	AGE (20-29=1,others=-1)	- 205.841	- 0.440/0.146	0.002
	CONSTANT		- 1.874/0.150	

Pattern	Number of patients	Observed proportion of LAP +	Predicted probability of LAP +
4-5 areas, MC-LD, other ages	56	0.36	0.39
1-3 areas, MC-LD, 20-29 yrs	29	0.21	0.10
1-3 areas, MC-LD, other ages	63	0.21	0.22
4-5 areas, LP-NS, other ages	110	0.20	0.17
4-5 areas, MC-LD, 20-29 yrs	26	0.19	0.21
1-3 areas, LP-NS, other ages	94	0.07	0.08
4-5 areas, LP-NS, 20-29 yrs	84	0.07	0.08
1-3 areas, LP-NS, 20-29 yrs	82	0.01	0.04

Table V-11. Prognostic factors of laparotomy findings in CS IIIA or CS IIIB patients (N=1,310)

Patients with PS I-II after laparotomy: n = 274   (20.9 %)
(207/756 (27.3%) in CSIIIA, and 67/554 (12.1%) in CSIIIB)

STEPWISE LOGISTIC REGRESSION

Parameters included in the model (number of dummy variables) = sex, age (4), mediastinal involvement (2), number of lymph node areas involved (3), histological subtype (2), extra nodal localization.

Step	Variable (codes)	log. likelihood	Coeff/s.e.	p value
0		- 663.744		
1	B SYMPTOMS (A=-1, B=1)	- 640.671	- 0.486/0.080	< 0.001
2	# LYMPH NODES INVOLVED (2-4=-1, 5+=1)	- 626.999	- 0.537/0.099	< 0.001
3	MEDIASTINAL INVOLVEMENT (NO=-1, YES=1)	- 615.987	+ 0.262/0.076	< 0.001
4	HISTOLOGY (LP-NS=-1, MC-LD-uncl.=1)	- 611.106	- 0.247/0.084	0.002
5	AGE (15-49=-1, 50+=1)	- 607.348	- 0.349/0.135	0.006
	CONSTANT		- 2.200/0.160	

Pattern	Number of patients	Observed proportion of PS I-II	Predicted probability of PS I-II
No B Symptoms, 2-4 areas, MED+, LP-NS, <50yrs	200	0.42	0.42
No B Symptoms, 2-4 areas, <50yrs	313	0.26	0.30
LP-NS, <50yrs <u>and</u> 2 of 3 other parameters present	211	0.23	0.30-0.36
No B Symptoms, 2-4 areas			
No B Symptoms, LP-NS, <50yrs	281	0.15	0.21-0.25
2-4 areas <u>and</u> (LP-NS or <50yrs)			
Others	282	0.06	0.01-0.18

Part VI - *Sixième partie*

RESPONSE TO INITIAL THERAPY
DESCRIPTION BY CLINICAL AND PATHOLOGICAL STAGE

EFFICACITE DU TRAITEMENT INITIAL
DESCRIPTION EN FONCTION DU STADE CLINIQUE ET DU STADE
PATHOLOGIQUE

Response to initial therapy study

Response to initial therapy was analyzed by clinical stage, and, within each stage, by type of therapy (Tables VI-1 to VI-9).

Relationships between mediastinal involvement, initial therapy or treatment period and response are given in Table VI-10.

The characteristics of patients who failed to achieve a complete remission, all therapies given, are detailed in Tables VI-11 and VI-12.

Then the factors associated with a high probability of failure were searched through a stepwise multiple logistic regression taking into account the clinical stage and whether a staging laparotomy was performed or not (Tables VI-14 to VI-17).

In any stage in patients without staging laparotomy age above 50 displayed prognostic significance in association with the presence of B symptoms (stages II and III) or initial disease location (stage IV).

When *biological parameters* were included in the model, only ESR > 50 or serum albumin < 25th percentile displayed any significant prognostic value.

- In clinical stage I patients, when ESR was considered, it was the only prognostic factor to reach a significant level ($p<0.001$).

- In clinical stage II patients, when serum albumin was entered in the model, ESR was the only prognostic factor to reach a significant level ($p<0.001$). When systemic symptoms were excluded from the analysis, age ($p=0.001$), ESR ($p=0.012$) and serum albumin ($p<0.001$) were associated with response to initial therapy.

- In clinical stage III patients, parameters retained by the model were either ESR > 50 ($p<0.001$) and age > 50 ($p=0.001$), or serum albumin < 25th percentile ($p<0.01$). When systemic symptoms were excluded from the analysis, age ($p<0.001$), ESR ($p=0.001$) and serum albumin ($p=0.004$) were associated with response to initial therapy.

- In clinical stage IV patients none of the above variables were significantly associated with a high failure rate. When systemic symptoms were excluded from the analysis, age ($p<0.001$), infradiaphragmatic presentation ($p<0.001$) and serum albumin ($p<0.001$) were associated with response to initial therapy.

In patients who underwent a *staging laparotomy* only presence of B symptoms was associated with a high probability of failure to achieve a complete remission. None of the biological parameters were found to be of prognostic value. When systemic symptoms where excluded from the analysis the following findings were observed:

- In PS I-II patients, ESR ($p<0.001$) and infradiaphragmatic presentation ($p=0.04$) were associated with response to initial therapy.

- In PS III patients, ESR ($p=0.001$) and the number of lymph node areas involved ($p=0.007$) were associated with response to initial therapy.

- In PS IV patients, ESR ($p<0.001$) and the serum albumin ($p<0.001$) were associated with response to initial therapy.

When *initial therapy* (i.e. radiotherapy, chemotherapy, or both) was taken into account in the analysis the results were modified as follows:

- In clinical stage II patients, age and B symptoms were prognostic only in patients treated without staging laparotomy and without combined modality treatments.

- In clinical stage III patients, age and B symptoms were prognostic only in patients treated without staging laparotomy but with combination chemotherapy.

- In clinical stage IV patients, age and disease topography were prognostic only in patients treated without staging laparotomy and without combined modality treatments. In those treated with combination chemotherapy, the only factor found was the presence of B symptoms ($p < 0.01$).

Table VI-1. Response to initial therapy for CS I patients (N=2,986)

Type of therapy	Number of patients at risk	CR	(%)
1 - NOT LAPAROTOMIZED PATIENTS (n=1,598)			
RT alone			
IF irradiation	298	290	(97)
Mantle or inverted Y RT	467	462	(99)
STNI or TNI	200	198	(99)
RT + vinblastine			
IF irradiation	6	6	
Mantle or inverted Y RT	70	70	(100)
STNI or TNI	20	20	
Combination CT			
MOPP-like	48	41	(85)
Others	2	2	
RT + Combination CT			
IF irradiation + MOPP-like	177	169	(95)
+ ADM containing	42	40	(95)
M or inverted Y RT + MOPP-like	126	123	(98)
+ ADM containing	15	15	
+ Alternated CT	3	3	
STNI or TNI + MOPP-like	81	81	(100)
Not available or not treated	43		
2 - PATIENTS WITH NEGATIVE LAPAROTOMY (n=1,017)			
RT alone			
IF irradiation	124	120	(97)
Mantle or inverted Y RT	355	353	(99)
STNI or TNI	386	385	(99)
RT + single or bi-agent CT			
Mantle or inverted Y RT	2	2	
STNI or TNI	18	18	
RT + Combination CT			
IF irradiation + MOPP-like	55	52	(95)
M or inverted Y RT + MOPP-like	51	51	(100)
+ Alternated CT	1	1	
STNI or TNI + MOPP-like	7	7	
Not available or not treated	18		

Table VI-1. Response to initial therapy for CS I patients (N=2,986) (continued)

Type of therapy		Number of patients at risk	CR	(%)
3 – PATIENTS WITH POSITIVE LAPAROTOMY (PS III-IV) (n=367)				
RT alone				
Mantle or inverted Y RT	PS III	2	2	
STNI or TNI	PS III	80	75	(94)
RT + single or bi-agent CT				
STNI or TNI	PS III	5	5	
Combination CT				
MOPP-like	PS III	65	58	(89)
	PS IV	12	10	
Alternated CT	PS III	9	6	
RT + Combination CT				
IF irradiation + MOPP-like	PS III	18	17	
	PS IV	1	0	
+ Alternated CT	PS III	5	3	
	PS IV	1	1	
M or inverted Y RT + MOPP-like	PS III	36	34	(94)
	PS IV	3	2	
+ ADM containing	PS III	5	5	
+ Alternated CT	PS III	5	5	
	PS IV	1	1	
STNI or TNI + MOPP-like	PS III	70	70	(100)
	PS IV	1	0	
+ ADM containing	PS III	5	5	
+ Alternated CT	PS III	1	1	
Not available or not treated		42		

Table VI-2. Treatment Summary for CS I patients (N=2,986)

Laparotomy	Treatment type	Number of patients at risk	CR	(%)
NO	RT +/- single or bi-agent CT	1,083	1,072	(99)
	Combination CT	51	43	(84)
	RT + Combination CT	447	434	(97)
PS I	RT +/- single or bi-agent CT	891	882	(99)
	RT + Combination CT	114	112	(98)
PS III-IV	RT +/- single or bi-agent CT	89	84	(94)
	Combination CT	91	79	(87)
	RT + Combination CT	179	172	(96)

Table VI-2. Treatment Summary for CS IA patients (N=2,707) (continued)

Laparotomy	Treatment type	Number of patients at risk	CR	(%)
NO	RT +/- single or bi-agent CT	1,020	1,010	(99)
	Combination CT	26	22	(85)
	RT + Combination CT	378	215	(57)
PS I	RT +/- single or bi-agent CT	847	839	(99)
	RT + Combination CT	90	89	(99)
PS III-IV	RT +/- single or bi-agent CT	80	76	(95)
	Combination CT	74	66	(89)
	RT + Combination CT	158	152	(96)
All patients	RT +/- single or bi-agent CT	1,947	1,908	(98)
	Combination CT	100	88	(88)
	RT + Combination CT	626	607	(97)
All patients	Patients treated 1960-69	230	228	(99)
	1970-79	1,504	1,474	(98)
	1980 +	949	930	(98)

Table VI-3. Response to initial therapy for CS II patients (N=6,105)

Type of therapy	Number of patients at risk	CR	(%)
1 - NOT LAPAROTOMIZED PATIENTS (N=3,016)			
RT alone			
IF irradiation	189	169	(89)
Mantle or inverted Y RT	650	616	(95)
STNI or TNI	407	395	(97)
RT + single or bi-agent CT			
IF irradiation	16	10	(63)
Mantle or inverted Y RT + vinblastine	67	65	(97)
+ others	22	16	(73)
STNI or TNI + vinblastine	19	18	(95)
+ others	13	13	(100)
Combination CT			
MOPP-like	292	192	(66)
ADM containing	6	5	
Alternated CT	17	6	
RT + Combination CT			
IF irradiation + MOPP-like	298	280	(94)
+ ADM containing	43	43	(100)
+ Alternated CT	2	2	
M or inverted Y RT + MOPP-like	460	421	(92)
+ ADM containing	130	127	(98)
+ Alternated CT	88	73	(83)
STNI or TNI + MOPP-like	205	200	(98)
+ ADM containing	2	2	
+ Alternated CT	6	6	
Not available or not treated	84		

Table VI-3. Response to initial therapy for CS II patients (N=6,105) (continued)

Type of therapy	Number of patients		
	at risk	CR	(%)
2 - PATIENTS WITH NEGATIVE LAPAROTOMY (n=2,124)			
RT alone			
IF irradiation	135	127	(94)
Mantle or inverted Y RT	469	443	(94)
STNI or TNI	939	930	(99)
RT + single or bi-agent CT			
Mantle or inverted Y RT + vinblastine	4	4	
STNI or TNI + vinblastine	5	5	
+ others	8	8	
Combination CT			
MOPP-like	46	21	(46)
Alternated CT	3	2	
RT + Combination CT			
IF irradiation + MOPP-like	130	119	(92)
+ ADM containing	2	2	
M or inverted Y RT + MOPP-like	188	185	(98)
+ ADM containing	1	1	
+ Alternated CT	25	23	(92)
STNI or TNI + MOPP-like	117	117	(100)
+ ADM containing	13	13	
+ Alternated CT	1	1	
Not available or not treated	38		

Table VI-3. Response to initial therapy for CS II patients (N=6,105)
(continued)

Type of therapy		Number of patients at risk	CR	(%)
3 – PATIENTS WITH POSITIVE LAPAROTOMY (PS III-IV) (n=949)				
RT alone				
Mantle or inverted Y RT	PS III	4	4	
	PS IV	1	0	
STNI or TNI	PS III	262	252	(96)
	PS IV	3	3	
RT + single or bi-agent CT				
IF irradiation	PS IV	1	1	
Mantle or inverted Y RT	PS III	1	1	
STNI or TNI	PS III	8	8	
Combination CT				
MOPP-like	PS III	141	106	(75)
	PS IV	36	26	(72)
Alternated CT	PS III	12	9	
	PS IV	7	6	
RT + Combination CT				
IF irradiation + MOPP-like	PS III	47	41	(87)
	PS IV	2	2	
+ Alternated CT	PS III	7	6	
	PS IV	1	1	
M or inverted Y RT + MOPP-like	PS III	72	63	(87)
	PS IV	5	5	
+ ADM containing	PS III	8	8	
+ Alternated CT	PS III	12	11	
	PS IV	2	2	
STNI or TNI + MOPP-like	PS III	266	257	(97)
	PS IV	8	8	
+ Alternated CT	PS III	2	2	
Not available or not treated		41		

Table VI-4. Treatment Summary for CS II patients (N=6,105)

Laparotomy	Treatment type	Number of patients		
		at risk	CR	(%)
NO	RT +/- single or bi-agent CT	1,391	1,308	(94)
	Combination CT	325	205	(63)
	RT + Combination CT	1,282	1,192	(93)
PS II	RT +/- single or bi-agent CT	1,569	1,522	(97)
	Combination CT	51	24	(48)
	RT + Combination CT	486	471	(97)
PS III-IV	RT +/- single or bi-agent CT	282	271	(96)
	Combination CT	198	149	(75)
	RT + Combination CT	454	427	(94)

Table VI-4. Treatment Summary for CS IIA patients (N=4,406) (continued)

Laparotomy	Treatment type	Number of patients		
		at risk	CR	(%)
NO	RT +/- single or bi-agent CT	1,153	1,095	(95)
	Combination CT	93	70	(75)
	RT + Combination CT	810	761	(94)
PS II	RT +/- single or bi-agent CT	1,327	1,301	(98)
	Combination CT	14	9	
	RT + Combination CT	293	284	(97)
PS III-IV	RT +/- single or bi-agent CT	253	245	(97)
	Combination CT	116	90	(78)
	RT + Combination CT	314	301	(96)
All patients	RT +/- single or bi-agent CT	2,733	2,651	(97)
	Combination CT	233	177	(76)
	RT + Combination CT	1,417	1,346	(95)
All patients	Patients treated 1960-69	396	384	(97)
	1970-79	2,476	2,352	(95)
	1980 +	1,510	1,419	(94)

Table VI-5. Treatment Summary for CS IB and IIB patients (N=1,974)

Laparotomy	Treatment type	Number of patients at risk	CR	(%)
NO	RT +/- single or bi-agent CT	301	274	(91)
	Combination CT	257	157	(61)
	RT + Combination CT	540	497	(92)
PS I-II	RT +/- single or bi-agent CT	286	266	(93)
	Combination CT	38	16	(42)
	RT + Combination CT	217	206	(95)
PS III-IV	RT +/- single or bi-agent CT	38	34	(90)
	Combination CT	98	71	(72)
	RT + Combination CT	161	147	(91)
All patients	RT +/- single or bi-agent CT	625	575	(92)
	Combination CT	393	244	(62)
	RT + Combination CT	918	854	(93)
All patients	Patients treated 1960-69	165	153	(93)
	1970-79	1,066	927	(87)
	1980 +	721	869	(83)

Table VI-6. Response to initial therapy for CS III patients (N=3,347)

Type of therapy	Number of patients at risk	CR	(%)
1 - NOT LAPAROTOMIZED PATIENTS (n=1,994)			
RT alone			
IF irradiation	10	8	
Mantle or inverted Y RT	19	12	(63)
STNI or TNI	182	155	(85)
RT + single or bi-agent CT			
IF irradiation	18	13	(72)
Mantle or inverted Y RT	7	3	
STNI or TNI	23	18	(78)
Combination CT			
MOPP-like	830	581	(70)
ADM containing	4	4	
Alternated CT	134	88	(66)
RT + Combination CT			
IF irradiation + MOPP-like	224	188	(84)
+ ADM containing	18	18	(100)
+ Alternated CT	78	65	(83)
M or inverted Y RT + MOPP-like	74	54	(73)
+ ADM containing	2	2	
+ Alternated CT	17	15	(88)
STNI or TNI + MOPP-like	237	215	(91)
+ ADM containing	18	17	(94)
+ Alternated CT	10	10	
Not available or not treated	89		

Table VI-6. Response to initial therapy for CS III patients (N=3,347) (continued)

Type of therapy	Number of patients		
	at risk	CR	(%)
2 - PATIENTS WITH NEGATIVE LAPAROTOMY			
* PS I or PS II (n=274)			
RT alone			
IF irradiation	17	15	(88)
Mantle or inverted Y RT	48	45	(94)
STNI or TNI	139	137	(99)
Combination CT	3	3	
RT + Combination CT			
IF irradiation + MOPP-like	23	21	(91)
+ Alternated CT	1	1	
M or inverted Y RT + MOPP-like	4	3	
STNI or TNI + MOPP-like	26	26	(100)
+ ADM containing	10	10	
+ Alternated CT	1	1	
Not available or not treated	2		
* PS III patients (n=899)			
RT alone			
IF irradiation	3	2	
Mantle or inverted Y RT	3	3	
STNI or TNI	213	199	(93)
RT + single or bi-agent CT			
STNI or TNI	3	3	
Combination CT			
MOPP-like	215	166	(77)
Alternated CT	19	17	(89)
RT + Combination CT			
IF irradiation + MOPP-like	105	90	(86)
+ ADM containing	1	1	
+ Alternated CT	11	10	
M or inverted Y RT + MOPP-like	19	15	(79)
+ Alternated CT	15	15	(100)
STNI or TNI + MOPP-like	219	207	(95)
+ ADM containing	37	37	(100)
+ Alternated CT	6	6	
Not available or not treated	31		

Table VI-6. Response to initial therapy for CS III patients (N=3,347) (continued)

Type of therapy	Number of patients		
	at risk	CR	(%)

3 - PATIENTS WITH POSITIVE LAPAROTOMY (PS IV) (n=139)

RT alone			
Mantle or inverted Y RT	1	0	
STNI or TNI	3	3	
Combination CT			
MOPP-like	74	51	(69)
ADM containing	1	1	
Alternated CT	6	4	
RT + Combination CT			
IF irradiation + MOPP-like	8	3	
+ Alternated CT	2	1	
M or inverted Y RT + MOPP-like	1	0	
+ Alternated CT	1	1	
STNI or TNI + MOPP-like	31	29	(94)
+ ADM containing	1	1	
+ Alternated CT	4	4	
Not available or not treated	6		

Table VI-7. Treatment Summary for CS III patients (N=3,347)

Laparotomy	Treatment type	Number of patients		
		at risk	CR	(%)
NO	RT +/- single or bi-agent CT	261	232	(89)
	Combination CT	982	687	(70)
	RT + Combination CT	725	624	(86)
PS I-II	RT +/- single or bi-agent CT	204	198	(97)
	Combination CT	3	3	
	RT + Combination CT	66	63	(95)
PS III	RT +/- single or bi-agent CT	221	206	(93)
	Combination CT	236	184	(78)
	RT + Combination CT	427	464	(92)
PS IV	RT +/- single or bi-agent CT	4	3	
	Combination CT	82	57	(70)
	RT + Combination CT	50	41	(82)

Table VI-7. Treatment Summary for CS III patients (N=3,347) (continued)

Laparotomy	Treatment type	Number of patients at risk	CR	(%)
* CLINICAL STAGE IIIA	**(n=1,558)**			
NO	RT +/- single or bi-agent CT	163	135	(83)
	Combination CT	314	245	(78)
	RT + Combination CT	316	275	(87)
PS I-II	RT +/- single or bi-agent CT	175	173	(99)
	Combination CT	2	2	
	RT + Combination CT	29	29	(100)
PS III	RT +/- single or bi-agent CT	171	162	(95)
	Combination CT	92	72	(78)
	RT + Combination CT	223	205	(92)
PS IV	RT +/- single or bi-agent CT	1	1	
	Combination CT	41	31	(76)
	RT + Combination CT	17	15	
All patients	RT +/- single or bi-agent CT	514	473	(92)
	Combination CT	449	350	(78)
	RT + Combination CT	585	527	(90)
All patients	Patients treated 1960-69	108	99	(92)
	1970-79	933	812	(87)
	1980 +	509	443	(87)
* CLINICAL STAGE IIIB	**(n=1,779)**			
NO	RT +/- single or bi-agent CT	100	78	(78)
	Combination CT	687	447	(65)
	RT + Combination CT	415	349	(84)
PS I-II	RT +/- single or bi-agent CT	29	24	(83)
	Combination CT	1	1	
	RT + Combination CT	37	34	(92)
PS III	RT +/- single or bi-agent CT	50	44	(88)
	Combination CT	143	113	(79)
	RT + Combination CT	204	188	(92)
PS IV	RT +/- single or bi-agent CT	3	2	
	Combination CT	41	26	(63)
	RT + Combination CT	33	26	(79)
All patients	RT +/- single or bi-agent CT	182	147	(81)
	Combination CT	872	584	(67)
	RT + Combination CT	689	599	(87)
All patients	Patients treated 1960-69	130	101	(78)
	1970-79	987	760	(77)
	1980 +	641	481	(75)

Table VI-8. Response to initial therapy for CS IV patients (N=1,870)

Type of therapy	Number of patients at risk	CR	(%)
1 - NOT LAPAROTOMIZED PATIENTS (n=1,543)			
RT alone			
IF irradiation	6	4	
Mantle or inverted Y RT	7	4	
STNI or TNI	11	10	
RT + single or bi-agent CT	15	4	(27)
Combination CT			
MOPP-like	794	458	(58)
ADM containing	6	6	
Alternated CT	159	106	(67)
RT + Combination CT			
IF irradiation + MOPP-like	104	61	(59)
+ ADM containing	2	1	
+ Alternated CT	60	52	(87)
M or inverted Y RT + MOPP-like	47	36	(77)
+ ADM containing	1	0	
+ Alternated CT	14	14	(100)
STNI or TNI + MOPP-like	72	69	(96)
+ ADM containing	7	7	
+ Alternated CT	10	10	
Not available or not treated	140		
2 - PATIENTS WITH PATHOLOGICAL STAGE I-II (n=17)			
RT alone			
IF irradiation (n=1)			
Mantle or inverted Y RT (n=2)	7	6	
STNI or TNI (n=4)			
RT + Combination CT			
IF irradiation + MOPP-like	7	5	
Others	3	2	

Table VI-8. Response to initial therapy for CS IV patients (N=1,870) (continued)

Type of therapy	Number of patients		
	at risk	CR	(%)

3 - PATIENTS WITH PATHOLOGICAL STAGE III   (n=45)

RT alone
    Mantle or inverted Y RT (n=1)
    STNI or TNI (n=2)

| | 3 | 2 | |

Combination CT
    MOPP-like

| | 25 | 11 | (44) |

RT + Combination CT
    IF irradiation + MOPP-like
    M or inverted Y RT + Alternated CT
    STNI or TNI + MOPP-like

	10	8	
	1	1	
	2	2	

Not available or not treated

| | 4 | | |

4 - PATIENTS WITH PATHOLOGICAL STAGE IV   (n=262)

RT alone
    IF irradiation (n=1)
    STNI or TNI   (n=2)

| | 3 | 2 | |

Combination CT
    MOPP-like
    Alternated CT

| | 193 | 131 | (68) |
| | 8 | 8 | |

RT + Combination CT
    IF irradiation + MOPP-like
                  + Alternated CT
    M or inverted Y RT + MOPP-like
                    + Alternated CT
    STNI or TNI + MOPP-like
              + ADM containing
              + Alternated CT

	13	9	
	3	2	
	4	2	
	3	3	
	12	12	
	4	4	
	2	2	

Not available or not treated

| | 13 | | |

Table VI-9. Treatment Summary for CS IV patients (N=1,870)

Laparotomy	Treatment type	Number of patients		
		at risk	CR	(%)
NO	RT +/- single or bi-agent CT	54	26	(48)
	Combination CT	1,061	594	(56)
	RT + Combination CT	390	296	(76)
PS I-III	RT +/- single or bi-agent CT	10	8	
	Combination CT	26	21	(81)
	RT + Combination CT	23	18	(78)
PS IV	RT +/- single or bi-agent CT	3	2	
	Combination CT	207	141	(68)
	RT + Combination CT	45	37	(82)
All patients	RT +/- single or bi-agent CT	67	36	(54)
	Combination CT	1,294	763	(59)
	RT + Combination CT	458	353	(77)
All patients	Patients treated 1960-69	60	42	(70)
	1970-79	1,031	639	(62)
	1980 +	751	473	(63)

Table VI-10. Treatment summary for patients with mediastinal involvement (N=3,159)*

Laparotomy	Treatment type	Number of patients		
		at risk	CR	(%)
* CLINICAL STAGE IIA (n=1,459)				
Not bulky (N=1,018)	RT +/- single/bi-agent CT	615	603	(98)
	Combination CT	28	21	(75)
	RT + Combination CT	363	352	(97)
	1960-69	50	47	(94)
	1970-79	542	526	(97)
	1980 +	416	399	(96)
Bulky (N=441)	RT +/- single/bi-agent CT	172	169	(98)
	Combination CT	17	13	
	RT + Combination CT	249	229	(92)
	1960-69	24	25	(96)
	1970-79	210	202	(96)
	1980 +	205	187	(91)
* CLINICAL STAGE IB - IIB (n=684)				
Not bulky (N=386)	RT +/- single/bi-agent CT	109	152	(94)
	Combination CT	43	38	(88)
	RT + Combination CT	226	212	(94)
	1960-69	19	17	
	1970-79	200	184	(92)
	1980 +	161	151	(94)
Bulky (N=298)	RT +/- single/bi-agent CT	54	50	(93)
	Combination CT	38	16	(42)
	RT + Combination CT	204	184	(90)
	1960-69	8	8	
	1970-79	142	126	(89)
	1980 +	142	116	(82)

Patients for whom all information relative to mediastinal involvement was available

Table VI-10. Treatment summary for patients with mediastinal involvement (N=3,159)* (continued)

Laparotomy	Treatment type	Number of patients		
		at risk	CR	(%)
* CLINICAL STAGE IIIA (n=263)				
Not bulky (N=195)	RT +/- single/bi-agent CT	53	51	(96)
	Combination CT	42	31	(74)
	RT + Combination CT	99	90	(91)
	1960-69	7	7	
	1970-79	105	99	(94)
	1980 +	82	66	(80)
Bulky (N=68)	RT +/- single/bi-agent CT	17	15	
	Combination CT	9	8	
	RT + Combination CT	42	34	(81)
	1960-69	5	5	
	1970-79	31	27	(87)
	1980 +	32	29	(91)
* CLINICAL STAGE IIIB - IV (n=753)				
Not bulky (N=509)	RT +/- single/bi-agent CT	24	21	(88)
	Combination CT	257	172	(67)
	RT + Combination CT	218	181	(83)
	1960-69	30	23	(77)
	1970-79	209	155	(74)
	1980 +	265	199	(75)
Bulky (N=244)	RT +/- single/bi-agent CT	8	6	
	Combination CT	103	64	(62)
	RT + Combination CT	131	111	(85)
	1960-69	10	6	
	1970-79	82	58	(71)
	1980 +	151	116	(77)

Patients for whom all information relative to mediastinal involvement was available

Table VI-11. Initial characteristics of the patients who failed to achieve a complete remission

Characteristics		Number of patients	(% of total)
SEX	Males	1,217	(14.2)
	Females	651	(11.6)
AGE	mean (SD)	39.8 (17.2)	
	range	15-87	
	15-19	159	(9.6)
	20-29	542	(10.9)
	30-39	352	(10.9)
	40-49	244	(13.4)
	50-59	246	(19.2)
	60-69	210	(24.9)
	70 +	114	(33.9)
HISTOLOGY	LP	72	(7.1)
	NS	1,014	(11.8)
	MC	553	(14.8)
	LD	158	(37.4)
	unclassified	68	(19.3)
TOPOGRAPHY	above diaphragm	580	(6.3)
	below	85	(14.5)
	above and below	1,227	(25.3)
CLINICAL STAGE	I	78	(2.6)
	II	469	(7.7)
	III	623	(18.8)
	IV without BM involvement	528	(36.7)
	with BM involvement	167	(39.1)
NUMBER OF LYMPH NODE AREAS INVOLVED	0	98	(46.2)
	1	220	(6.7)
	2	594	(12.8)
	3	272	(10.8)
	4	204	(13.8)
	5 +	467	(23.6)
MEDIASTINUM	not involved	815	(11.9)
	not bulky	909	(14.4)
	bulky	144	(13.3)
EXTRA LOCALIZATION E+	absent	1,655	(13.1)
	present	212	(13.6)
SYSTEMIC SYMPTOMS	absent	609	(6.8)
	present	1,251	(24.4)

Table VI-11. Initial characteristics of the patients who failed to achieve a complete remission (continued)

Characteristics		Number of patients	(% of total)
E.S.R. number available		1,327	(15.3)
mean (SD)		61.7 (37.6)	
0- 9		95	(5.6)
10-19		102	(8.0)
20-29		115	(12.3)
30-39		119	(13.7)
40-49		116	(15.9)
50-59		128	(19.3)
60-69		108	(19.3)
70-79		105	(24.5)
80-89		101	(26.8)
90-99		86	(28.6)
100 +		252	(30.8)
SERUM L.D.H.	number available	296	(16.6)
	< 25th percentile	52	(13.1)
	25-75th percentile	152	(15.0)
	> 75th percentile	92	(25.0)
ALKALINE PHOSPHATASE	number available	1,052	(13.9)
	< 25th percentile	178	(10.9)
	25-75th percentile	489	(12.0)
	> 75th percentile	385	(20.4)
SERUM ALBUMIN	number available	1,044	(19.6)
	< 25th percentile	418	(38.5)
	25-75th percentile	501	(18.5)
	> 75th percentile	125	(8.2)
HEMOGLOBIN number available		1,667	(16.0)
mean (SD)		7.4 (1.3)	
< 3.9		13	(37.1)
4.0-4.9		47	(39.5)
5.0-5.9		146	(34.4)
6.0-6.9		403	(28.3)
7.0-7.9		473	(18.4)
8.0-8.9		402	(12.1)
9.0-9.9		150	(7.2)
10.0 +		33	(7.4)

Table VI-11. Initial characteristics of the patients who failed to achieve a complete remission (continued)

Characteristics		Number of patients	(% of total)
TREATMENT PERIOD 1960-1969		84	(7.7)
1970-1979		1,040	(13.0)
1980 +		744	(14.6)
LAPAROTOMY-SPLENECTOMY		451	(7.5)
Laparotomy findings	PS I	10	(0.9)
	PS II	100	(4.3)
	PS III	205	(9.7)
	PS IV	146	(27.2)
TREATMENT			
No treatment or surgery alone		17	(48.6)
RT alone		216	(3.8)
Single or bi-agent CT		19	(76.0)
RT + single or bi-agent CT		41	(11.6)
Combination CT : MOPP-like		1,004	(34.6)
ADM containing		1	(5.6)
Alternated		127	(33.1)
RT + Combination CT : MOPP-like		351	(9.1)
ADM containing		9	(2.2)
Alternated		51	(12.3)
Not specified		51	(33.3)
TOTAL FAIL		1,868	

Table VI-12. Distribution of the patients (all clinical stages) who failed to achieve a complete remission according to age and hemoglobin level

AGE	HEMOGLOBIN*	TREATMENT TYPE	N	(% of total)
<50 yrs	normal	RT +/- single/bi-agent CT	89	(3.5)
		Combination CT	282	(26.5)
		RT + Combination	132	(6.4)
	abnormal	RT +/- single/bi-agent CT	34	(7.0)
		Combination CT	439	(37.3)
		RT + Combination CT	164	(15.9)
50+ yrs	normal	RT +/- single/bi-agent CT	38	(7.7)
		Combination CT	111	(32.8)
		RT + Combination CT	36	(10.3)
	abnormal	RT +/- single/bi-agent CT	36	(33.0)
		Combination CT	224	(46.0)
		RT + Combination CT	43	(23.9)

* normal if 8.0+ mmol/l in males and 7.0+ mmol/l in females; abnormal if decreased

Table VI-13. Distribution of the patients who failed to achieve a complete remission by pathological stage and treatment

PATHOLOGICAL STAGE	TREATMENT TYPE	N	(% of total)
PS I	RT +/- single/bi-agent CT	7	(0.8)
	Combination CT	0/2	
	RT + Combination CT	4	(3.3)
PS II	RT +/- single/bi-agent CT	51	(2.9)
	Combination CT	29	(51.8)
	RT + Combination CT	21	(3.8)
PS III	RT +/- single/bi-agent CT	31	(5.3)
	Combination CT	103	(20.9)
	RT + Combination CT	69	(6.6)
PS IV	RT +/- single/bi-agent CT	3/12	
	Combination CT	105	(30.2)
	RT + Combination CT	21	(16.7)

Table VI-14. Prognostic factors of response to initial treatment in CS I patients (N=1,509) without staging laparotomy

Patients who failed to achieve a complete remission: n = 39   (2.6 %)

STEPWISE LOGISTIC REGRESSION

Parameters included in the analysis (number of dummy variables) = sex, age (4), mediastinal involvement (2), histological subtype (2), extra nodal localization, systemic symptoms, topography.

Step	Variable (codes)	log. likelihood	Coeff/s.e.	p value
0		- 106.08		
1	AGE (<50=-1, 50+=1)	- 103.37	- 0.489/0.219	0.020
2	HISTOLOGY (LP-NS=-1, MC-LD-uncl.=1)	- 100.74	- 0.511/0.232	0.022
	CONSTANT		3.703/0.233	

Pattern	number of patients	observed proportion of CR	predicted probability of CR
AGE 50+ yrs, MC-LD	114	0.95	0.94
AGE 50+ yrs, LP-NS	121	0.97	0.98
AGE <50 yrs, MC-LD	319	0.97	0.98
AGE <50 yrs, LP-NS	462	0.99	0.99

Table VI-15. Prognostic factors of response to initial treatment in CS II patients (N=2,880) without staging laparotomy

Patients who failed to achieve a complete remission: n = 276 (9.6 %)

STEPWISE LOGISTIC REGRESSION

Parameters included in the analysis (number of dummy variables) = sex, age (4), mediastinal involvement (2), histological subtype (2), extra nodal localization, systemic symptoms, number of lymph node areas involved (3), topography.

Step	Variable (codes)	log. likelihood	Coeff/s.e.	p value
0		− 582.00		
1	SYSTEMIC SYMPTOMS (absent=−1, present=1)	− 569.00	− 0.401/0.082	< 0.001
2	AGE (<50=−1, 50+=1)	− 561.73	− 0.400/0.099	< 0.001
	CONSTANT		2.194/0.099	

Pattern	number of patients	observed proportion of CR	predicted probability of CR
AGE 50+ yrs, SYMPTOMS present	115	0.82	0.80
AGE 50+ yrs, SYMPTOMS absent	170	0.88	0.90
AGE <50 yrs, SYMPTOMS present	611	0.90	0.90
AGE <50 yrs, SYMPTOMS absent	1,354	0.95	0.95

Table VI-16. Prognostic factors of response to initial treatment in CS III patients (N=1,856) without staging laparotomy

Patients who failed to achieve a complete remission: n = 440 (23.7%)

STEPWISE LOGISTIC REGRESSION

Parameters included in the analysis (number of dummy variables) = sex, age (4), mediastinal involvement (2), histological subtype (2), extra nodal localization, systemic symptoms, number of lymph node areas involved (3).

Step	Variable (codes)	log. likelihood	Coeff/s.e.	p value
0		− 714.53		
1	SYSTEMIC SYMPTOMS (absent=−1, present=1)	− 705.65	− 0.297/0.073	< 0.001
2	AGE (<50=−1, 50+=1)	− 701.52	− 0.214/0.073	0.004
	CONSTANT		1.322/0.079	

Pattern	number of patients	observed proportion of CR	predicted probability of CR
SYMPTOMS present, AGE 50+ yrs	215	0.69	0.69
SYMPTOMS present, AGE <50 yrs	655	0.77	0.77
SYMPTOMS absent, AGE 50+ yrs	121	0.80	0.80
SYMPTOMS absent, AGE <50 yrs	400	0.86	0.86

Table VI-17. Prognostic factors of response to initial treatment in CS IV patients (N=1,839)

Patients who failed to achieve a complete remission: n = 674 (36.7%)

STEPWISE LOGISTIC REGRESSION

Parameters included in the analysis (number of dummy variables) = sex, age (4), mediastinal involvement (2), histological subtype (2), extra nodal localization, systemic symptoms, number of lymph node areas involved (3), bone marrow involvement, topography.

Step	Variable (codes)	log. likelihood	Coeff/s.e.	p value
0		− 1208.35		
1	AGE (<50=−1, 50+=1)	− 1194.39	− 0.267/0.053	< 0.001
2	TOPOGRAPHY (one side=−1, both sides=1)	− 1187.67	− 0.269/0.076	< 0.001
	CONSTANT		0.634/0.079	

Pattern	number of patients	observed proportion of CR	predicted probability of CR
AGE 50+ yrs, both sides	462	0.53	0.52
AGE 50+ yrs, one side	50	0.58	0.65
AGE <50 yrs, both sides	1,113	0.65	0.65
AGE <50 yrs, one side	214	0.78	0.76

Table VI-18. Prognostic factors of response to initial treatment in CS I-II-III-IV patients (N=5,954) with staging laparotomy

Patients who failed to achieve a complete remission:

PS I-II	110/3,382	3.3%
PS III	197/2,094	9.4%
PS IV	128/478	26.8%

STEPWISE LOGISTIC REGRESSION

Parameters included in the analysis (number of dummy variables) = sex, age (4), mediastinal involvement (2), histological subtype (2), extra nodal localization, systemic symptoms, number of lymph node areas involved (3), topography.

In these three categories of patients, ie PS I-II, PS III, and PS IV, the only parameter which significantly ($p<0.001$) predicts treatment response was the **presence of systemic symptoms**.

Pattern	number of patients	observed proportion of CR	predicted probability of CR
PS I-II patients			
SYSTEMIC SYMPTOMS present	615	0.90	0.90
SYSTEMIC SYMPTOMS absent	2,767	0.98	0.98
PS III patients			
SYSTEMIC SYMPTOMS present	680	0.86	0.86
SYSTEMIC SYMPTOMS absent	1,414	0.93	0.93
PS IV patients			
SYSTEMIC SYMPTOMS present	304	0.69	0.69
SYSTEMIC SYMPTOMS absent	174	0.81	0.81

Part VII - *Septième partie*

PROGNOSTIC STUDY OF RELAPSE-FREE SURVIVAL BY CLINICAL STAGE

ANALYSE PRONOSTIQUE DE LA DUREE DE SURVIE SANS RECHUTE EN FONCTION DU STADE CLINIQUE

Relapse-free survival prognostic study

In this chapter, only patients who achieved a complete remission by initial therapy are considered in the analysis, e.g. 11,904 patients out of 13,772 (86.4%) treated patients for whom response to initial treatment was available.

The prognostic value on relapse-free survival was estimated separately (univariate) for each variable by clinical stage and presence or absence of systemic symptoms with stratification on treatment period, type of initial therapy and staging laparotomy (Tables VII-1 to VII-6) using the logrank test.

Then crude 5-year and 10-year relapse-free survival rates are given according to clinical stage, presence or absence of B symptoms, and by initial treatment type (Tables VII-8 to VII-12).

Crude relapse-free survival curves are also provided for the entire cohort according to period of start of first therapy (Figure VII-1), sex (Figure VII-2), age at diagnosis (Figure VII-3), histological subtypes (Figure VII-4), clinical stage and B symptoms (Figure VII-5), or by stage (Figures VII-6 to VII-12 for early stages, and Figures VII-13 to VII-15 for advanced stages).

Prognostic factors by stage

1) Regression model allowing all variables simultaneously

The results from proportional hazards survival analysis are given by stage and presence or absence of B symptoms, overall and according to whether the patients were submitted to staging laparotomy (Tables VII-13 to VII-21).

In *clinical stage I patients,* besides staging laparotomy, histological subtypes, sex, age above 40, topography and B symptoms were significantly associated with a higher risk of relapse (Table VII-13). The laparotomy significance seems to reflect the better results observed after therapy adapted to laparotomy findings.

In these patients when biological parameters were included in the model, ESR was significantly associated with clinical outcome, as was hemoglobin.

- Coefficients of risk (s.d.) were:

ESR	1-20	0		
ESR	20-39	0.40	(0.12)	$p=0.001$
ESR	40-59	0.65	(0.16)	$p<0.001$
ESR	60+	0.86	(0.18)	$p<0.001$

with sex, age, and histology still displaying significant prognostic value, as does extra nodal localization (E+) ($p<0.05$).

For hemoglobin, the coefficients of risk (s.d.) were:

Hb	< 7.0	1.07 (0.22)	$p<0.001$
Hb	7.0-8.9	0.59 (0.11)	$p<0.001$
Hb	9.0 +	0	

with sex, age, and histology still displaying significant prognostic value, as does extra nodal localization (E+) ($p<0.05$).

The prognostic significance of ESR and hemoglobin values was also observed in clinical stage I patients without staging laparotomy, while in those who were laparotomized only ESR above 60 or Hb below 7.0 were marginally significant ($p=0.05$). In this latter group, data of only 749 and 958 patients were available, respectively.

The same conclusions were observed in clinical stage IA patients (Table VII-14).

In *clinical stage II patients*, besides staging laparotomy, histological subtypes, B symptoms, sex, and the number of lymph node areas involved were significantly associated with a higher risk of relapse (Table VII-15). Like in clinical stage I patients, laparotomy significance seems to reflect the better results observed after therapy adapted to laparotomy findings.

In these patients, when biological parameters were included in the model ESR (N = 3,122), hemoglobin (N = 3,606), and serum albumin (N = 1,680) were significantly associated with clinical outcome.

- For ESR, the coefficients of risk (s.d.) were:

ESR	1-20	0	
ESR	20-39	0.45 (0.10)	$p<0.001$
ESR	40-59	0.44 (0.11)	$p<0.001$
ESR	60+	0.57 (0.10)	$p<0.001$

with sex still displaying significant prognostic value in addition to mediastinal involvement ($p<0.05$).

For hemoglobin, the coefficients of risk (s.d.) were:

Hb	< 7.0	0.45 (0.13)	$p<0.01$
Hb	7.0-8.9	0.27 (0.09)	$p<0.01$
Hb	9.0 +	0	

with sex, histology, age ($p<0.05$) and B symptoms still displaying significant prognostic value as did mediastinal involvement ($p<0.05$) and the number of lymph node areas involved ($p<0.05$).

For serum albumin, the coefficients of risk (s.d.) were:

SA	< 25th	0.43	(0.15)	p<0.01
SA	25-75th	0.21	(0.10)	p<0.05
SA	> 75th	0		

with histology still displaying significant prognostic value in addition to mediastinal involvement (p<0.01).

The significant prognostic value of ESR and serum albumin was also observed in clinical stage II patients with or without staging laparotomy. In patients without staging laparotomy, two other factors presented with significant coefficient of risk: sex (p<0.05) and B symptoms (p<0.05); sex was the only factor of prognostic importance (p<0.05) in laparotomized patients. In addition to serum albumin the factors which were associated with a higher risk of relapse were histology (p<0.01) and mediastinal involvement (p<0.01).

In *clinical stage IIA patients* the results were quite different (Table VII-16). In these patients, when ESR was considered in the model it appeared as the only prognostic factor on relapse occurrence (p<0.001). When hemoglobin was included, age (p<0.01) and histological types MC-LD (p<0.05) were also associated with a higher risk. No major modifications in the results were observed when serum albumin was considered.

In *clinical stage IB-IIB patients*, histology was the only prognostic factor observed (Table VII-17). After ESR inclusion in the model the results were the following:

SEX	Males	0		
	Females	-0.41	(0.13)	p<0.01
# of LYMPH NODES				
	2, 3, 4	0		
	5	0.60	(0.25)	p<0.05
MEDIASTINUM				
	not involved	0		
	involved	0.32	(0.16)	p<0.05

but ESR was no longer a significant prognostic factor.

Similar results were obtained when hemoglobin was included but Hb < 7.0 displayed an independent prognostic significant value (p<0.05), as did serum albumin < 25th percentile (p<0.01).

In *clinical stage III patients* overall, ESR did not appear as a prognostic factor nor were hemoglobin and serum albumin, and when included in the model, only slightly modified the results given in Table VII-18, inducing a decrease in the significance levels.

In *clinical stage IIIA patients*, when ESR was taken into account, only ESR above 60 reached the 0.05 level. Two other variables were also significantly associated with an increase in relapse risk: age above 50 (p<0.05) and mediastinal involvement (p<0.05). Other biological parameters were of no prognostic value.

In *clinical stage IIIB patients*, sex was the only significant factor on relapse-free survival, whatever the variables included in the model (Table VII-20).

In *clinical stage IV patients*, none of the variables studied were associated with an increase in risk of relapse (Table VII-21). This finding was also observed when biological factors were included in the model.

2) Stepwise regression model

The results from stepwise regression model are given in Tables VII-14a, VII-16a, VII-17a, VII-19a, VII-20a and VII-21a, by clinical stage and presence or absence of B symptoms.

In comparison with previous analyses including all the variables in the model simultaneously (see above), slight changes were observed:

- In clinical stage IA patients, the prognostic value of histology disappeared (Table VII-14a), possibly a consequence of stratification on staging laparotomy.

- In clinical stage IIA patients, only unfavorable histological subtypes remained significant (Table VII-16a).

- In clinical stage IB-IIB patients, again the prognostic significance of histology disappeared (Table VII-17a).

- No modifications were observed in clinical stage IIIA patients (Table VII-19a).

- In clinical stage IIIB patients, the prognostic value of the number of lymph node areas involved was no longer observed (Table VII-20a).

- In clinical stage IV patients, age above 60 years at diagnosis remained the only significant factor (Table VII-21a).

When biological parameters were included in the models one at the time, the following were observed:

- Accelerated ESR was the major prognostic indicator in clinical stages IA, IIA, and IIIA patients. In these two last groups it was the only predictive factor that remained statistically significant.

- When hemoglobin was included in the model, it was significant for clinical stages IA, IB-IIB, and IIIA patients. In the latter group it was the only factor that remained statistically significant.

- Decreased serum albumin level was only predictive in clinical stage IB-IIB patients where it preceded sex.

None of the other biological parameters were found to be prognostic.

Relapse characteristics

Relapse characteristics are shown in Table VII-22. The median time from start of therapy to failure was, in any stage, less than 24 months. Nevertheless, late relapses, beyond 10 years, were observed in all stages.

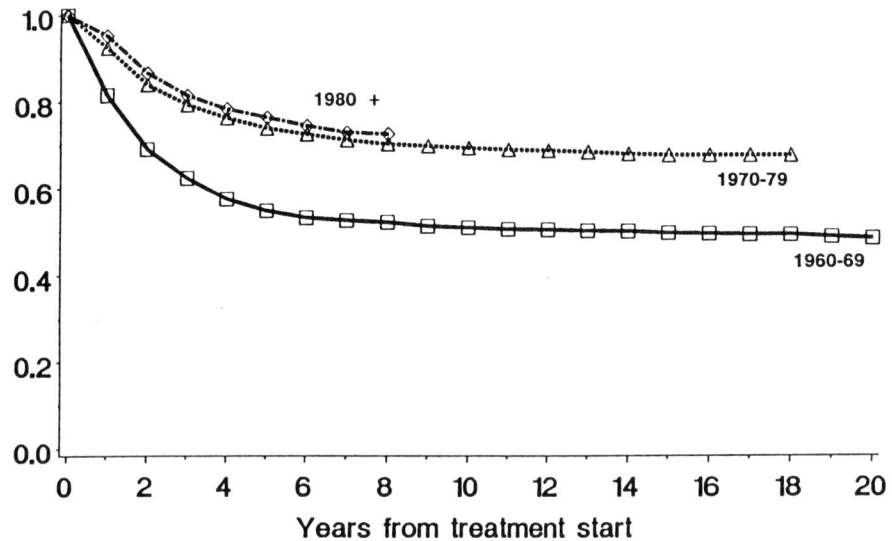

Figure VII-1: *All stages. Relapse-free survival by treatment period. (1960-69 : 1,008 pts; 1970-79 : 6,970 pts; 1980+ : 4,338 pts).*

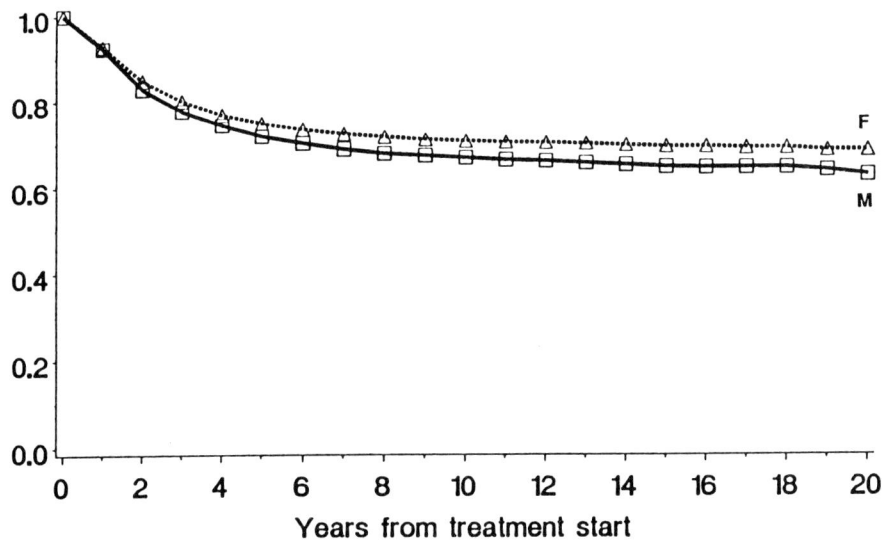

Figure VII-2: *All stages. Relapse-free survival by sex. (Males : 7,368 pts; Females : 4,948 pts).*

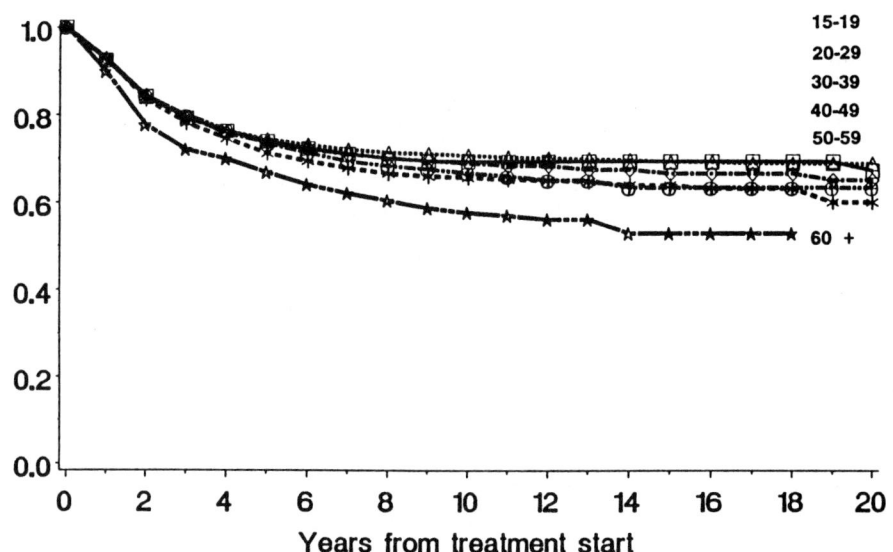

Figure VII-3: *All stages. Relapse-free survival by age at Hodgkin disease diagnosis. (15-19 yrs: 1,503 pts; 20-29 yrs: 4,449 pts; 30-39 yrs: 2,880 pts; 40-49 yrs: 1,579 pts; 50-59 yrs: 1,034 pts; 60+ yrs: 856 pts).*

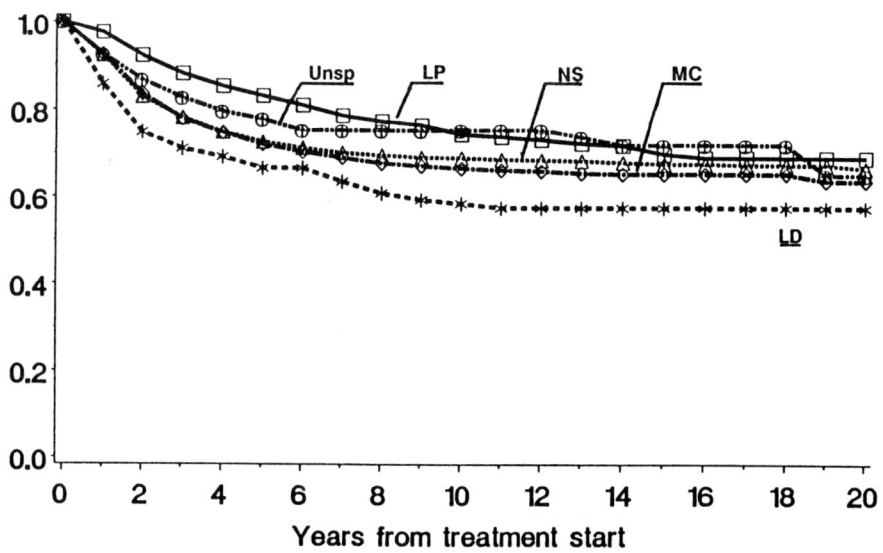

Figure VII-4: *All stages. Relapse-free survival by histological type. (LP: 938 pts; NS: 7,596 pts; MC: 3,183 pts; LD: 264 pts; Type unspecified: 285 pts).*

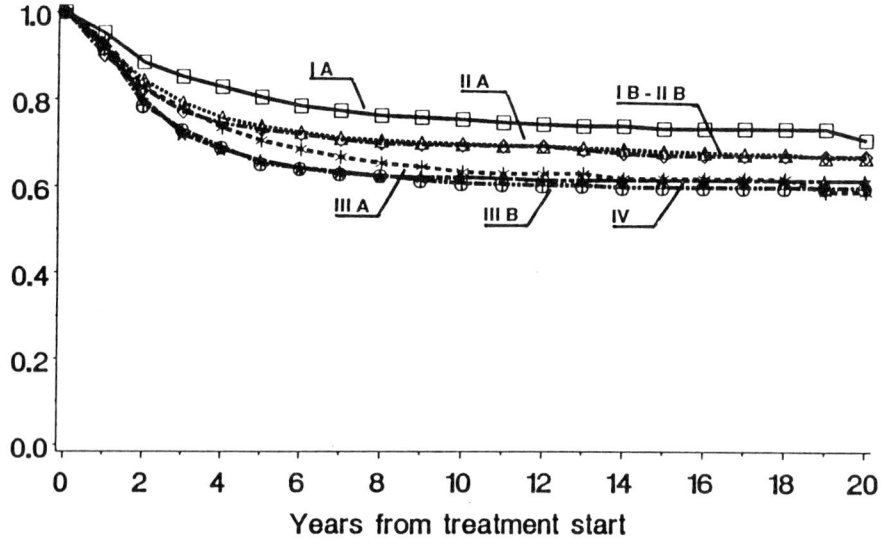

Figure VII-5 : *All stages. Relapse-free survival by clinical stage and presence or absence of B symptoms. (IA : 2,625 pts; IIA : 4,165 pts; IB-IIB : 1,679 pts; IIIA : 1,349 pts; IIIB : 1,339 pts; IV : 1,143 pts).*

Table VII-1. Prognostic value on relapse-free survival for CS IA patients who achieved a complete remission (N=2,625) *

Parameter		Patients at risk	Relative risk of relapse	p value (heterogeneity)
SEX	males	1,775	1.0	
	females	850	0.80	0.015
AGE	15-19	244	1.0	
	20-29	847	0.89	
	30-39	601	1.02	
	40-49	382	1.35	
	50-59	283	1.12	
	60+	266	1.38	0.011
HISTOLOGY	LP	427	1.0	
	NS	1,237	1.50	
	MC	881	1.77	
	LD	16	1.63	0.001
TOPOGRAPHY	above diaphragm	2,487	1.0	
	below	128	0.52	0.007
MEDIASTINUM	not involved	2,366	1.0	
	involved	247	0.94	> 0.20
EXTRA LOCALIZATION E +	absent	2,420	1.0	
	present	205	0.86	> 0.20
E.S.R.	0-19	1,185	1.0	
	20-39	341	1.36	
	40-59	154	2.03	
	60+	101	2.23	< 0.001
L.D.H.	<25th percentile	68	1.0	
	25-75th	106	1.28	> 0.20
	>75th	8		
ALKALINE PHOSPHATASE	<25th percentile	399	1.0	
	25-75th	732	1.12	
	>75th	170	1.05	> 0.20
ALBUMIN	<25th percentile	38	1.86	
	25-75th	457	1.29	
	>75th	473	1.0	0.04
HEMOGLOBIN	abnormal**	147	2.05	
	normal	1,772	1.0	< 0.001

* with stratification on period, treatment and staging laparotomy
** Hb < 8.0 mmol/l in males and < 7.0 mmol/l in females

Table VII-2. Prognostic value on relapse-free survival for CS IIA patients who achieved a complete remission (N=4,165) *

Parameter		Patients at risk	Relative risk of relapse	p value (heterogeneity)
SEX	males	2,117	1.0	
	females	2,048	0.92	0.15
AGE	15-19	622	1.0	
	20-29	1,718	0.94	
	30-39	1,033	1.08	
	40-49	432	1.00	
	50-59	209	1.17	
	60+	147	1.28	> 0.20
HISTOLOGY	LP	234	1.0	
	NS	3,013	1.38	
	MC	774	1.61	
	LD	58	2.04	0.005
TOPOGRAPHY	above diaphragm	3,941	1.0	
	below	223	1.61	0.11
MEDIASTINUM	not involved	1,346	1.0	
	involved	2,805	0.96	> 0.20
EXTRA LOCALIZATION E +	absent	3,670	1.0	
	present	495	1.06	> 0.20
# OF LYMPH NODE AREAS INVOLVED	2	2,343	1.0	
	3	1,109	1.17	
	4	454	1.27	
	5+	236	1.38	0.006
E.S.R.	0-19	934	1.0	
	20-39	655	1.61	
	40-59	408	1.65	
	60+	412	1.82	< 0.001
L.D.H.	<25th percentile	101	1.0	
	25-75th	282	1.0	
	>75th	61	1.19	> 0.20
ALKALINE PHOSPHATASE	<25th percentile	485	1.0	
	25-75th	1,283	1.05	
	>75th	371	1.22	> 0.20
ALBUMIN	<25th percentile	99	1.29	
	25-75th	660	1.27	
	>75th	483	1.0	0.081
HEMOGLOBIN	abnormal**	363	1.27	
	normal	2,344	1.0	0.024

* with stratification on period, treatment and staging laparotomy
** Hb < 8.0 mmol/l in males and < 7.0 mmol/l in females

Table VII-3. Prognostic value on relapse-free survival for CS IB and CS IIB patients who achieved a complete remission (N=1,679) *

Parameter		Patients at risk	Relative risk of relapse	p value (heterogeneity)
SEX	males	952	1.0	
	females	727	0.72	0.001
AGE	15-19	211	1.0	
	20-29	634	1.10	
	30-39	385	1.17	
	40-49	224	1.28	
	50-59	130	1.00	
	60+	92	1.17	> 0.20
HISTOLOGY	LP	74	1.0	
	NS	1,167	2.42	
	MC	361	2.73	
	LD	36	2.98	0.008
TOPOGRAPHY	above diaphragm	1,555	1.0	
	below	123	1.13	> 0.20
MEDIASTINUM	not involved	545	1.0	
	involved	1,131	1.17	0.12
EXTRA LOCALIZATION E +	absent	1,448	1.0	
	present	231	1.16	> 0.20
# OF LYMPH NODE AREAS INVOLVED	1	253	1.0	
	2	652	1.12	
	3	433	1.19	
	4	209	1.13	
	5+	122	1.90	0.018
E.S.R.	0-19	183	1.0	
	20-39	160	1.41	
	40-59	204	1.15	
	60+	435	1.53	0.064
L.D.H.	<25th percentile	37	1.0	
	25-75th	119	0.84	
	>75th	42	0.80	> 0.20
ALKALINE PHOSPHATASE	<25th percentile	187	1.0	
	25-75th	536	0.91	
	>75th	265	0.94	> 0.20
ALBUMIN	<25th percentile	127	1.92	
	25-75th	298	1.22	
	>75th	134	1.0	0.008
HEMOGLOBIN	abnormal**	428	1.56	
	normal	702	1.0	< 0.001

* with stratification on period, treatment and staging laparotomy
** Hb < 8.0 mmol/l in males and < 7.0 mmol/l in females

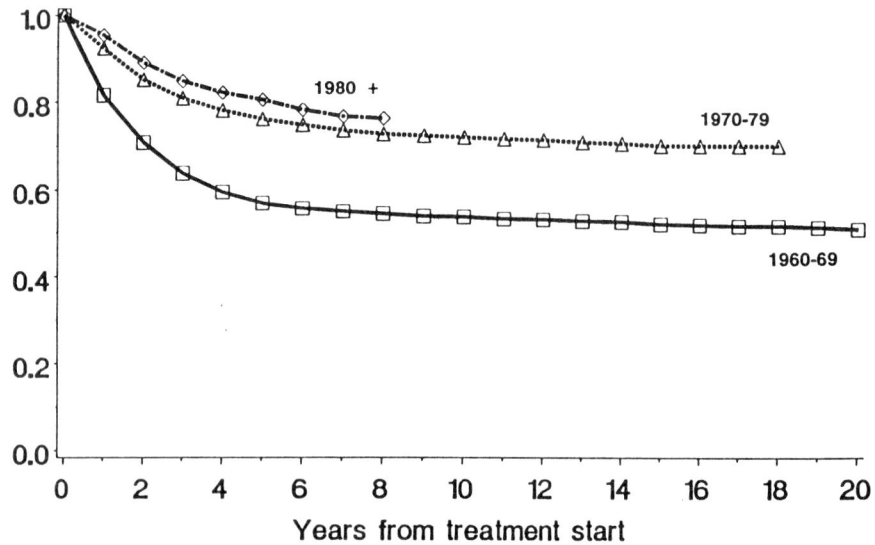

Figure VII-6: *Clinical stages I-II. Relapse-free survival by treatment period. (1960-69 : 766 pts; 1970-79 : 4,762 pts; 1980+ : 2,942 pts).*

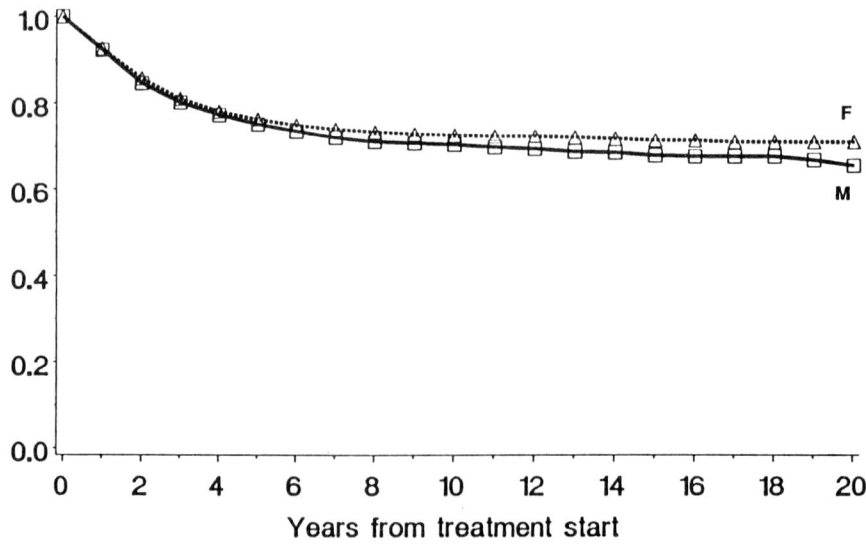

Figure VII-7: *Clinical stages I-II. Relapse-free survival by sex. (Males : 4,844 pts; Females : 3,626 pts).*

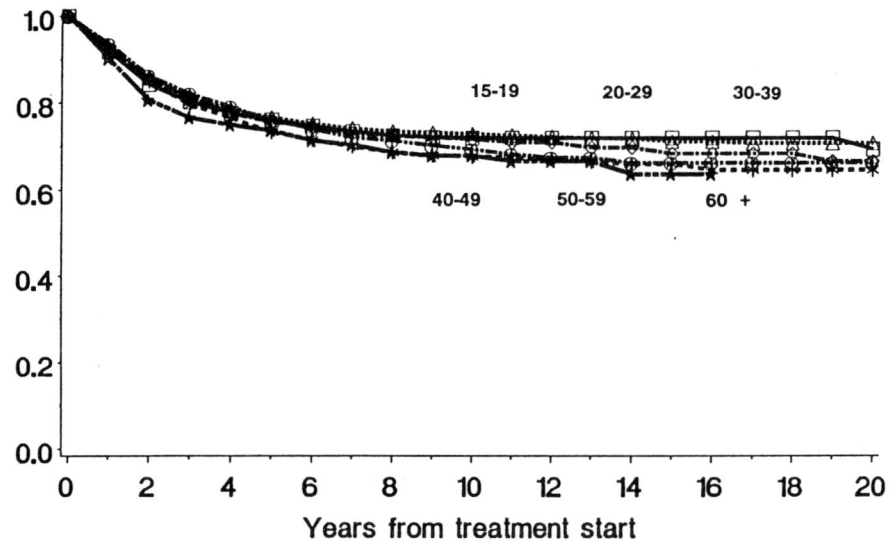

Figure VII-8 : *Clinical stages I-II. Relapse-free survival by age at Hodgkin disease diagnosis. (15-19 yrs: 1,077 pts; 20-29 yrs : 3,199 pts; 30-39 yrs : 2,019 pts; 40-49 yrs : 1,038 pts; 50-59 yrs : 623 pts; 60+ yrs : 505 pts).*

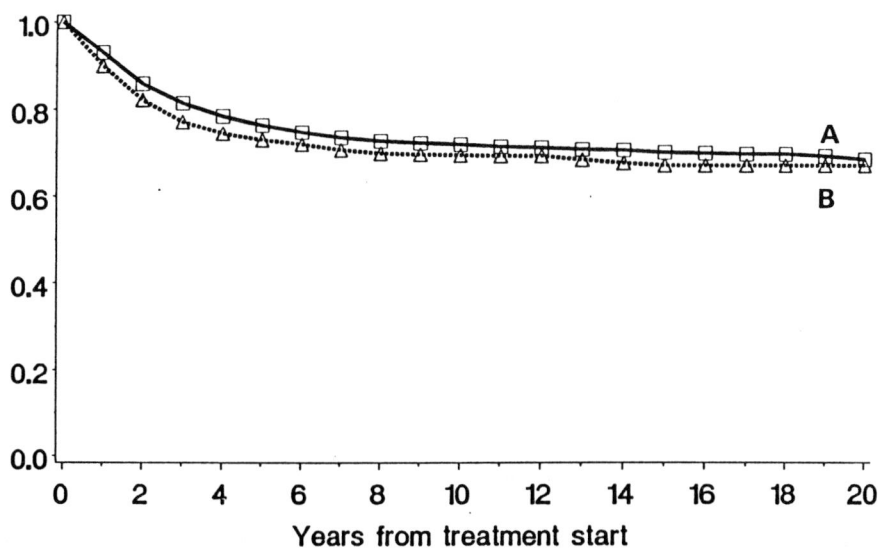

Figure VII-9 : *Clinical stages I-II. Relapse-free survival by presence or absence of B symptoms. (A : 6,790 pts; B : 1,679 pts).*

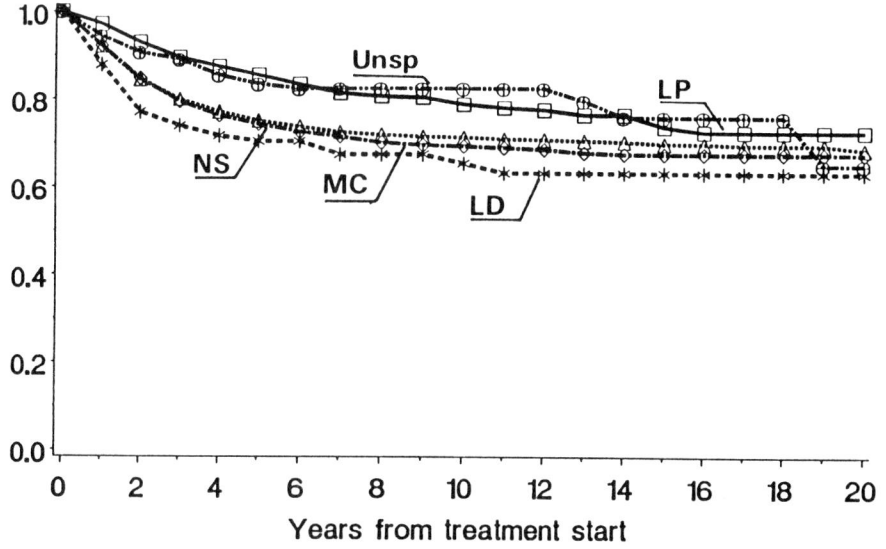

Figure VII-10 : *Clinical stages I-II. Relapse-free survival by histological type. (LP : 735 pts; NS : 5,417 pts; MC : 2,016 pts; LD : 110 pts; Type unspecified : 145 pts).*

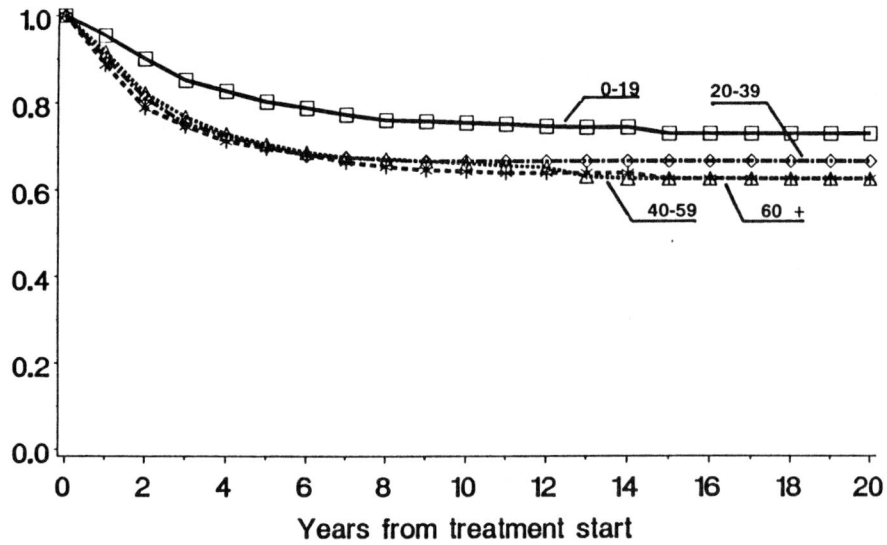

Figure VII-11 : *Clinical stages I-II. Relapse-free survival by ESR level. (0-19 mm : 1,616 pts; 20-39 mm : 1,842 pts; 40-59 mm : 698 pts; 60+ mm : 202 pts).*

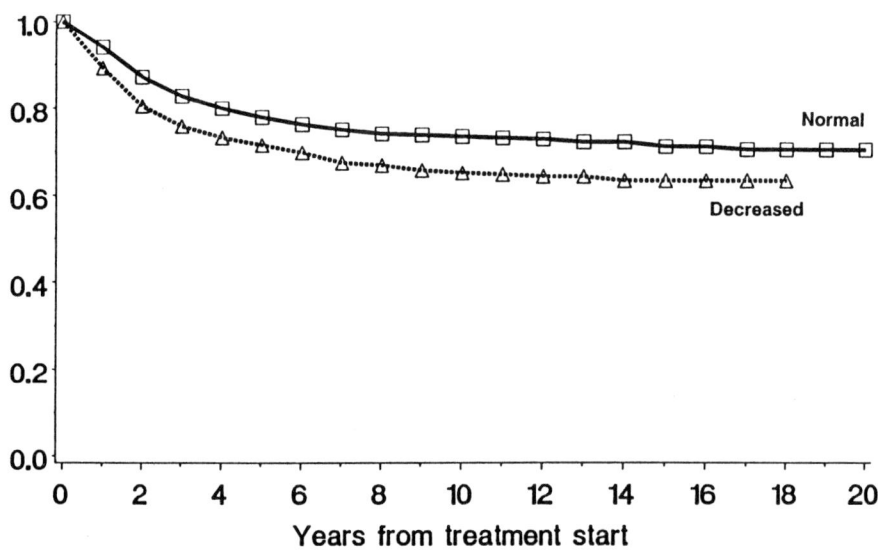

Figure VII-12 : *Clinical stages I-II. Relapse-free survival by hemoglobin level. (Normal : 4,843 pts; Abnormal, < 8.0 mmol/l in males and < 7.0 mmol/l in females: 949 pts).*

Table VII-4. Prognostic value on relapse-free survival for CS IIIA patients who achieved a complete remission (N=1,349) *

Parameter			Patients at risk	Relative risk of relapse	p value (heterogeneity)
SEX	males		873	1.0	
	females		476	0.88	> 0.20
AGE	15-19		161	1.0	
	20-29		473	0.78	
	30-39		286	0.80	
	40-49		189	0.84	
	50-59		128	1.11	
	60+		110	1.13	0.14
HISTOLOGY	LP		115	1.0	
	NS		738	1.38	
	MC		441	1.39	
	LD		25	2.12	0.12
MEDIASTINUM	not involved		683	1.0	
	involved		656	1.17	0.12
EXTRA LOCALIZATION E +	absent		1,267	1.0	
	present		82	0.97	> 0.20
# OF LYMPH NODE AREAS INVOLVED	2		523	1.0	
	3		244	1.50	
	4		241	1.57	
	5+		333	1.82	< 0.001
E.S.R.	0-19		295	1.0	
	20-39		179	1.11	
	40-59		117	1.19	
	60+		115	1.67	0.03
L.D.H.	<25th percentile		34	1.0	
	25-75th		97	0.36	
	>75th		31	1.04	> 0.20
ALKALINE PHOSPHATASE	<25th percentile		144	1.0	
	25-75th		381	1.12	
	>75th		98	1.72	0.07
ALBUMIN	<25th percentile		56	1.53	
	25-75th		304	1.26	
	>75th		175	1.0	0.20
HEMOGLOBIN	abnormal**		184	1.48	
	normal		752	1.0	0.005

* with stratification on period, treatment and staging laparotomy
** Hb < 8.0 mmol/l in males and < 7.0 mmol/l in females

Table VII-5. Prognostic value on relapse-free survival for CS IIIB patients who achieved a complete remission (N=1,337) *

Parameter			Patients at risk	Relative risk of relapse	p value (heterogeneity)
SEX	males		924	1.0	
	females		413	0.73	0.003
AGE	15-19		142	1.0	
	20-29		446	1.04	
	30-39		326	1.04	
	40-49		174	1.01	
	50-59		133	0.84	
	60+		113	1.60	0.07
HISTOLOGY	LP		48	1.0	
	NS		771	1.66	
	MC		408	1.63	
	LD		57	2.02	> 0.20
MEDIASTINUM	not involved		510	1.0	
	involved		820	1.22	0.05
EXTRA LOCALIZATION E +	absent		1,228	1.0	
	present		108	0.87	> 0.20
# OF LYMPH NODE AREAS INVOLVED	2		354	1.0	
	3		249	1.21	
	4		215	1.31	
	5+		511	1.42	0.06
E.S.R.	0-19		100	1.0	
	20-39		124	0.65	
	40-59		149	1.06	
	60+		380	0.84	0.09
L.D.H.	<25th percentile		48	1.0	
	25-75th		110	1.40	
	>75th		55	1.37	> 0.20
ALKALINE PHOSPHATASE	<25th percentile		138	1.0	
	25-75th		364	0.99	
	>75th		239	1.20	> 0.20
ALBUMIN	<25th percentile		144	0.81	
	25-75th		257	0.66	
	>75th		78	1.0	0.11
HEMOGLOBIN	abnormal**		535	1.15	
	normal		460	1.0	0.20

* with stratification on period, treatment and staging laparotomy
** Hb < 8.0 mmol/l in males and < 7.0 mmol/l in females

Table VII-6. Prognostic value on relapse-free survival for CS IV patients who achieved a complete remission (N=1,146) *

Parameter		Patients at risk	Relative risk of relapse	p value (heterogeneity)
SEX	males	718	1.0	
	females	428	0.78	0.03
AGE	15-19	121	1.0	
	20-29	329	1.34	
	30-39	249	1.33	
	40-49	174	1.34	
	50-59	147	1.21	
	60+	126	1.90	0.10
HISTOLOGY	LP	38	1.0	
	NS	666	0.63	
	MC	317	0.54	
	LD	70	0.68	0.09
TOPOGRAPHY	above diaphragm	195	1.0	
	below	949	0.90	> 0.20
MEDIASTINUM	not involved	443	1.0	
	involved	693	0.88	> 0.20
EXTRA LOCALIZATION E +	absent	923	1.0	
	present	223	1.15	> 0.20
B SYMPTOMS	absent	275	1.0	
	present	867	1.17	> 0.20
# OF LYMPH NODE AREAS INVOLVED	0	114	1.01	
	1	180	1.0	
	2	185	0.99	
	3	202	0.94	
	4	149	1.12	
	5+	311	1.29	> 0.20
BONE MARROW INVOLVEMENT	No	634	1.0	
	Yes	260	1.16	> 0.20

* with stratification on period, treatment and staging laparotomy

Table VII-6. Prognostic value on relapse-free survival for CS IV patients who achieved a complete remission (N=1,146) *
(continued)

Parameter		Patients at risk	Relative risk of relapse	p value (heterogeneity)
E.S.R.	0-19	90	1.0	
	20-39	112	0.69	
	40-59	115	0.89	
	60+	277	0.90	> 0.20
L.D.H.	<25th percentile	56	1.0	
	25-75th	144	0.79	
	>75th	79	1.09	> 0.20
ALKALINE PHOSPHATASE	<25th percentile	96	1.0	
	25-75th	275	1.49	
	>75th	360	1.41	> 0.20
ALBUMIN	<25th percentile	202	1.64	
	25-75th	236	1.81	
	>75th	66	1.0	0.10
HEMOGLOBIN	abnormal**	535	0.99	
	normal	409	1.0	< 0.20

* *with stratification on period, treatment and staging laparotomy*
** *Hb < 8.0 mmol/l in males and < 7.0 mmol/l in females*

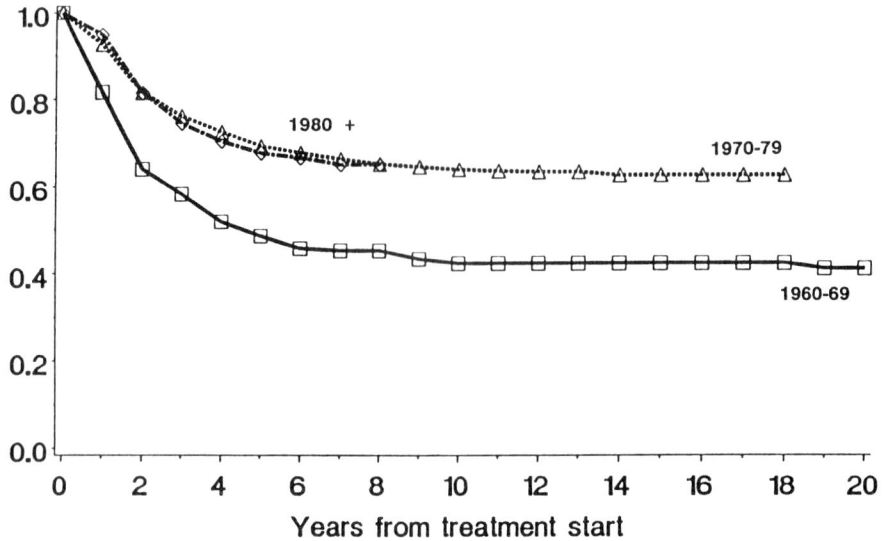

Figure VII-13 : *Clinical stages III-IV. Relapse-free survival by treatment period. (1960-69 : 241 pts; 1970-79 : 2,204 pts; 1980+ : 1,396 pts).*

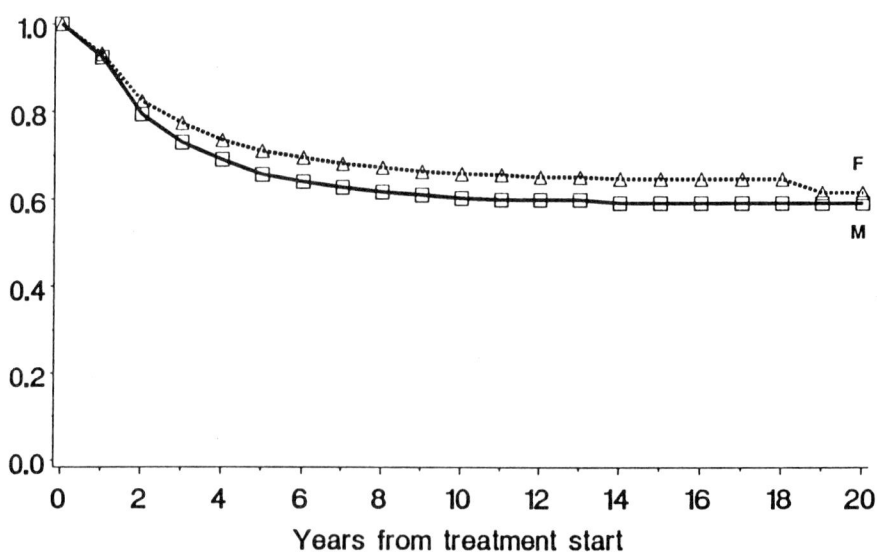

Figure VII-14 : *Clinical stages III-IV. Relapse-free survival by sex. (Males : 2,521 pts; Females : 1,320 pts).*

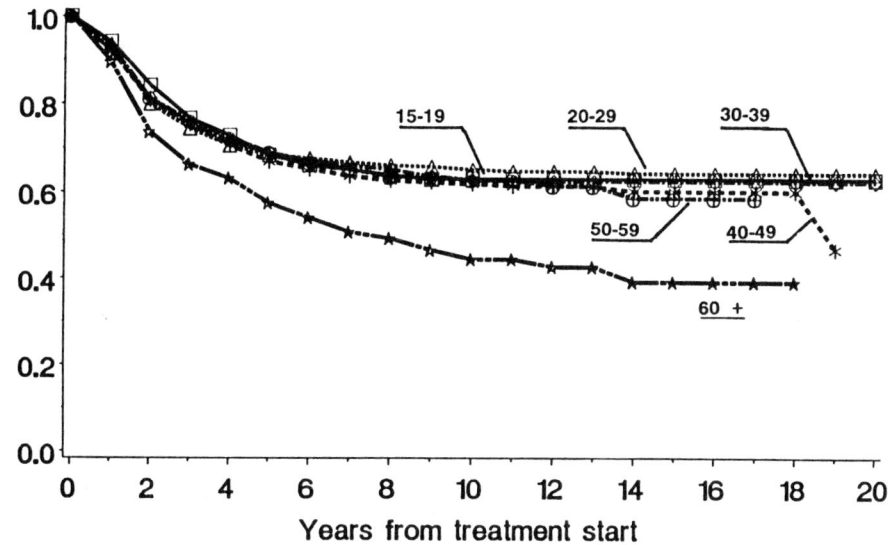

Figure VII-15 : *Clinical stages III-IV. Relapse-free survival by age at Hodgkin disease diagnosis. (15-19 yrs: 426 pts; 20-29 yrs : 1,249 pts; 30-39 yrs : 861 pts; 40-49 yrs : 539 pts; 50-59 yrs : 411 pts; 60+ yrs : 350 pts).*

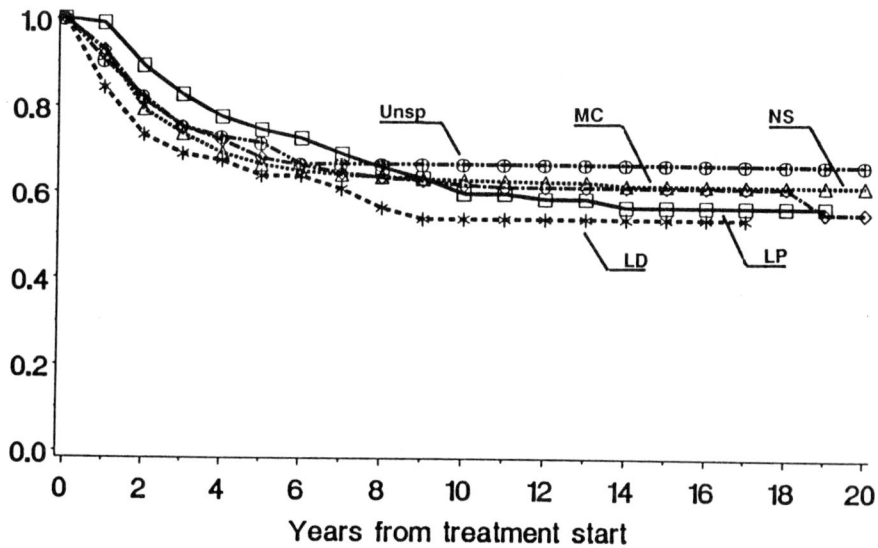

Figure VII-16 : *Clinical stages III-IV. Relapse-free survival by histological type. (LP : 202 pts; NS : 2,178 pts; MC : 1,166 pts; LD : 153 pts; Type unspecified : 140 pts).*

Table VII-7. Relapse-free survival for CS IA patients who achieved a complete remission

Treatment type		Patients at risk	Relapse-free survival at 5-yrs(s.e.)	10-yrs(s.e.)
All patients		2,622	.80 (.01)	.75 (.01)
No laparotomy		1,396	.77 (.01)	.71 (.01)
Laparotomy		1,226	.85 (.01)	.80 (.01)
NO LAPAROTOMY :				
RT alone	IF irradiation	291	.65 (.03)	.59 (.03)
	Mantle or inverted Y RT	446	.70 (.02)	.63 (.03)
	STNI or TNI	181	.79 (.03)	.75 (.04)
RT + single or bi-agent CT		85	.91 (.03)	.76 (.05)
Combination CT	MOPP-like	24	.59 (.11)	
	Others	2	–	
RT + Combination CT				
	IF irradiation + MOPP	157	.91 (.02)	.86 (.04)
	+ Others	41	.93 (.04)	
	Mantle or inverted Y RT + MOPP-like	98	.94 (.03)	.86 (.05)
	+ Others	8	–	
	STNI or TNI + MOPP-like	74	.93 (.03)	.89 (.04)
	+ Others	0		
LAPAROTOMY *(all PS patients)* **:**				
RT alone	IF irradiation	125	.72 (.04)	.64 (.05)
	Mantle or inverted Y RT	341	.87 (.02)	.83 (.02)
	STNI or TNI	434	.85 (.02)	.79 (.02)
RT + single or bi-agent CT		23	.87 (.07)	
Combination CT	MOPP-like	66	.83 (.05)	
	Others	5	–	
RT + Combination CT				
	IF irradiation + MOPP-like	69	.89 (.04)	
	+ Others	2	–	
	Mantle or inverted Y RT + MOPP-like	75	.91 (.04)	
	+ Others	11	–	
	STNI or TNI + MOPP-like	65	.92 (.04)	
	+ Others	6	–	

Table VII-8. Relapse-free survival for CS IIA patients who achieved a complete remission

Treatment type		Patients at risk	Relapse-free survival at 5-yrs(s.e.)	10-yrs(s.e.)
All patients		4,156	.74 (.01)	.70 (.01)
No laparotomy		1,925	.72 (.01)	.68 (.01)
Laparotomy		2,231	.75 (.01)	.71 (.01)

NO LAPAROTOMY :

Treatment type		Patients at risk	5-yrs(s.e.)	10-yrs(s.e.)
RT alone	IF irradiation	150	.60 (.04)	.57 (.04)
	Mantle or inverted Y RT	524	.57 (.02)	.51 (.02)
	STNI or TNI	314	.77 (.03)	.76 (.03)
RT + single or bi-agent CT		103	.63 (.05)	.59 (.05)
Combination CT	MOPP-like	62	.69 (.07)	
	Others	5	-	
RT + Combination CT				
IF irradiation + MOPP		197	.86 (.03)	.83 (.03)
+ Others		33	-	
Mantle or inverted Y RT + MOPP-like		259	.89 (.03)	.77 (.03)
+ Others		116	.88 (.05)	
STNI or TNI + MOPP-like		135	.89 (.03)	.86 (.03)
+ Others		6	-	

LAPAROTOMY *(all PS patients)* :

Treatment type		Patients at risk	5-yrs(s.e.)	10-yrs(s.e.)
RT alone	IF irradiation	122	.66 (.04)	.60 (.05)
	Mantle or inverted Y RT	401	.68 (.02)	.63 (.03)
	STNI or TNI	994	.73 (.02)	.68 (.02)
RT + single or bi-agent CT		21	-	
Combination CT	MOPP-like	85	.78 (.05)	
	Others	10	-	
RT + Combination CT				
IF irradiation + MOPP-like		101	.83 (.04)	.81 (.04)
+ Others		4	-	
Mantle or inverted Y RT + MOPP-like		161	.91 (.02)	.88 (.03)
+ Others		40	-	
STNI or TNI + MOPP-like		224	.87 (.02)	.84 (.03)
+ Others		36	.90 (.06)	

Table VII-9. Relapse-free survival for CS IB-IIB patients who achieved a complete remission

Treatment type	Patients at risk	Relapse-free survival at 5-yrs(s.e.)	10-yrs(s.e.)
All patients	1,674	.73 (.01)	.69 (.01)
No laparotomy	935	.70 (.02)	.66 (.02)
Laparotomy	739	.76 (.02)	.74 (.02)

NO LAPAROTOMY :

Treatment type	Patients at risk	5-yrs(s.e.)	10-yrs(s.e.)
RT alone IF irradiation	26	.40 (.10)	
Mantle or inverted Y RT	114	.43 (.05)	.43 (.05)
STNI or TNI	99	.59 (.05)	.52 (.05)
RT + single or bi-agent CT	33	.49 (.09)	
Combination CT MOPP-like	151	.72 (.04)	
Others	6	–	
RT + Combination CT			
IF irradiation + MOPP	101	.78 (.04)	
+ Others	13	–	
Mantle or inverted Y RT + MOPP-like	194	.82 (.03)	.78 (.04)
+ Others	94	.91 (.03)	
STNI or TNI + MOPP-like	76	.86 (.04)	
+ Others	2	–	

LAPAROTOMY *(all PS patients)* **:**

Treatment type	Patients at risk	5-yrs(s.e.)	10-yrs(s.e.)
RT alone IF irradiation	5	–	
Mantle or inverted Y RT	66	.48 (.06)	
STNI or TNI	222	.67 (.03)	.64 (.03)
RT + single or bi-agent CT	8	–	
Combination CT MOPP-like	71	.81 (.05)	.75 (.06)
Others	10	–	
RT + Combination CT			
IF irradiation + MOPP-like	69	.82 (.05)	
+ Others	9	–	
Mantle or inverted Y RT + MOPP-like	107	.85 (.04)	
+ Others	8	–	
STNI or TNI + MOPP-like	140	.90 (.03)	.87 (.03)
+ Others	12	–	

Table VII-10. Relapse-free survival for CS IIIA patients who achieved a complete remission

Treatment type		Patients at risk	Relapse-free survival at 5-yrs(s.e.)	10-yrs(s.e.)
All patients		1,349	.71 (.01)	.63 (.01)
No laparotomy		655	.67 (.02)	.57 (.02)
Laparotomy		684	.74 (.02)	.69 (.02)
NO LAPAROTOMY :				
RT alone	IF irradiation	4	–	
	Mantle or inverted Y RT	9	–	
	STNI or TNI	108	.55 (.05)	.46 (.05)
RT + single or bi-agent CT		12	–	
Combination CT	MOPP-like	233	.64 (.04)	.58 (.04)
	Others	10	–	
RT + Combination CT				
IF irradiation + MOPP		96	.70 (.05)	
+ Others		16	–	
Mantle or inverted Y RT + MOPP-like		22	–	
+ Others		11	–	
STNI or TNI + MOPP-like		111	.79 (.04)	.69 (.05)
+ Others				
LAPAROTOMY *(all PS patients)* :				
RT alone	IF irradiation	16	.75 (.11)	
	Mantle or inverted Y RT	42	.79 (.07)	
	STNI or TNI	276	.64 (.03)	.60 (.03)
RT + single or bi-agent CT		2	–	
Combination CT	MOPP-like	89	.72 (.05)	.66 (.06)
	Others	9	6	
RT + Combination CT				
IF irradiation + MOPP-like		53	.80 (.06)	.78 (.06)
+ Others		3	–	
Mantle or inverted Y RT + MOPP-like		10	.88 (.11)	
+ Others		13	–	
STNI or TNI + MOPP-like		135	.87 (.03)	.83 (.03)
+ Others		28	.81 (.08)	

Table VII-11. Relapse-free survival for CS IIIB patients who achieved a complete remission

Treatment type	Patients at risk	Relapse-free survival at 5-yrs(s.e.)	10-yrs(s.e.)
All patients	1,338	.65 (.01)	.61 (.02)
No laparotomy	876	.63 (.02)	.57 (.02)
Laparotomy	462	.68 (.02)	.66 (.02)

NO LAPAROTOMY :

RT alone IF irradiation	4	–	
Mantle or inverted Y RT	3	–	
STNI or TNI	47	.32 (.07)	
RT + single or bi-agent CT	22	.67 (.10)	
Combination CT MOPP-like	347	.66 (.03)	.58 (.03)
Others	82	.62 (.06)	
RT + Combination CT			
IF irradiation + MOPP	97	.58 (.05)	.56 (.06)
+ Others	67	.75 (.06)	
Mantle or inverted Y RT + MOPP-like	36	.65 (.08)	
+ Others	6	–	
STNI or TNI + MOPP-like	109	.72 (.05)	.62 (.06)
+ Others	14	–	

LAPAROTOMY *(all PS patients)* :

RT alone IF irradiation	0		
Mantle or inverted Y RT	6	–	
STNI or TNI	63	.43 (.06)	
RT + single or bi-agent CT	1	–	
Combination CT MOPP-like	123	.76 (.04)	.74 (.04)
Others	12	–	
RT + Combination CT			
IF irradiation + MOPP-like	61	.67 (.06)	.67 (.06)
+ Others	10	–	
Mantle or inverted Y RT + MOPP-like	8	–	
+ Others	2	–	
STNI or TNI + MOPP-like	124	.76 (.04)	.72 5.04)
+ Others	29	.83 (.07)	

Table VII-12. Relapse-free survival for CS IV patients who achieved a complete remission

Treatment type		Patients at risk	Relapse-free survival at 5-yrs(s.e.)	10-yrs(s.e.)
All patients		1,214	.66 (.02)	.62 (.02)
No laparotomy		951	.65 (.02)	.60 (.02)
Laparotomy		263	.68 (.03)	.65 (.03)
NO LAPAROTOMY :				
RT alone	IF irradiation	4	–	
	Mantle or inverted Y RT	8	–	
	STNI or TNI	10	–	
RT + single or bi-agent CT		5	–	
Combination CT	MOPP-like	477	.62 (.02)	.56 (.03)
	Others	114	.67 (.06)	
RT + Combination CT				
IF irradiation + MOPP		62	.64 (.07)	
+ Others		54	.57 (.09)	
Mantle or inverted Y RT + MOPP-like		39	.76 (.07)	
+ Others		15	–	
STNI or TNI + MOPP-like		73	.84 (.04)	.84 (.04)
+ Others		17	–	
LAPAROTOMY *(all PS patients)* **:**				
RT alone	IF irradiation	2	–	
	Mantle or inverted Y RT	3	–	
	STNI or TNI	5	–	
RT + single or bi-agent CT		0	–	
Combination CT	MOPP-like	168	.67 (.04)	.63 (.04)
	Others	11	–	
RT + Combination CT				
IF irradiation + MOPP-like		22	.63 (.11)	
+ Others		2	–	
Mantle or inverted Y RT + MOPP-like		3	–	
+ Others		5	–	
STNI or TNI + MOPP-like		26	.66 (.10)	
+ Others		9	–	

Table VII-13. Proportional hazards model on relapse-free survival for 2,783 CS I patients who achieved a complete remission (1). Results for a model allowing all the variables simultaneously

Variables	All patients coeff./s.e. RR[2]	without laparotomy coeff./s.e. RR	with laparotomy coeff./s.e. RR
SEX			
M	0 1.0[3]	0 1.0	0 1.0
F	-0.27/0.09 0.76**[4]	-0.25/0.12 0.78*	-0.21/0.15 0.81
AGE			
<40 yrs	0 1.0	0 1.0	0 1.0
40+ yrs	0.26/0.09 1.30**	0.24/0.11 1.27*	0.27/0.14 1.31+
HISTOLOGY			
LP	0 1.0	0 1.0	0 1.0
NS	0.51/0.14 1.67***	0.36/0.16 1.43*	0.76/0.25 2.13**
MC-LD	0.58/0.14 1.79***	0.47/0.16 1.60**	0.70/0.25 2.01**
TOPOGRAPHY			
supra-D	0 1.0	0 1.0	0 1.0
infra-D	-0.54/0.23 0.58**	-0.66/0.30 0.52*	-0.14/0.37 0.87
MEDIASTINAL INVOLVEMENT			
no	0 1.0	0 1.0	0 1.0
yes	-0.06/0.15 0.94	-0.18/0.19 0.83	0.18/0.22 1.20
EXTRA LOCALIZATION E +			
absent	0 1.0	0 1.0	0 1.0
present	-0.27/0.17 0.76	-0.21/0.22 0.81	-0.28/0.28 0.76
SYSTEMIC SYMPTOMS			
absent	0 1.0	0 1.0	0 1.0
present	0.41/0.14 1.51**	0.49/0.18 1.64**	0.23/0.24 1.25
LAPAROTOMY			
no	0 1.0		
yes	-0.39/0.09 0.67***		
LAPAROTOMY FINDINGS[5]			
PS I			0 1.0
PS III-IV			1.0 /0.18 2.72***
Global chi-square	77.3	33.2	60.9
p value (df)	<0.0001 (9)	0.0008 (8)	<0.0001 (9)

(1) after adjustment on initial therapy (i.e. RT with or w/o single or bi-agent CT, combination CT, or RT + combination CT) and treatment period (i.e. 1960-69, 1970-79 and 1980+)
(2) relative risk RR = exp (regression coefficient)
(3) reference category
*(4) p value : + < 0.10, * < 0.05, ** < 0.01, *** < 0.001*
(5) no PS II were observed

Table VII-14. Proportional hazards model on relapse-free survival for 2,542 CS IA patients who achieved a complete remission (1). Results for a model allowing all the variables simultaneously

Variables	All patients coeff./s.e.	RR[2]	without laparotomy coeff./s.e.	RR	with laparotomy coeff./s.e.	RR
SEX						
M	0	1.0[3]	0	1.0	0	1.0
F	-0.27/0.10	0.76**[4]	-0.23/0.12	0.80+	-0.26/0.16	0.77+
AGE						
<40 yrs	0	1.0	0	1.0	0	1.0
40+ yrs	0.31/0.09	1.37***	0.29/0.11	1.33**	0.32/0.15	1.38*
HISTOLOGY						
LP	0	1.0	0	1.0	0	1.0
NS	0.48/0.14	1.62***	0.34/0.17	1.40*	0.76/0.26	2.13**
MC-LD	0.56/0.14	1.76***	0.44/0.17	1.56**	0.69/0.26	2.0 **
TOPOGRAPHY						
supra-D	0	1.0	0	1.0	0	1.0
infra-D	-0.64/0.25	0.53**	-0.85/0.34	0.43*	-0.17/0.37	0.85
MEDIASTINAL INVOLVEMENT						
no	0	1.0	0	1.0	0	1.0
yes	-0.13/0.16	0.88	-0.19/0.21	0.82	0.0/0.26	1.0
EXTRA LOCALIZATION E +						
absent	0	1.0	0	1.0	0	1.0
present	-0.16/0.18	0.85	-0.05/0.23	1.05	-0.38/0.32	0.69
LAPAROTOMY						
no	0	1.0				
yes	-0.39/0.10	0.68***				
LAPAROTOMY FINDINGS[5]						
PS I					0	1.0
PS III-IV					1.04/0.18	2.82***
Global chi-square	68.8		24.8		59.4	
p value (df)	<0.0001 (8)		0.0008 (7)		<0.0001 (8)	

(1) after adjustment on initial therapy (i.e. RT with or w/o single or bi-agent CT, combination CT, or RT + combination CT) and treatment period (i.e. 1960-69, 1970-79 and 1980+)
(2) relative risk RR = exp (regression coefficient)
(3) reference category
(4) p value : + < 0.10, * < 0.05, ** < 0.01, *** < 0.001
(5) no PS II were observed

Table VII-14a. Stepwise proportional hazards model on relapse-free survival for 2,542 CS IA patients who achieved a complete remission (1)

Step no	Variable	Log likelihood	Coeff./s.e.	RR[2]
0		- 2985.249		
1	AGE 40+ yrs	- 2980.193	0.30/0.09	1.35 ***[3]
2	TOPOGRAPHY Infra-D	- 2974.981	-0.75/0.25	0.47 **
3	FEMALE GENDER	- 2971.60	-0.24/0.10	0.78 **

(1) after adjustment on initial therapy (i.e. RT with or w/o single or bi-agent CT, combination CT, or RT + combination CT), treatment period (i.e. 1960-69, 1970-79 and 1980+), and staging laparotomy (performed or not performed)
(2) relative risk RR = exp (regression coefficient)
*(3) p value : ** < 0.01, *** < 0.001*

Table VII-15. Proportional hazards model on relapse-free survival for 5,414 CS II patients who achieved a complete remission (1). Results for a model allowing all the variables simultaneously

Variables	All patients coeff./s.e.	RR[2]	without laparotomy coeff./s.e.	RR	with laparotomy coeff./s.e.	RR
SEX						
M	0	1.0[3]	0	1.0	0	1.0
F	-0.16/0.05	0.85**[4]	-0.17/0.08	0.85**	-0.15/0.08	0.86+
AGE						
<50 yrs	0	1.0	0	1.0	0	1.0
50+ yrs	0.17/0.09	1.18+	0.17/0.11	1.18	0.17/0.16	1.19
HISTOLOGY						
LP	0	1.0	0	1.0	0	1.0
NS	0.45/0.14	1.57***	0.40/0.18	1.49*	0.58/0.21	1.78**
MC-LD	0.58/0.14	1.78***	0.67/0.18	1.95***	0.48/0.22	1.61*
TOPOGRAPHY						
supra-D	0	1.0	0	1.0	0	1.0
infra-D	0.18/0.11	1.20+	0.10/0.15	1.10	0.42/0.18	1.52*
# OF LYMPH NODES INVOLVED						
2, 3, 4	0	1.0	0	1.0	0	1.0
5 +	0.31/0.10	1.37**	0.43/0.17	1.54**	0.23/0.13	1.25+
MEDIASTINAL INVOLVEMENT						
no	0	1.0	0	1.0	0	1.0
yes	0.06/0.07	1.06	0.06/0.09	1.06	0.04/0.10	1.04
EXTRA LOCALIZATION E +						
absent	0	1.0	0	1.0	0	1.0
present	0.12/0.08	1.13	-0.10/0.12	0.91	0.34/0.11	1.41**
SYSTEMIC SYMPTOMS						
absent	0	1.0	0	1.0	0	1.0
present	0.24/0.06	1.27***	0.33/0.09	1.39***	0.19/0.09	1.21*
LAPAROTOMY						
no	0	1.0				
yes	-0.21/0.06	0.81***				
LAPAROTOMY FINDINGS						
PS II					0	1.0
PS III-IV					0.45/0.09	1.56***
Global chi-square	72.2		59.7		57.4	
p value (df)	<0.0001 (10)		<0.001 (9)		<0.0001 (10)	

(1) after adjustment on initial therapy (i.e. RT with or w/o single or bi-agent CT, combination CT, or RT + combination CT) and treatment period (i.e. 1960-69, 1970-79 and 1980+)
(2) relative risk RR = exp (regression coefficient)
(3) reference category
(4) p value : + < 0.10, * < 0.05, ** < 0.01, *** < 0.001

Table VII-16. Proportional hazards model on relapse-free survival for 4,038 CS IIA patients who achieved a complete remission (1). Results for a model allowing all the variables simultaneously

Variables	All patients coeff./s.e.	RR(2)	without laparotomy coeff./s.e.	RR	with laparotomy coeff./s.e.	RR
SEX						
M	0	1.0(3)	0	1.0	0	1.0
F	-0.09/0.08	0.92	-0.07/0.09	0.94	-0.10/0.09	0.91
AGE						
<50 yrs	0	1.0	0	1.0	0	1.0
50+ yrs	0.25/0.11	1.28*(4)	0.29/0.13	1.33*	0.17/0.18	1.18
HISTOLOGY						
LP	0	1.0	0	1.0	0	1.0
NS	0.34/0.15	1.41*	0.20/0.20	1.22	0.55/0.23	1.72*
MC-LD	0.48/0.15	1.62**	0.47/0.20	1.60*	0.49/0.24	1.63*
TOPOGRAPHY						
supra-D	0	1.0	0	1.0	0	1.0
infra-D	0.22/0.13	1.24+	0.12/0.18	1.13	0.50/0.20	1.65*
# OF LYMPH NODES INVOLVED						
2, 3, 4	0	1.0	0	1.0	0	1.0
5 +	0.22/0.13	1.25*	-0.07/0.28	0.93	0.27/0.15	1.31+
MEDIASTINAL INVOLVEMENT						
no	0	1.0	0	1.0	0	1.0
yes	0.05/0.08	1.05	0.01/0.11	1.01	0.11/0.11	1.11
EXTRA LOCALIZATION E +						
absent	0	1.0	0	1.0	0	1.0
present	0.03/0.10	1.03	-0.19/0.16	0.83	0.21/0.13	1.24+
LAPAROTOMY						
no	0	1.0				
yes	-0.14/0.07	0.87*				
LAPAROTOMY FINDINGS						
PS II					0	1.0
PS III-IV					0.52/0.10	1.68***
Global chi-square	32.2		19.6		46.4	
p value (df)	0.0002 (9)		0.012 (8)		<0.0001 (9)	

(1) after adjustment on initial therapy (i.e. RT with or w/o single or bi-agent CT, combination CT, or RT + combination CT) and treatment period (i.e. 1960-69, 1970-79 and 1980+)
(2) relative risk RR = exp (regression coefficient)
(3) reference category
*(4) p value : + < 0.10, * < 0.05, ** < 0.01, *** < 0.001*

Table VII-16a. Stepwise proportional hazards model on relapse-free survival for 4,038 CS IIA patients who achieved a complete remission [1]

Step no	Variable	Log likelihood	Coeff./s.e.	RR[2]
0		− 6573.418		
1	HISTOLOGY MC + LD	− 6569.855	0.20/0.07	1.22 **[3]

[1] after adjustment on initial therapy (i.e. RT with or w/o single or bi-agent CT, combination CT, or RT + combination CT), treatment period (i.e. 1960-69, 1970-79 and 1980+), and staging laparotomy (performed or not performed)
[2] relative risk RR = exp (regression coefficient)
[3] p value : ** < 0.01, *** < 0.001

Table VII-17. Proportional hazards model on relapse-free survival for 1,617 CS IB-IIB patients who achieved a complete remission (1). Results for a model allowing all the variables simultaneously

Variables	All patients coeff./s.e.	RR[2]	without laparotomy coeff./s.e.	RR	with laparotomy coeff./s.e.	RR
SEX						
M	0	1.0[3]	0	1.0	0	1.0
F	-0.35/0.10	0.70***[4]	-0.36/0.13	0.70**	-0.32/0.16	0.73*
AGE						
<40 yrs	0	1.0	0	1.0	0	1.0
40+ yrs	0.08/0.11	1.09	0.09/0.14	1.09	0.07/0.20	1.07
HISTOLOGY						
LP	0	1.0	0	1.0	0	1.0
NS	0.96/0.30	2.60**	1.07/0.39	2.91**	0.81/0.49	2.25+
MC-LD	1.0 /0.31	2.73***	1.23/0.40	3.42**	0.58/0.50	1.79
TOPOGRAPHY						
supra-D	0	1.0	0	1.0	0	1.0
infra-D	0.23/0.21	1.26	0.19/0.25	1.21	0.32/0.40	1.38
# OF LYMPH NODES INVOLVED						
1 to 4	0	1.0	0	1.0	0	1.0
5 +	0.50/0.16	1.64**	-0.91/0.22	2.48***	0.14/0.24	1.15
MEDIASTINAL INVOLVEMENT						
no	0	1.0	0	1.0	0	1.0
yes	0.18/0.12	1.20	0.22/0.16	1.24	0.07/0.20	1.08
EXTRA LOCALIZATION E +						
absent	0	1.0	0	1.0	0	1.0
present	0.09/0.14	1.09	-0.21/0.19	0.81	0.53/0.20	1.70**
LAPAROTOMY						
no	0	1.0				
yes	-0.43/0.11	0.65***				
LAPAROTOMY FINDINGS						
PS I - II					0	1.0
PS III-IV					0.21/0.20	1.24
Global chi-square	52.0		43.8		17.2	
p value (df)	<0.0001 (9)		<0.0001 (8)		0.0463 (9)	

(1) after adjustment on initial therapy (i.e. RT with or w/o single or bi-agent CT, combination CT, or RT + combination CT) and treatment period (i.e. 1960-69, 1970-79 and 1980+)
(2) relative risk RR = exp (regression coefficient)
(3) reference category
*(4) p value : + < 0.10, * < 0.05, ** < 0.01, *** < 0.001*

Table VII-17a. Stepwise proportional hazards model on relapse-free survival for 1,617 CS IB - CS IIB patients who achieved a complete remission *(1)*

Step no	Variable	Log likelihood	Coeff./s.e.	RR[2]
0		- 2115.441		
1	FEMALE GENDER	- 2109.624	-0.32/0.10	0.72 **[3]
2	5+ LYMPH NODE AREAS INVOLVED	- 2105.618	0.49/0.16	1.64 **

(1) after adjustment on initial therapy (i.e. RT with or w/o single or bi-agent CT, combination CT, or RT + combination CT), treatment period (i.e. 1960-69, 1970-79 and 1980+), and staging laparotomy (performed or not performed)
(2) relative risk RR = exp (regression coefficient)
*(3) p value : ** < 0.01, *** < 0.001*

Table VII-18. Proportional hazards model on relapse-free survival for 2,568 CS III patients who achieved a complete remission [1]. Results for a model allowing all the variables simultaneously

Variables	All patients coeff./s.e. RR[2]		without laparotomy coeff./s.e. RR		with laparotomy coeff./s.e. RR	
SEX						
M	0	1.0[3]	0	1.0	0	1.0
F	-0.26/0.08	0.77***[4]	-0.28/0.10	0.75**	-0.19/0.12	0.83
AGE						
<50 yrs	0	1.0	0	1.0	0	1.0
50+ yrs	0.32/0.09	1.37***	0.26/0.11	1.29*	0.42/0.16	1.52**
HISTOLOGY						
LP	0	1.0	0	1.0	0	1.0
NS	0.37/0.16	1.45*	0.16/0.19	1.17	0.79/0.31	2.21**
MC-LD	0.38/0.16	1.46*	0.25/0.19	1.28	0.61/0.31	1.84*
# OF LYMPH NODES INVOLVED						
2 or 3	0	1.0	0	1.0	0	1.0
4 +	0.28/0.07	1.32***	0.27/0.09	1.31**	0.23/0.12	1.26*
MEDIASTINAL INVOLVEMENT						
no	0	1.0	0	1.0	0	1.0
yes	0.19/0.08	1.21*	0.22/0.10	1.38**	0.07/0.12	1.07
EXTRA LOCALIZATION E +						
absent	0	1.0	0	1.0	0	1.0
present	-0.11/0.14	0.90	-0.27/0.21	0.77	-0.01/0.21	0.99
SYSTEMIC SYMPTOMS						
absent	0	1.0	0	1.0	0	1.0
present	0.20/0.08	1.22**	0.12/0.09	1.13	0.31/0.12	1.36*
LAPAROTOMY						
no	0	1.0				
yes	-0.25/0.08	0.78**				
LAPAROTOMY FINDINGS						
PS III					0	1.0
PS I-II					-0.89/0.16	0.41***
PS IV					0.59/0.19	1.81**
Global chi-square	77.8		36.1		82.2	
p value (df)	<0.0001 (9)		<0.0001 (8)		<0.0001 (10)	

(1) *after adjustment on initial therapy (i.e. RT with or w/o single or bi-agent CT, combination CT, or RT + combination CT) and treatment period (i.e. 1960-69, 1970-79 and 1980+)*
(2) *relative risk RR = exp (regression coefficient)*
(3) *reference category*
(4) *p value : + < 0.10, * < 0.05, ** < 0.01, *** < 0.001*

Table VII-19. Proportional hazards model on relapse-free survival for 1,301 CS IIIA patients who achieved a complete remission (1). Results for a model allowing all the variables simultaneously

Variables	All patients coeff./s.e.	RR[2]	without laparotomy coeff./s.e.	RR	with laparotomy coeff./s.e.	RR
SEX						
M	0	1.0[3]	0	1.0	0	1.0
F	-0.16/0.11	0.85	-0.17/0.15	0.84	-0.07/0.16	0.93
AGE						
<50 yrs	0	1.0	0	1.0	0	1.0
50+ yrs	0.42/0.13	1.52***[4]	0.35/0.17	1.42*	0.45/0.20	1.58*
HISTOLOGY						
LP	0	1.0	0	1.0	0	1.0
NS	0.34/0.19	1.40+	0.0 /0.24	1.0	0.79/0.32	2.21*
MC-LD	0.36/0.19	1.43+	0.14/0.24	1.15	0.68/0.33	1.98*
# OF LYMPH NODES INVOLVED						
2 or 3	0	1.0	0	1.0	0	1.0
4 +	0.38/0.10	1.46***	0.36/0.15	1.43*	0.39/0.16	1.48**
MEDIASTINAL INVOLVEMENT						
no	0	1.0	0	1.0	0	1.0
yes	0.15/0.11	1.16	0.46/0.15	1.58**	-0.07/0.16	0.93
EXTRA LOCALIZATION E +						
absent	0	1.0	0	1.0	0	1.0
present	-0.10/0.21	0.90	-0.18/0.29	0.83	-0.18/0.34	0.84
LAPAROTOMY						
no	0	1.0				
yes	-0.25/0.11	0.78*				
LAPAROTOMY FINDINGS						
PS III					0	1.0
PS I-II					-0.82/0.19	0.44***
PS IV					0.59/0.29	1.80*
Global chi-square	40.0		19.2		46.0	
p value (df)	<0.0001 (8)		0.0076 (7)		<0.0001 (9)	

(1) *after adjustment on initial therapy (i.e. RT with or w/o single or bi-agent CT, combination CT, or RT + combination CT) and treatment period (i.e. 1960-69, 1970-79 and 1980+)*
(2) *relative risk RR = exp (regression coefficient)*
(3) *reference category*
(4) *p value : + < 0.10, * < 0.05, ** < 0.01, *** < 0.001*

Table VII-19a. Stepwise proportional hazards model on relapse-free survival for 1,301 CS IIIA patients who achieved a complete remission [1]

Step no	Variable	Log likelihood	Coeff./s.e.	RR[2]
0		-1892.812		
1	4+ LYMPH NODE AREAS INVOLVED	-1887.598	0.36/0.11	1.44 **[3]
2	AGE 50+ yrs	-1883.992	0.35/0.13	1.42 **

[1] after adjustment on initial therapy (i.e. RT with or w/o single or bi-agent CT, combination CT, or RT + combination CT), treatment period (i.e. 1960-69, 1970-79 and 1980+), and staging laparotomy (performed or not performed)
[2] relative risk RR = exp (regression coefficient)
[3] p value : ** < 0.01, *** < 0.001

Table VII-20. Proportional hazards model on relapse-free survival for 1,267 CS IIIB patients who achieved a complete remission (1). Results for a model allowing all the variables simultaneously

Variables	All patients coeff./s.e.	RR[2]	without laparotomy coeff./s.e.	RR	with laparotomy coeff./s.e.	RR
SEX						
M	0	1.0[3]	0	1.0	0	1.0
F	-0.37/0.11	0.69***[4]	-0.36/0.13	0.70**	-0.33/0.20	0.72+
AGE						
<50 yrs	0	1.0	0	1.0	0	1.0
50+ yrs	0.25/0.13	1.28+	0.24/0.15	1.27	0.37/0.30	1.45
HISTOLOGY						
LP	0	1.0	0	1.0	0	1.0
NS	0.44/0.30	1.55	0.32/0.32	1.38	0.52/1.02	1.68
MC-LD	0.42/0.30	1.52	0.38/0.32	1.46	0.21/1.03	1.23
# OF LYMPH NODES INVOLVED						
2 or 3	0	1.0	0	1.0	0	1.0
4 +	0.20/0.10	1.22*	0.22/0.12	1.24+	-0.03/0.20	0.97
MEDIASTINAL INVOLVEMENT						
no	0	1.0	0	1.0	0	1.0
yes	0.24/0.11	1.27*	0.24/0.13	1.27+	0.29/0.20	1.33
EXTRA LOCALIZATION E +						
absent	0	1.0	0	1.0	0	1.0
present	0.16/0.19	0.85	-0.36/0.30	0.70	0.13/0.28	1.14
LAPAROTOMY						
no	0	1.0				
yes	-0.24/0.11	0.79*				
LAPAROTOMY FINDINGS						
PS III					0	1.0
PS I-II					-0.98/0.30	0.38**
PS IV					0.52/0.27	1.69*
Global chi-square	30.1		17.7		27.0	
p value (df)	0.0002 (8)		0.0135 (7)		0.0014 (9)	

(1) after adjustment on initial therapy (i.e. RT with or w/o single or bi-agent CT, combination CT, or RT + combination CT) and treatment period (i.e. 1960-69, 1970-79 and 1980+)
(2) relative risk RR = exp (regression coefficient)
(3) reference category
(4) p value : + < 0.10, * < 0.05, ** < 0.01, *** < 0.001

Table VII-20a. Stepwise proportional hazards model on relapse-free survival for 1,267 CS IIIB patients who achieved a complete remission [1]

Step no	Variable	Log likelihood	Coeff./s.e.	RR[2]
0		− 2049.262		
1	FEMALE GENDER	− 2044.645	−0.37/0.11	0.69 **[3]
2	AGE 60+ yrs	− 2040.365	0.55/0.16	1.74 **
3	MEDIASTINAL INVOLVEMENT	− 2036.843	0.28/0.11	1.32 **

(1) after adjustment on initial therapy (i.e. RT with or w/o single or bi-agent CT, combination CT, or RT + combination CT), treatment period (i.e. 1960-69, 1970-79 and 1980+), and staging laparotomy (performed or not performed)
(2) relative risk RR = exp (regression coefficient)
*(3) p value : ** < 0.01, *** < 0.001*

Table VII-21. Proportional hazards model on relapse-free survival for 819 CS IV patients who achieved a complete remission (1). Results for a model allowing all the variables simultaneously

Variables	All patients coeff./s.e.	RR[(2)]	without laparotomy coeff./s.e.	RR	with laparotomy coeff./s.e.	RR
SEX						
M	0	1.0[(3)]	0	1.0	0	1.0
F	-0.17/0.14	0.84	-0.15/0.15	0.86	-0.66/0.40	0.52+
AGE						
<50 yrs	0	1.0	0	1.0	0	1.0
50+ yrs	0.27/0.15	1.31+[(4)]	0.32/0.16	1.37*	-0.18/0.44	0.84
HISTOLOGY						
LP	0	1.0	0	1.0	0	1.0
NS	-0.18/0.28	0.83	-0.09/0.31	0.92	-0.24/0.80	0.79
MC-LD	-0.53/0.28	0.59+	-0.49/0.31	0.61	-0.62/0.80	0.54
TOPOGRAPHY						
one side	0	1.0	0	1.0	0	1.0
both side	-0.24/0.18	0.79	-0.32/0.19	0.72+	0.41/0.51	1.50
# OF LYMPH NODES INVOLVED						
1 to 4	0	1.0	0	1.0	0	1.0
5 +	0.21/0.14	1.23	0.33/0.16	1.39*	-0.66/0.41	0.52+
MEDIASTINAL INVOLVEMENT						
no	0	1.0	0	1.0	0	1.0
yes	-0.12/0.15	0.89	0.17/0.17	0.85	-0.05/0.36	0.95
EXTRA LOCALIZATION E +						
absent	0	1.0	0	1.0	0	1.0
present	0.23/0.15	1.25	0.23/0.17	1.26	0.09/0.42	1.10
SYSTEMIC SYMPTOMS						
absent	0	1.0	0	1.0	0	1.0
present	0.21/0.17	1.24	0.24/0.19	1.28	-0.02/0.39	0.98
BM INVOLVEMENT						
absent	0	1.0	0	1.0	0	1.0
present	0.25/0.15	1.28+	0.21/0.16	1.23	0.21/0.48	1.23
LAPAROTOMY						
no	0	1.0				
yes	-0.20/0.17	0.82				
LAPAROTOMY FINDINGS						
PS IV					0	1.0
PS I-II-III					-0.20/0.44	0.82
Global chi-square	21.9		21.7		8.1	
p value (df)	0.0249 (11)		0.0168 (10)		0.71 (11)	

(1) *after adjustment on initial therapy (i.e. RT with or w/o single or bi-agent CT, combination CT, or RT + combination CT) and treatment period (i.e. 1960-69, 1970-79 and 1980+)*
(2) *relative risk RR = exp (regression coefficient)*
(3) *reference category*
(4) *p value : + < 0.10, * < 0.05, ** < 0.01, *** < 0.001*

Table VII-21a. Stepwise proportional hazards model on relapse-free survival for 819 CS IV patients who achieved a complete remission [1]

Step no	Variable	Log likelihood	Coeff./s.e.	RR[2]
0		− 1222.973		
1	AGE 50+ yrs	− 1217.902	0.57/0.17	1.78 ***[3]

(1) after adjustment on initial therapy (i.e. RT with or w/o single or bi-agent CT, combination CT, or RT + combination CT), treatment period (i.e. 1960-69, 1970-79 and 1980+), and staging laparotomy (performed or not performed)
(2) relative risk RR = exp (regression coefficient)
*(3) p value : ** < 0.01, *** < 0.001*

Table VII-22. Relapse characteristics by clinical stage

Clinical stage	IA	IIA	IB-IIB	IIIA	IIIB	IV
# of patients who relapsed (%)	564 (21.5)	1,134 (27.2)	460 (27.4)	422 (31.3)	439 (32.8)	403 (35.2)
Delay from start of medical therapy						
1st year	109	300	146	70	94	70
2nd	175	315	131	148	163	148
3rd	79	198	86	56	75	88
4th	54	125	38	49	37	42
5th	47	70	18	34	33	25
6th	39	41	11	19	12	12
7th	19	35	13	15	6	7
8th	17	16	6	11	5	6
9th	6	9	3	6	8	0
10th	4	6	1	6	3	3
11th +	15	19	7	6	3	2
median (months)	23	21	18	23	20	21
range (years)	0-16	0-16	0-15	0-16	0-14	0-12
Type of relapse (R)						
true nodal R. infield	11	12	6	10	32	10
" outfield	41	87	60	57	48	30
" in+outfield	11	21	13	7	14	7
extension nodal R.	111	161	73	51	31	18
nodal R. unspecified	35	141	49	61	53	33
true extra nodal R.	56	127	53	21	36	43
other extra nodal R.	19	67	29	28	33	31
nodal + extra nodal R.	79	217	88	69	84	65
other R. unspecified	201	301	89	20	108	166

Part VIII - *Huitième partie*

PROGNOSTIC STUDY OF OVERALL SURVIVAL BY CLINICAL STAGE

ANALYSE PRONOSTIQUE DE LA SURVIE GLOBALE EN FONCTION DU STADE CLINIQUE

Overall survival prognostic study

The prognostic value on overall survival was estimated separately (univariate) for each variable by clinical stage and presence or absence of systemic symptoms with stratification on treatment period, type of initial therapy and staging laparotomy (Tables VIII-1 to VIII-6) using the logrank test.

Then crude 5-year and 10-year overall survival rates are given according to stage, presence or absence of systemic symptoms, and by initial treatment type (Tables VIII-7 to VIII-12). Also crude overall survival rates are given by treatment period and summarized by initial treatment type.

Crude survival curves are also provided for the entire cohort according to period of start of first therapy (Figure VIII-1), sex (Figure VIII-2), age at diagnosis (Figure VIII-3), histological subtypes (Figure VIII-4), clinical stage and B symptoms (Figures VIII-5 and VIII-6), or by stage (Figures VIII-7 to VIII-11 for early stages, and Figures VIII-12 to VIII-15 for advanced stages).

Prognostic factors by stage

Stepwise regression model

The results from proportional hazards survival analysis on the overall material are given in Table VIII-13. Its main purpose is to study the prognostic value of clinical stage. In this table, and in the tables to follow, results are expressed in three ways: *i)* all causes of death taken together; and causes of death subgrouped into *ii)* those due to disease progression or failure, or treatment related; and *iii)* those due to other causes.

In this analysis, two parameters were not included in the model, i.e. response to initial treatment and occurrence of further relapse, since the aim of the study was to predict survival using initial patient characteristics only.

In this model, where B symptoms were included as an independent factor, it was observed that B symptoms appeared at the first step in the regression, immediately followed by age, advanced stages, and unfavorable histological types when the end point was death due to Hodgkin disease (Table VIII-13b). By contrast, when death due to other causes was considered in the model, the most important factor remained age at diagnosis. Sex and B symptoms were of less importance (Table VIII-13c).

These findings are rather constant when the analysis is repeated according to clinical stage and B symptoms (Tables VIII-19).

When *biological parameters* were included in the model, one at the time, the following were observed when the end-point was Hodgkin disease-free survival:

- Accelerated ESR had no influence in most of the groups. It had an influence in clinical stage IB-IIB where it came in second position after the number of lymph node areas involved. It had also an influence in stage IIIB where it appeared at the third step after age.

- Decreased hemoglobin level was significantly associated with a poor survival in stages IA, IB-IIB, IIIB and IV patients but never it appeared at the first step.

- Elevated alkaline phosphatase was never prognostic except in clinical stage IB-IIB patients where it appeared at second step after topography.

- Decreased serum albumin level was only predictive in stage IIIB patients where it was preceded by age.

- Finally, elevated LDH was predictive in clinical stage IV patients only.

Cumulative incidence of death by type of initial treatment

The 10-year crude cumulative incidence of death by treatment category are given in Table VIII-20. In this table the rates are calculated from the date of start of first therapy. Most of patients who did not achieve a complete remission following initial therapy died as did 50% of those who relapsed.

In patients who never relapsed after achieving a complete remission 12.3% died. The most important cause of death was intercurrent diseases (in which cardiac failures are included).

In patients who relapsed, survival after relapse was relatively poor (Table VIII-21, and Figures VIII-16 and VIII-17). Most died from disease progression or treatment related deaths, but deaths from second cancer were not negligible.

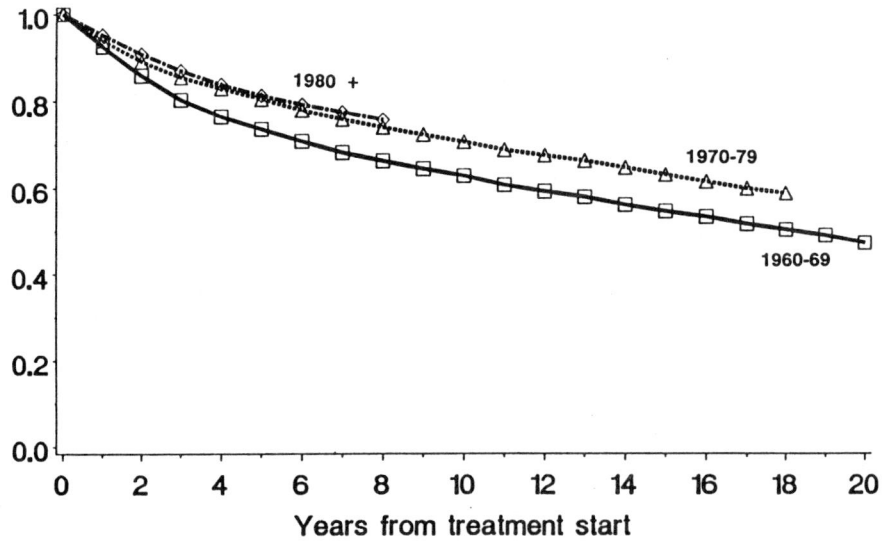

Figure VIII-1 : *All stages. Overall survival by treatment period. (1960-69 : 1,115 pts; 1970-79 : 8,104 pts; 1980+ : 5,096 pts).*

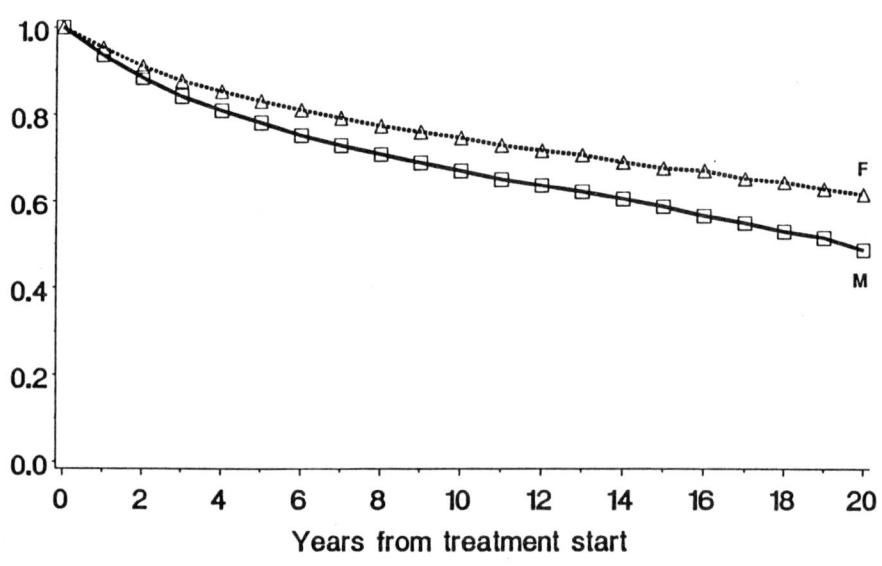

Figure VIII-2 : *All stages. Overall survival by sex. (Males : 8,671 pts; Females : 5,644 pts).*

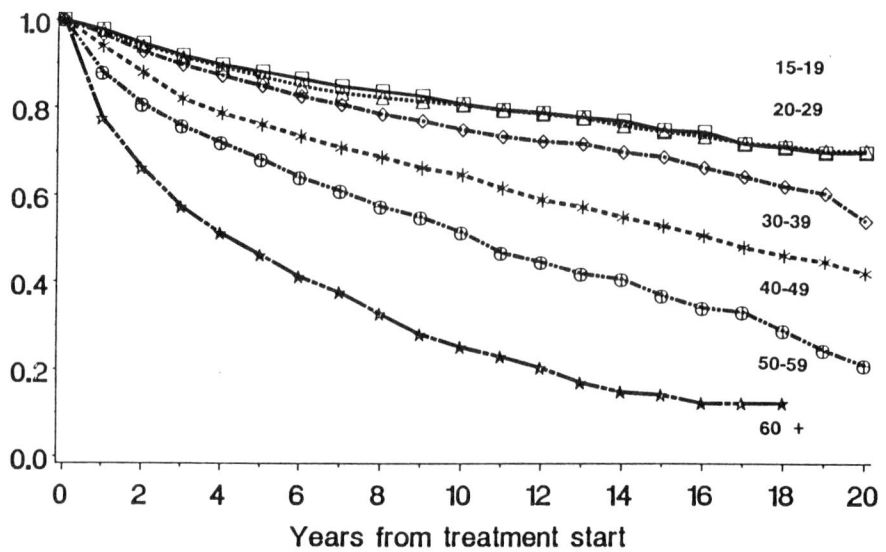

Figure VIII-3 : *All stages. Overall survival by age at Hodgkin disease diagnosis. (15-19 yrs: 1,684 pts; 20-29 yrs : 5,026 pts; 30-39 yrs : 3,254 pts; 40-49 yrs : 1,837 pts; 50-59 yrs : 1,292 pts; 60+ yrs : 1,198 pts).*

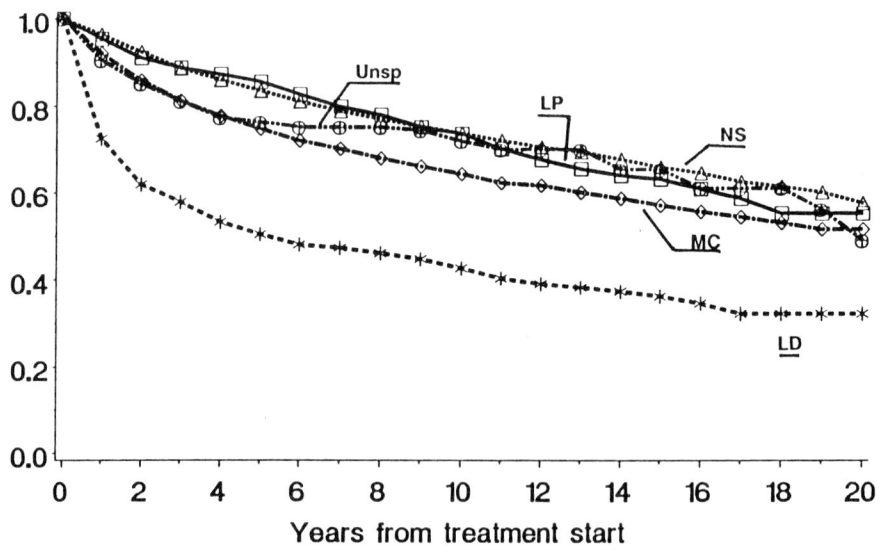

Figure VIII-4 : *All stages. Overall survival by histological type. (LP : 1,012 pts; NS : 8,684 pts; MC : 3,778 pts; LD : 429 pts; Type unspecified : 358 pts).*

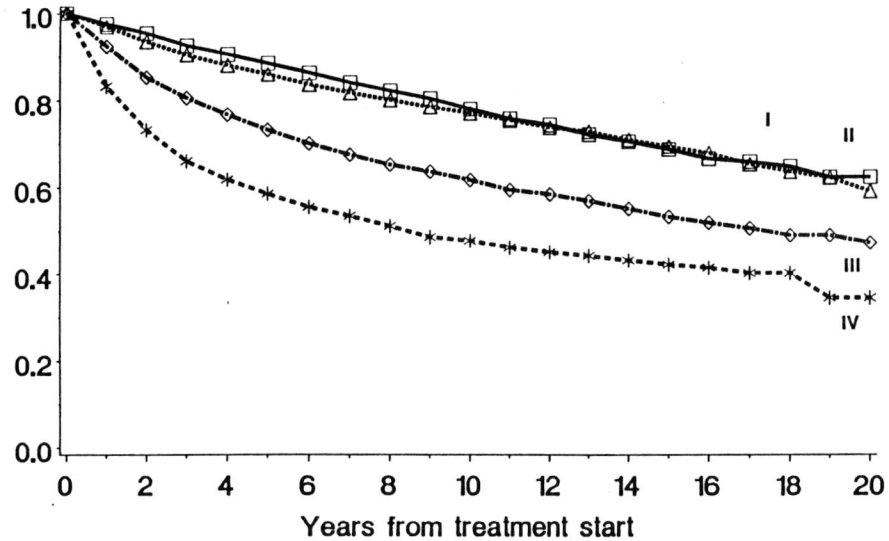

Figure VIII-5: *All stages. Overall survival by clinical stage. (I : 2,986 pts; II : 6,104 pts; III : 3,347 pts; IV : 1,870 pts).*

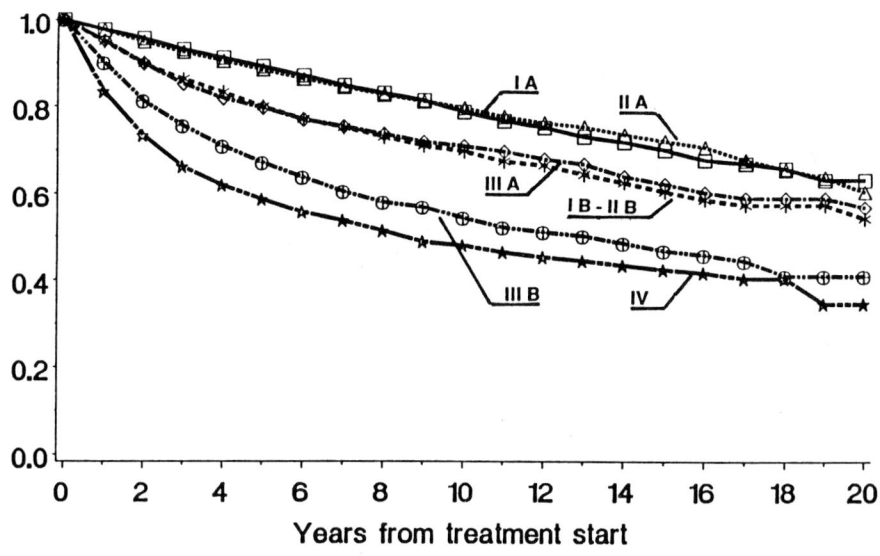

Figure VIII-6: *All stages. Overall survival by clinical stage and presence or absence of systemic symptoms. (IA : 2,707 pts; IIA : 4,406 pts; IB-IIB : 1,974 pts; IIIA : 1,558 pts; IIIB : 1,779 pts; IV : 1,860 pts).*

Table VIII-1. Prognostic value on overall survival for CS IA patients (N=2,696) *

Parameter		Patients at risk	Relative risk of death	p value (heterogeneity)
SEX	males	1,827	1.0	
	females	869	0.68	< 0.001
AGE	15-19	248	1.0	
	20-29	870	1.51	
	30-39	612	1.94	
	40-49	390	3.71	
	50-59	293	6.03	
	60+	281	12.64	< 0.001
HISTOLOGY	LP	432	1.0	
	NS	1,262	0.94	
	MC	912	1.26	
	LD	23	4.49	< 0.001
	unclassified	51		
TOPOGRAPHY	above diaphragm	2,551	1.0	
	below	135	0.83	> 0.20
MEDIASTINUM	not involved	2,427	1.0	
	involved	257	0.65	0.013
EXTRA LOCALIZATION E +	absent	2,486	1.0	
	present	210	0.94	> 0.20
E.S.R.	0-19	1,200	1.0	
	20-39	350	1.52	
	40-59	164	1.85	
	60+	108	2.09	< 0.001
L.D.H.	<25th percentile	69	1.0	
	25-75th	114	1.33	
	>75th	9	0.49	> 0.20
ALKALINE PHOSPHATASE	<25th percentile	412	1.0	
	25-75th	752	1.40	
	>75th	180	1.54	0.06
ALBUMIN	<25th percentile	39	2.03	
	25-75th	473	1.72	
	>75th	479	1.0	< 0.001
HEMOGLOBIN	abnormal**	156	1.65	
	normal	1,820	1.0	0.002

* with stratification on period, treatment and staging laparotomy
** Hb < 8.0 mmol/l in males and < 7.0 mmol/l in females

Table VIII-2. Prognostic value on overall survival for CS IIA patients (N=4,395) *

Parameter			Patients at risk	Relative risk of death	p value (heterogeneity)
SEX	males		2,254	1.0	
	females		2,141	0.73	< 0.001
AGE	15-19		658	1.0	
	20-29		1,796	1.0	
	30-39		1,073	1.25	
	40-49		454	1.99	
	50-59		231	3.52	
	60+		179	6.59	< 0.001
HISTOLOGY	LP		244	1.0	
	NS		3,181	0.79	
	MC		813	1.18	
	LD		66	1.82	< 0.001
	unclassified		69		
TOPOGRAPHY	above diaphragm		4,146	1.0	
	below		247	1.61	< 0.001
MEDIASTINUM	not involved		1,434	1.0	
	involved		2,945	0.66	< 0.001
EXTRA LOCALIZATION E +	absent		3,874	1.0	
	present		520	1.16	0.18
# OF LYMPH NODE AREAS INVOLVED	2		2,491	1.0	
	3		1,160	1.06	
	4		469	1.02	
	5+		248	1.07	> 0.20
E.S.R.	0-19		967	1.0	
	20-39		698	1.25	
	40-59		444	1.33	
	60+		450	1.34	0.05
L.D.H.	<25th percentile		108	1.0	
	25-75th		301	1.02	
	>75th		64	1.0	> 0.20
ALKALINE PHOSPHATASE	<25th percentile		505	1.0	
	25-75th		1,355	1.07	
	>75th		401	1.37	0.10
ALBUMIN	<25th percentile		116	1.62	
	25-75th		725	1.13	
	>75th		508	1.0	0.05
HEMOGLOBIN	abnormal**		410	1.23	
	normal		2,489	1.0	0.08

* with stratification on period, treatment and staging laparotomy
** Hb < 8.0 mmol/l in males and < 7.0 mmol/l in females

Table VIII-3. Prognostic value on overall survival for CS IB-IIB patients (N=1,968) *

Parameter		Patients at risk	Relative risk of death	p value (heterogeneity)
SEX	males	1,128	1.0	
	females	840	0.76	0.003
AGE	15-19	240	1.0	
	20-29	738	1.06	
	30-39	452	1.31	
	40-49	250	1.81	
	50-59	157	2.01	
	60+	127	5.27	< 0.001
HISTOLOGY	LP	77	1.0	
	NS	1,357	1.34	
	MC	430	1.74	
	LD	55	2.65	< 0.001
	unclassified	41		
TOPOGRAPHY	above diaphragm	1,808	1.0	
	below	159	1.55	0.002
MEDIASTINUM	not involved	644	1.0	
	involved	1,320	0.89	0.19
EXTRA LOCALIZATION E +	absent	1,701	1.0	
	present	267	1.17	> 0.20
# OF LYMPH NODE AREAS INVOLVED	1	277	1.0	
	2	808	1.14	
	3	488	0.95	
	4	240	1.06	
	5+	143	1.34	> 0.20
E.S.R.	0-19	204	1.0	
	20-39	191	1.25	
	40-59	241	1.14	
	60+	549	1.66	0.007
L.D.H.	<25th percentile	44	1.0	
	25-75th	139	2.70	
	>75th	44	2.37	0.16
ALKALINE PHOSPHATASE	<25th percentile	217	1.0	
	25-75th	606	0.88	
	>75th	310	1.23	0.06
ALBUMIN	<25th percentile	190	2.12	
	25-75th	374	1.23	
	>75th	152	1.0	< 0.001
HEMOGLOBIN	abnormal**	545	1.52	
	normal	826	1.0	< 0.001

* with stratification on period, treatment and staging laparotomy
** Hb < 8.0 mmol/l in males and < 7.0 mmol/l in females

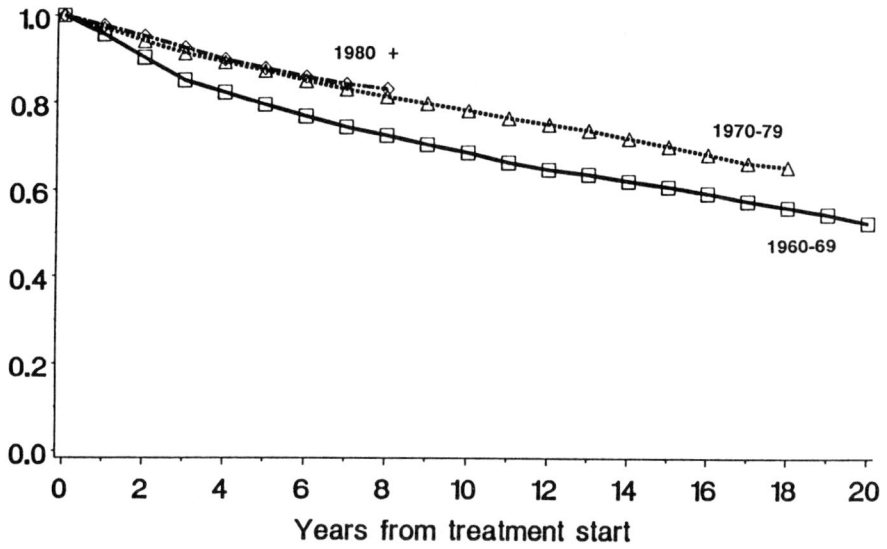

Figure VIII-7 : *Clinical stages I-II. Overall survival by treatment period. (1960-69 : 806 pts; 1970-79 : 5,094 pts; 1980+ : 3,190 pts).*

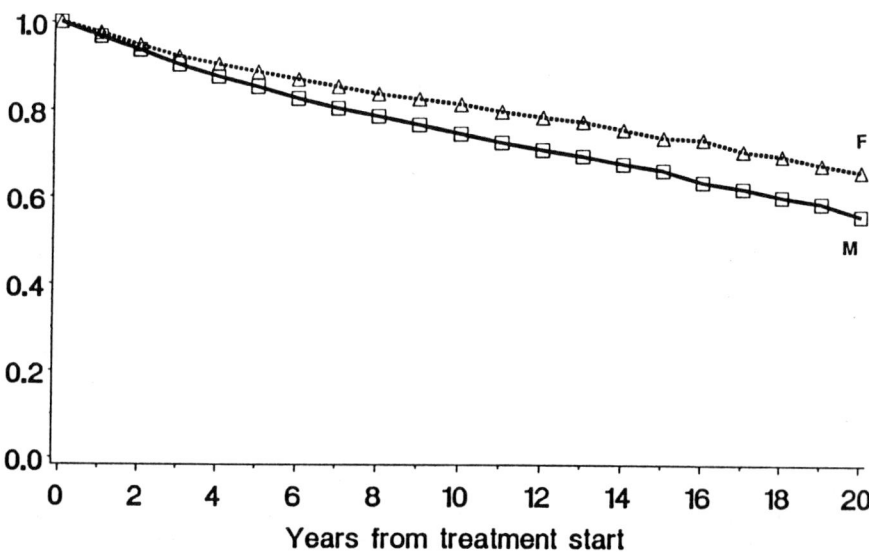

Figure VIII-8 : *Clinical stages I-II. Overall survival by sex. (Males : 5,227 pts; Females : 3,863 pts).*

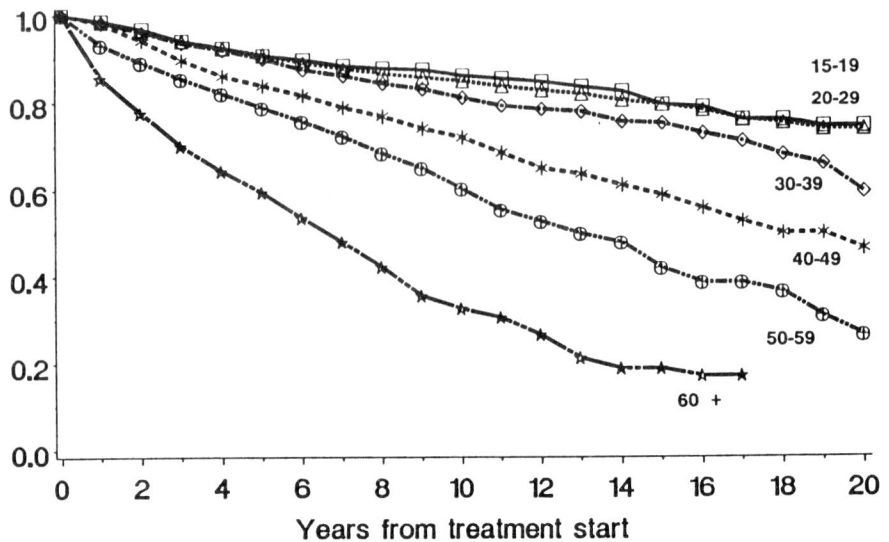

Figure VIII-9 : *Clinical stages I-II. Overall survival by age at Hodgkin disease diagnosis.*
(15-19 yrs: 1,152 pts; 20-29 yrs : 3,412 pts; 30-39 yrs : 2,140 pts; 40-49 yrs : 1,095 pts; 50-59 yrs : 683 pts; 60+ yrs : 591 pts).

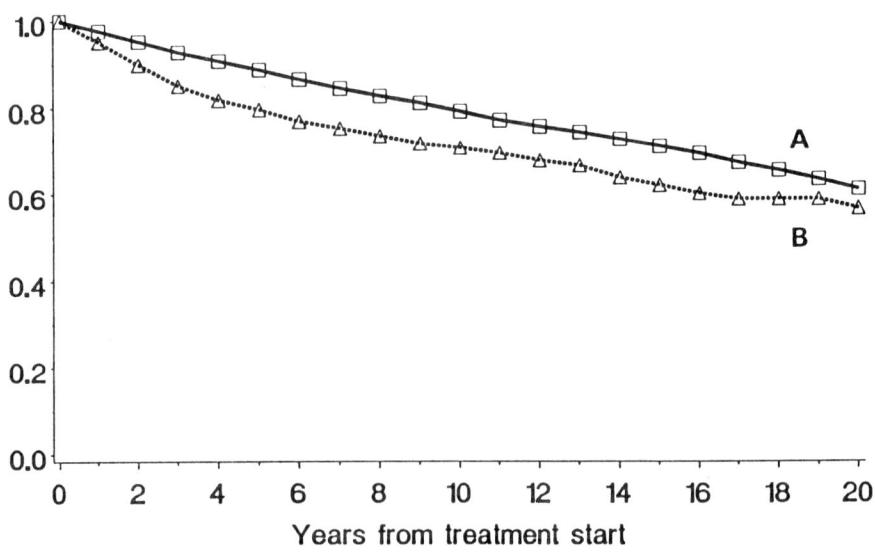

Figure VIII-10 : *Clinical stages I-II. Overall survival by presence or absence of B symptoms.*
(A : 7,113 pts; B : 1,974 pts).

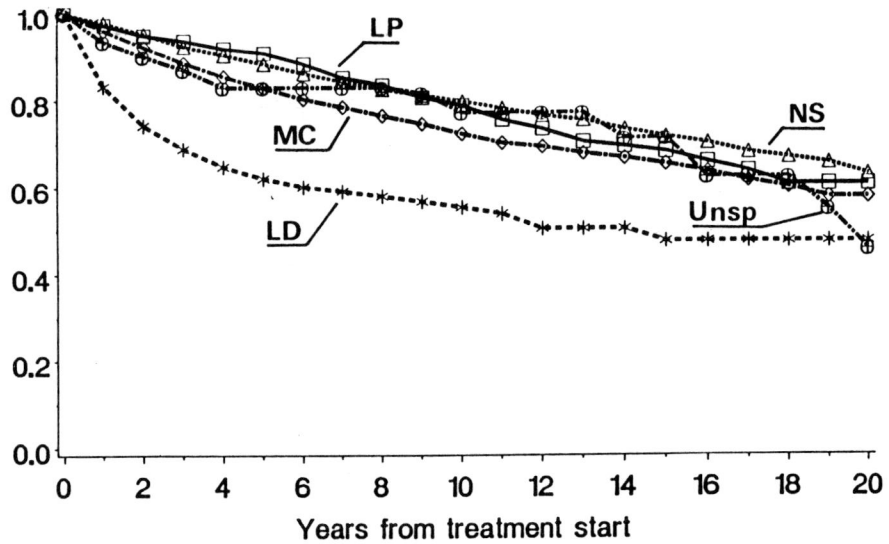

Figure VIII-11: *Clinical stages I-II. Overall survival by histological type. (LP : 754 pts; NS : 5,824 pts; MC : 2,158 pts; LD : 144 pts; Type unspecified : 162 pts).*

Table VIII-4. Prognostic value on overall survival for CS IIIA patients (N=1,558) *

Parameter		Patients at risk	Relative risk of death	p value (heterogeneity)
SEX	males	1,024	1.0	
	females	534	0.75	0.006
AGE	15-19	183	1.0	
	20-29	530	0.88	
	30-39	320	1.06	
	40-49	225	1.69	
	50-59	155	2.72	
	60+	143	3.80	< 0.001
HISTOLOGY	LP	131	1.0	
	NS	832	1.03	
	MC	526	1.31	
	LD	34	2.02	0.008
	unclassified	35		
MEDIASTINUM	not involved	780	1.0	
	involved	761	0.83	0.05
EXTRA LOCALIZATION E +	absent	1,464	1.0	
	present	94	0.94	> 0.20
# OF LYMPH NODE AREAS INVOLVED	2	597	1.0	
	3	271	1.16	
	4	269	0.98	
	5+	411	1.41	0.014
E.S.R.	0-19	331	1.0	
	20-39	215	1.21	
	40-59	139	1.49	
	60+	162	1.67	0.013
L.D.H.	<25th percentile	41	1.0	
	25-75th	116	1.80	
	>75th	38	1.59	> 0.20
ALKALINE PHOSPHATASE	<25th percentile	169	1.0	
	25-75th	450	0.95	
	>75th	122	1.22	> 0.20
ALBUMIN	<25th percentile	74	1.38	
	25-75th	377	1.03	
	>75th	209	1.0	> 0.20
HEMOGLOBIN	abnormal**	243	1.16	
	normal	880	1.0	> 0.20

* with stratification on period, treatment and staging laparotomy
** Hb < 8.0 mmol/l in males and < 7.0 mmol/l in females

Table VIII-5. Prognostic value on overall survival for CS IIIB patients (N=1,773) *

Parameter			Patients at risk	Relative risk of death	p value (heterogeneity)
SEX	males		1,202	1.0	
	females		571	0.86	0.06
AGE	15-19		170	1.0	
	20-29		576	1.31	
	30-39		410	1.52	
	40-49		233	2.28	
	50-59		199	3.02	
	60+		182	5.35	< 0.001
HISTOLOGY	LP		60	1.0	
	NS		1,001	0.90	
	MC		553	1.14	
	LD		89	1.56	< 0.001
	unclassified		69		
MEDIASTINUM	not involved		681	1.0	
	involved		1,080	0.86	0.05
EXTRA LOCALIZATION E +	absent		1,629	1.0	
	present		143	1.17	> 0.20
# OF LYMPH NODE AREAS INVOLVED	2		477	1.0	
	3		320	1.16	
	4		277	1.20	
	5+		687	1.22	> 0.20
E.S.R.	0-19		128	1.0	
	20-39		161	0.87	
	40-59		203	1.29	
	60+		560	1.25	0.04
L.D.H.	<25th percentile		61	1.0	
	25-75th		149	1.29	
	>75th		78	1.85	0.16
ALKALINE PHOSPHATASE	<25th percentile		194	1.0	
	25-75th		500	0.94	
	>75th		322	1.11	> 0.20
ALBUMIN	<25th percentile		236	1.73	
	25-75th		361	1.24	
	>75th		91	1.0	0.003
HEMOGLOBIN	abnormal**		761	1.26	
	normal		610	1.0	0.007

* with stratification on period, treatment and staging laparotomy
** Hb < 8.0 mmol/l in males and < 7.0 mmol/l in females

Table VIII-6. Prognostic value on overall survival for CS IV patients (N=1,868) *

Parameter			Patients at risk	Relative risk of death	p value (heterogeneity)
SEX		males	1,200	1.0	
		females	668	0.74	< 0.001
AGE		15-19	176	1.0	
		20-29	502	0.91	
		30-39	381	1.16	
		40-49	280	1.43	
		50-59	252	2.08	
		60+	276	3.33	< 0.001
HISTOLOGY		LP	64	1.0	
		NS	1,017	0.57	
		MC	536	0.85	
		LD	160	1.27	< 0.001
		unclassified	87		
TOPOGRAPHY		above diaphragm	265	1.0	
		above and/or below	1,599	1.34	0.006
MEDIASTINUM		not involved	753	1.0	
		involved	1,094	0.70	< 0.001
EXTRA LOCALIZATION E +		absent	1,518	1.0	
		present	350	1.04	> 0.20
B SYMPTOMS		absent	409	1.0	
		present	1,449	1.45	< 0.001
# OF LYMPH NODE AREAS INVOLVED		0	212	1.26	
		1	323	1.0	
		2	299	1.10	
		3	283	0.97	
		4	228	1.21	
		5+	514	1.22	0.13
BONE MARROW INVOLVEMENT		No	978	1.0	
		Yes	432	1.18	0.06

* with stratification on period, treatment and staging laparotomy

Table VIII-6. Prognostic value on overall survival for CS IV patients (continued) (N=1,868) *

Parameter		Patients at risk	Relative risk of death	p value (heterogeneity)
E.S.R.	0-19	155	1.0	
	20-39	190	0.80	
	40-59	200	0.80	
	60+	652	0.92	> 0.20
L.D.H.	<25th percentile	80	1.0	
	25-75th	211	0.71	
	>75th	143	1.10	0.05
ALKALINE PHOSPHATASE	<25th percentile	148	1.0	
	25-75th	434	1.26	
	>75th	580	1.31	0.16
ALBUMIN	<25th percentile	431	2.26	
	25-75th	402	1.40	
	>75th	96	1.0	< 0.001
HEMOGLOBIN	abnormal**	963	1.43	
	normal	600	1.0	< 0.001

* with stratification on period, treatment and staging laparotomy
** Hb < 8.0 mmol/l in males and < 7.0 mmol/l in females

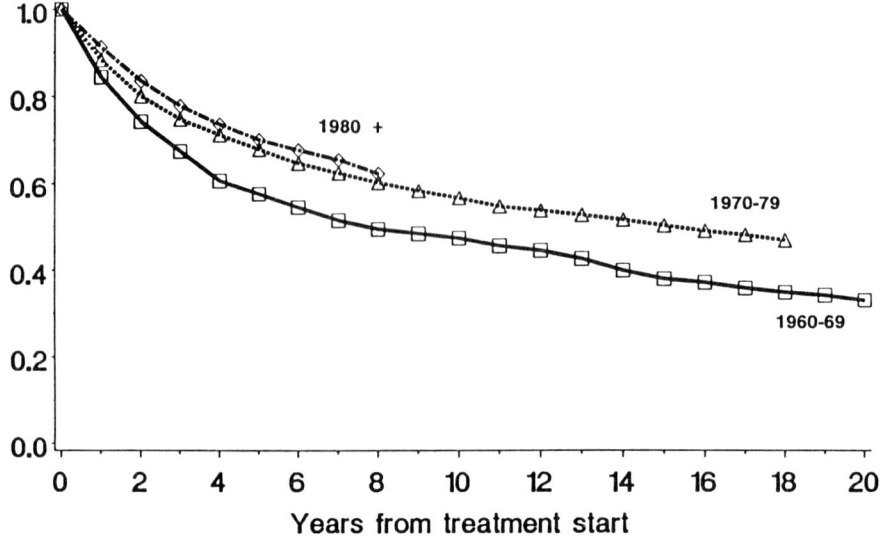

Figure VIII-12: *Clinical stages III-IV. Overall survival by treatment period. (1960-69 : 308 pts; 1970-79 : 3,004 pts; 1980+ : 1,905 pts).*

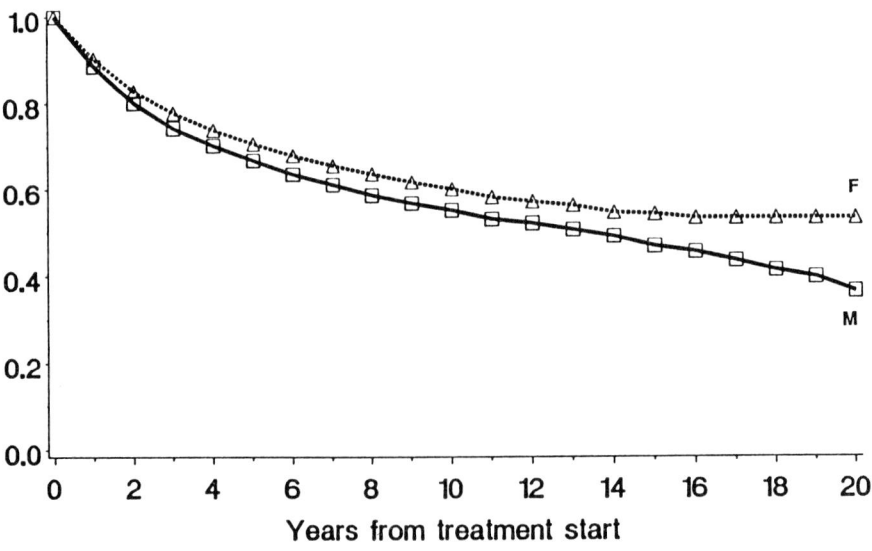

Figure VIII-13: *Clinical stages III-IV. Overall survival by sex. (Males : 3,440 pts; Females : 1,777 pts).*

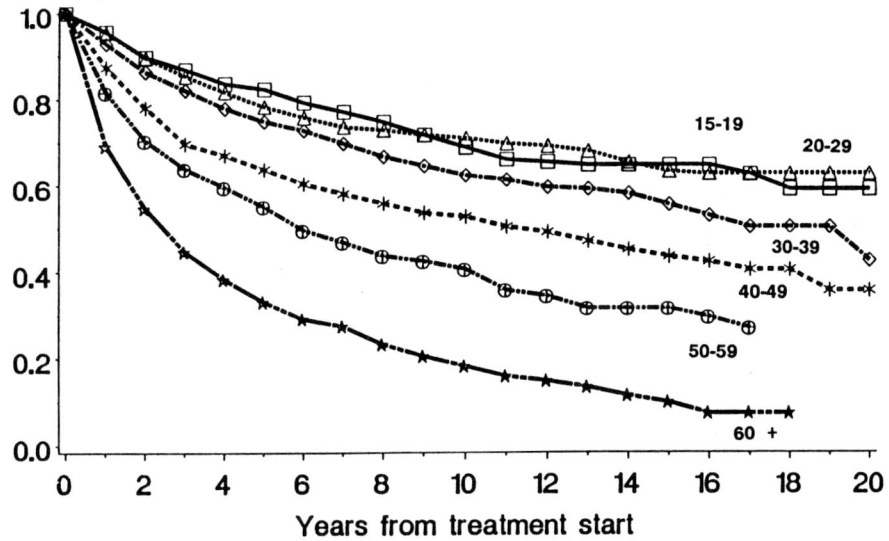

Figure VIII-14: *Clinical stages III-IV. Overall survival by age at Hodgkin disease diagnosis. (15-19 yrs: 532 pts; 20-29 yrs: 1,613 pts; 30-39 yrs: 1,113 pts; 40-49 yrs: 740 pts; 50-59 yrs: 609 pts; 60+ yrs: 604 pts).*

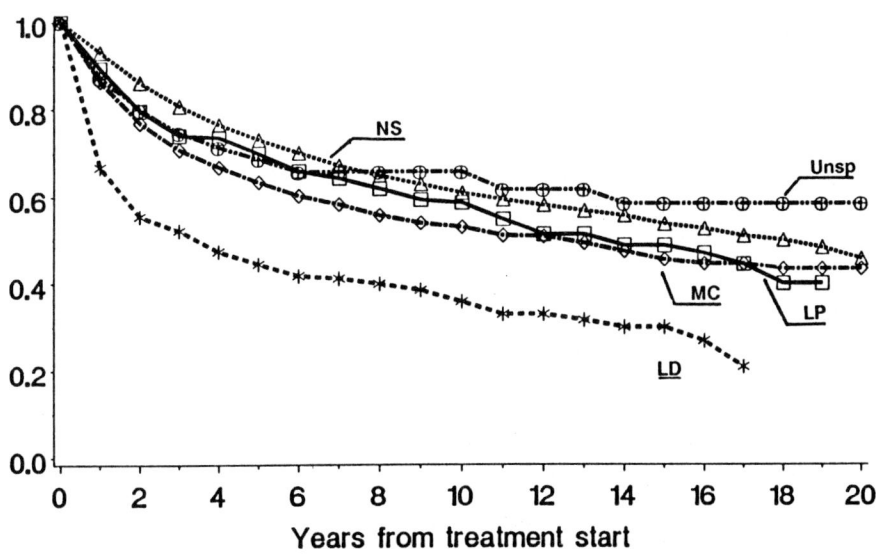

Figure VIII-15: *Clinical stages III-IV. Overall survival by histological type. (LP: 257 pts; NS: 2,858 pts; MC: 1,617 pts; LD: 284 pts; Type unspecified: 196 pts).*

Table VIII-7. Overall survival for CS IA patients (N=2,683)

Treatment type	Patients at risk	Overall survival at 5-yrs(s.e.)	10-yrs(s.e.)
No initial complete remission	58	.52 (.07)	
Initial complete remission and relapse	565	.75 (.02)	.56 (.02)
Initial complete remission, no relapse	2,060	.95 (.01)	.87 (.07)

NO COMPLETE REMISSION OR INITIAL COMPLETE REMISSION FOLLOWED BY A RELAPSE :

Treatment type	Patients at risk	5-yrs(s.e.)	10-yrs(s.e.)
RT alone IF irradiation	155	.69 (.04)	.55 (.04)
Mantle or inverted Y RT	209	.82 (.03)	.60 (.04)
STNI or TNI	116	.74 (.04)	.54 (.05)
RT + single or bi-agent CT	24	.58 (.10)	
Combination CT MOPP-like	31	.51 (.09)	
Others	2	–	
RT + Combination CT			
IF irradiation + MOPP	34	.78 (.08)	
+ Others	4	–	
Mantle or inverted Y RT + MOPP-like	18	.60 (.12)	
+ Others	0	–	
STNI or TNI + MOPP-like	14	.57 (.13)	
+ Others	2	–	

INITIAL COMPLETE REMISSION, NO FURTHER RELAPSE :

Treatment type	Patients at risk	5-yrs(s.e.)	10-yrs(s.e.)
RT alone IF irradiation	259	.94 (.02)	.84 (.03)
Mantle or inverted Y RT	577	.95 (.01)	.88 (.02)
STNI or TNI	498	.96 (.01)	.87 (.02)
RT + single or bi-agent CT	84	.93 (.03)	.84 (.04)
Combination CT MOPP-like	58	.86 (.05)	.82 (.06)
Others	5	–	
RT + Combination CT			
IF irradiation + MOPP-like	186	.98 (.01)	.96 (.02)
+ Others	38	.93 (.05)	
Mantle or inverted Y RT + MOPP-like	155	.91 (.02)	.84 (.04)
+ Others	19	–	
STNI or TNI + MOPP-like	125	.95 (.02)	.83 (.05)
+ Others	4	–	

Table VIII-7. Overall survival for CS IA patients (continued)

	Overall survival at		
	5-yrs(s.e.)	10-yrs(s.e.)	15-yrs(s.e.)
ALL PATIENTS (N=2,696)	.89 (.01)	.78 (.01)	.70 (.01)
patients at risk	1,821	900	288
TREATMENT PERIOD			
1960-69 (N=231)	.81 (.03)	.69 (.03)	.62 (.03)
patients at risk	186	151	124
1970-79 (N=1,516)	.90 (.01)	.79 (.01)	.70 (.02)
patients at risk	1,286	749	164
1980 + (N=949)	.90 (.01)		
patients at risk	349		
TREATMENT TYPE			
RT+/-single/bi-agent CT (N=1,953)	.89 (.01)	.78 (.01)	.69 (.02)
patients at risk	1,365	745	272
Combination CT (N=101)	.76 (.05)		
patients at risk	52		
RT + Combination CT (N=633)	.91 (.01)	.82 (.02)	
patients at risk	399	135	

Table VIII-8. Overall survival for CS IIA patients (N=4,380)

Treatment type	Patients at risk	Overall survival at 5-yrs(s.e.)	10-yrs(s.e.)
No initial complete remission	217	.45 (.04)	.34 (.04)
Initial complete remission and relapse	1,137	.77 (.01)	.58 (.02)
Initial complete remission, no relapse	3,026	.96 (.01)	.92 (.01)

NO COMPLETE REMISSION OR INITIAL COMPLETE REMISSION FOLLOWED BY A RELAPSE :

Treatment type	Patients at risk	5-yrs(s.e.)	10-yrs(s.e.)
RT alone IF irradiation	138	.78 (.04)	.59 (.04)
Mantle or inverted Y RT	411	.74 (.02)	.60 (.03)
STNI or TNI	384	.80 (.02)	.62 (.03)
RT + single or bi-agent CT	52	.69 (.06)	.45 (.07)
Combination CT MOPP-like	85	.65 (.06)	
Others	8	–	
RT + Combination CT			
IF irradiation + MOPP	70	.62 (.06)	
+ Others	5	–	
Mantle or inverted Y RT + MOPP-like	89	.50 (.06)	
+ Others	28	–	
STNI or TNI + MOPP-like	57	.58 (.07)	
+ Others	3	–	

INITIAL COMPLETE REMISSION, NO FURTHER RELAPSE :

Treatment type	Patients at risk	5-yrs(s.e.)	10-yrs(s.e.)
RT alone IF irradiation	158	.97 (.02)	.89 (.03)
Mantle or inverted Y RT	552	.96 (.01)	.90 (.02)
STNI or TNI	943	.97 (.01)	.94 (.01)
RT + single or bi-agent CT	79	.97 (.02)	.95 (.03)
Combination CT MOPP-like	108	.93 (.03)	.89 (.04)
Others	12	–	
RT + Combination CT			
IF irradiation + MOPP-like	249	.96 (.01)	.89 (.03)
+ Others	32	–	
Mantle or inverted Y RT + MOPP-like	360	.95 (.01)	.87 (.03)
+ Others	143	.98 (.02)	
STNI or TNI + MOPP-like	309	.96 (.01)	.93 (.02)
+ Others	39	.97 (.03)	

Table VIII-8. Overall survival for CS IIA patients (continued)

	Overall survival at		
	5-yrs(s.e.)	10-yrs(s.e.)	15-yrs(s.e.)
ALL PATIENTS (N=4,395)	.88 (.01)	.79 (.01)	.71 (.01)
patients at risk	3,014	1,514	138
TREATMENT PERIOD			
1960-69 (N=396)	.85 (.02)	.73 (.03)	.66 (.02)
patients at risk	333	281	237
1970-79 (N=2,488)	.88 (.01)	.79 (.01)	.70 (.02)
patients at risk	2,067	1,233	272
1980 + (N=1,511)	.90 (.01)		
patients at risk	614		
TREATMENT TYPE			
RT+/-single/bi-agent CT (N=2,738)	.89 (.01)	.79 (.01)	.72 (.02)
patients at risk	2,052	1,148	457
Combination CT (N=224)	.80 (.03)	.72 (.04)	
patients at risk	112	44	
RT + Combination CT (N=1,426)	.88 (.01)	.78 (.02)	.68 (.03)
patients at risk	849	321	44

Table VIII-9. Overall survival for CS IB-IIB patients (N=1,951)

Treatment type	Patients at risk	Overall survival at 5-yrs(s.e.)	10-yrs(s.e.)
No initial complete remission	272	.39 (.03)	.28 (.03)
Initial complete remission and relapse	460	.64 (.02)	.47 (.03)
Initial complete remission, no relapse	1,219	.94 (.01)	.89 (.01)

NO COMPLETE REMISSION OR INITIAL COMPLETE REMISSION FOLLOWED BY A RELAPSE :

Treatment type	Patients at risk	5-yrs(s.e.)	10-yrs(s.e.)
RT alone IF irradiation	23	.35 (.10)	
Mantle or inverted Y RT	124	.66 (.04)	.49 (.05)
STNI or TNI	136	.69 (.04)	.56 (.04)
RT + single or bi-agent CT	27	.42 (.10)	
Combination CT MOPP-like	189	.58 (.04)	
Others	18	-	
RT + Combination CT			
IF irradiation + MOPP	52	.39 (.07)	
+ Others	5	-	
Mantle or inverted Y RT + MOPP-like	76	.43 (.06)	
+ Others	14	-	
STNI or TNI + MOPP-like	39	.56 (.08)	
+ Others	5	-	

INITIAL COMPLETE REMISSION, NO FURTHER RELAPSE :

Treatment type	Patients at risk	5-yrs(s.e.)	10-yrs(s.e.)
RT alone IF irradiation	13	.76 (.12)	
Mantle or inverted Y RT	79	.92 (.03)	.87 (.04)
STNI or TNI	200	.94 (.02)	.92 (.02)
RT + single or bi-agent CT	23	.91 (.06)	
Combination CT MOPP-like	163	.97 (.02)	.89 (.04)
Others	11	-	
RT + Combination CT			
IF irradiation + MOPP-like	137	.91 (.03)	.80 (.05)
+ Others	19	-	
Mantle or inverted Y RT + MOPP-like	251	.95 (.01)	.91 (.02)
+ Others	94	.99 (.01)	
STNI or TNI + MOPP-like	184	.96 (.02)	.91 (.03)
+ Others	10	-	

Table VIII-9. Overall survival for CS IB-IIB patients (continued)

	Overall survival at		
	5-yrs(s.e.)	10-yrs(s.e.)	15-yrs(s.e.)
ALL PATIENTS (N=1,968)	.79 (.01)	.69 (.01)	.60 (.01)
patients at risk	1,134	565	151
TREATMENT PERIOD			
1960-69 (N=166)	.65 (.04)	.56 (.04)	.47 (.04)
patients at risk	105	87	67
1970-79 (N=1,081)	.80 (.01)	.70 (.02)	.62 (.02)
patients at risk	812	478	84
1980 + (N=721)	.81 (.02)		
patients at risk	217		
TREATMENT TYPE			
RT +/- single/bi-agent CT (N=630)	.78 (.02)	.68 (.02)	.57 (.02)
patients at risk	444	296	115
Combination CT (N=397)	.73 (.02)	.59 (.03)	
patients at risk	176	62	
RT + Combination CT (N=926)	.83 (.01)	.75 (.02)	.68 (.03)
patients at risk	512	207	30

Table VIII-10. Overall survival for CS IIIA patients (N=1,550)

Treatment type	Patients at risk	Overall survival at 5-yrs(s.e.)	10-yrs(s.e.)
No initial complete remission	201	.31 (.04)	.21 (.04)
Initial complete remission and relapse	429	.73 (.02)	.51 (.03)
Initial complete remission, no relapse	920	.93 (.01)	.87 (.01)

NO COMPLETE REMISSION OR INITIAL COMPLETE REMISSION FOLLOWED BY A RELAPSE :

Treatment type	Patients at risk	5-yrs(s.e.)	10-yrs(s.e.)
RT alone IF irradiation	9	-	
Mantle or inverted Y RT	21	.85 (.08)	
STNI or TNI	186	.74 (.03)	.57 (.04)
RT + single or bi-agent CT	17	-	
Combination CT MOPP-like	194	.51 (.04)	.31 (.05)
Others	10	-	
RT + Combination CT			
IF irradiation + MOPP	64	.52 (.06)	
+ Others	5	-	
Mantle or inverted Y RT + MOPP-like	14	.43 (.13)	
+ Others	3	-	
STNI or TNI + MOPP-like	75	.61 (.06)	.37 (.06)
+ Others	10	-	

INITIAL COMPLETE REMISSION, NO FURTHER RELAPSE :

Treatment type	Patients at risk	5-yrs(s.e.)	10-yrs(s.e.)
RT alone IF irradiation	12	1.0	
Mantle or inverted Y RT	35	.94 (.04)	.94 (.04)
STNI or TNI	224	.92 (.02)	.86 (.03)
RT + single or bi-agent CT	5	-	
Combination CT MOPP-like	218	.92 (.02)	.84 (.04)
Others	14	-	
RT + Combination CT			
IF irradiation + MOPP-like	106	.94 (.02)	.90 (.03)
+ Others	16	.93 (.07)	
Mantle or inverted Y RT + MOPP-like	25	.96 (.04)	
+ Others	23	-	
STNI or TNI + MOPP-like	195	.91 (.02)	.83 (.03)
+ Others	32	1.0	

Table VIII-10. Overall survival for CS IIIA patients (continued)

	Overall survival at		
	5-yrs(s.e.)	10-yrs(s.e.)	15-yrs(s.e.)
ALL PATIENTS (N=1,558)	.79 (.01)	.68 (.01)	.58 (.02)
patients at risk	954	507	159
TREATMENT PERIOD			
1960-69 (N=108)	.75 (.04)	.61 (.05)	.51 (.05)
patients at risk	79	63	44
1970-79 (N=940)	.78 (.01)	.66 (.02)	.57 (.02)
patients at risk	703	444	115
1980 + (N=510)	.83 (.02)		
patients at risk	172		
TREATMENT TYPE			
RT +/- single/bi-agent CT (N=511)	.83 (.02)	.72 (.02)	.63 (.03)
patients at risk	380	254	105
Combination CT (N=451)	.72 (.02)	.58 (.03)	
patients at risk	208	76	
RT + Combination CT (N=593)	.81 (.02)	.69 (.02)	.60 (.03)
patients at risk	366	177	43

Table VIII-11. Overall survival for CS IIIB patients (N=1,757)

Treatment type	Patients at risk	Overall survival at 5-yrs(s.e.)	10-yrs(s.e.)
No initial complete remission	419	.23 (.02)	
Initial complete remission and relapse	454	.59 (.02)	.32 (.03)
Initial complete remission, no relapse	884	.90 (.01)	.83 (.02)

NO COMPLETE REMISSION OR INITIAL COMPLETE REMISSION FOLLOWED BY A RELAPSE :

RT alone IF irradiation	7	–	
Mantle or inverted Y RT	12	–	
STNI or TNI	89	.46 (.05)	.26 (.05)
RT + single or bi-agent CT	17	.47 (.12)	
Combination CT MOPP-like	376	.38 (.03)	.19 (.03)
Others	73	.44 (.08)	
RT + Combination CT			
IF irradiation + MOPP	99	.41 (.05)	
+ Others	27	.56 (.11)	
Mantle or inverted Y RT + MOPP-like	35	.33 (.09)	
+ Others	1	–	
STNI or TNI + MOPP-like	79	.58 (.06)	.29 (.05)
+ Others	9	.89 (.11)	

INITIAL COMPLETE REMISSION, NO FURTHER RELAPSE :

RT alone IF irradiation	1	–	
Mantle or inverted Y RT	3	–	
STNI or TNI	39	.90 (.05)	.84 (.06)
RT + single or bi-agent CT	12	.92 (.08)	
Combination CT MOPP-like	320	.87 (.02)	.81 (.03)
Others	66	.95 (.03)	
RT + Combination CT			
IF irradiation + MOPP-like	99	.93 (.03)	.83 (.04)
+ Others	63	.93 (.05)	
Mantle or inverted Y RT + MOPP-like	27	.88 (.06)	.82 (.08)
+ Others	7	–	
STNI or TNI + MOPP-like	169	.89 (.03)	.80 (.03)
+ Others	35	.94 (.04)	

Table VIII-11. Overall survival for CS IIIB patients (continued)

	Overall survival at		
	5-yrs(s.e.)	10-yrs(s.e.)	15-yrs(s.e.)
ALL PATIENTS (N=1,773)	.65 (.01)	.51 (.01)	.42 (.02)
patients at risk	830	418	123
TREATMENT PERIOD			
1960-69 (N=131)	.53 (.04)	.42 (.04)	.33 (.04)
patients at risk	69	53	38
1970-79 (N=1,001)	.64 (.02)	.50 (.02)	.42 (.02)
patients at risk	612	365	85
1980 + (N=641)	.70 (.02)		
patients at risk	149		
TREATMENT TYPE			
RT +/- single/bi-agent CT (N=182)	.58 (.04)	.44 (.04)	.35 (.04)
patients at risk	102	66	36
Combination CT (N=879)	.61 (.02)	.47 (.02)	.40 (.03)
patients at risk	341	170	34
RT + Combination CT (N=699)	.74 (.02)	.58 (.02)	.49 (.03)
patients at risk	386	182	53

Table VIII-12. Overall survival for CS IV patients (N=1,832)

Treatment type	Patients at risk	Overall survival at 5-yrs(s.e.)	10-yrs(s.e.)
No initial complete remission	690	.19 (.02)	.09 (.01)
Initial complete remission and relapse	375	.58 (.03)	.30 (.03)
Initial complete remission, no relapse	767	.90 (.01)	.80 (.02)

NO COMPLETE REMISSION OR
INITIAL COMPLETE REMISSION FOLLOWED BY A RELAPSE :

RT alone IF irradiation	6	–	
Mantle or inverted Y RT	9	–	
STNI or TNI	13	–	
RT + single or bi-agent CT	14	–	
Combination CT MOPP-like	741	.33 (.02)	.17 (.02)
Others	90	.38 (.07)	
RT + Combination CT			
IF irradiation + MOPP	85	.23 (.05)	
+ Others	27	–	
Mantle or inverted Y RT + MOPP-like	25	.23 (.09)	
+ Others	8	–	
STNI or TNI + MOPP-like	23	.61 (.10)	
+ Others	6	–	

INITIAL COMPLETE REMISSION,
NO FURTHER RELAPSE :

RT alone IF irradiation	2	–	
Mantle or inverted Y RT	5	–	
STNI or TNI	6	–	
RT + single or bi-agent CT	2	–	
Combination CT MOPP-like	404	.88 (.02)	.78 (.02)
Others	93	.92 (.04)	
RT + Combination CT			
IF irradiation + MOPP-like	53	.88 (.05)	.85 (.06)
+ Others	39	.90 (.07)	
Mantle or inverted Y RT + MOPP-like	33	.87 (.03)	
+ Others	16	1.0	
STNI or TNI + MOPP-like	80	.89 (.04)	.79 (.05)
+ Others	20	.89 (.07)	

Table VIII-12. Overall survival for CS IV patients (continued)

	Overall survival at		
	5-yrs(s.e.)	10-yrs(s.e.)	15-yrs(s.e.)
ALL PATIENTS (N=1,868)	.56 (.01)	.43 (.01)	.36 (.02)
patients at risk	751	322	76
TREATMENT PERIOD			
1960-69 (N=62)	.36 (.06)		
patients at risk	22		
1970-79 (N=1,052)	.54 (.02)	.40 (.02)	.35 (.02)
patients at risk	544	304	63
1980 + (N=752)	.62 (.02)		
patients at risk	185		
TREATMENT TYPE			
RT +/- single/bi-agent CT (N=52)	.39 (.07)		
patients at risk	17		
Combination CT (N=1,317)	.53 (.01)	.39 (.02)	.32 (.02)
patients at risk	519	218	42
RT + Combination CT (N=461)	.67 (.02)	.55 (.03)	.51 (.03)
patients at risk	209	88	26

Table VIII-13. Stepwise proportional hazards model on survival for 13,425 CS I-IV patients *(1)*.

a) End point = death (all causes)

Step no	Variable	Log likelihood	Coeff./s.e.	RR[2]
0		− 21135.013		
1	AGE 60+ yrs	− 20811.156	1.63/0.06	5.09 ***[3]
2	B SYMPTOMS	− 20609.274	0.40/0.04	1.50 ***
3	AGE 50-59 yrs	− 20500.407	1.04/0.06	2.82 ***
4	AGE 40-49 yrs	− 20432.771	0.67/0.06	1.96 ***
5	CS IV	− 20375.546	0.94/0.07	2.55 ***
6	CS III	− 20311.566	0.68/0.06	1.96 ***
7	FEMALE GENDER	− 20287.101	−0.26/0.04	0.77 ***
8	HISTOLOGY = LD	− 20274.241	0.47/0.08	1.60 ***
9	AGE 30-39 yrs	− 20263.093	0.25/0.05	1.28 ***
10	CS II	− 20254.924	0.28/0.06	1.32 ***
11	HISTOLOGY = MC	− 20245.199	0.18/0.04	1.20 ***

(1) after adjustment on initial therapy (i.e. RT with or w/o single or bi-agent CT, combination CT, or RT + combination CT), treatment period (i.e. 1960-69, 1970-79 and 1980 +), and staging laparotomy (performed or not performed)
(2) relative risk RR = exp (regression coefficient)
*(3) p value : ** < 0.01, *** < 0.001*

Table VIII-13. Stepwise Proportional hazards model on survival for 13,425 CS I-IV patients (continued) *(1)*.

b) End point = death from Hodgkin Disease

Step no	Variable	Log likelihood	Coeff./s.e.	RR[2]
0		− 11400.414		
1	B SYMPTOMS	− 11213.090	0.50/0.06	1.65 ***[3]
2	AGE 60+ yrs	− 11116.644	1.17/0.08	3.21 ***
3	CS IV	− 11053.217	1.38/0.11	3.97 ***
4	CS III	− 10992.379	1.02/0.10	2.78 ***
5	HISTOLOGY = LD	− 10968.297	0.79/0.10	2.19 ***
6	HISTOLOGY = MC	− 10948.735	0.31/0.06	1.37 ***
7	AGE 50-59 yrs	− 10931.805	0.68/0.09	1.96 ***
8	CS II	− 10917.332	0.53/0.09	1.70 ***
9	AGE 40-49 yrs	− 10904.127	0.45/0.08	1.57 ***
10	AGE 30-39 yrs	− 10899.827	0.19/0.07	1.21 **
11	FEMALE GENDER	− 10896.048	−0.15/0.05	0.86 **

c) End point = death from other causes than Hodgkin Disease

Step no	Variable	Log likelihood	Coeff./s.e.	RR[2]
0		− 7037.439		
1	AGE 60+ yrs	− 6795.178	2.66/0.09	14.28 ***[3]
2	AGE 50-59 yrs	− 6699.270	1.78/0.10	5.92 ***
3	AGE 40-49 yrs	− 6637.138	1.24/0.10	3.44 ***
4	FEMALE GENDER	− 6614.136	−0.45/0.07	0.64 ***
5	AGE 30-39 yrs	− 6602.249	0.50/0.10	1.65 ***
6	B SYMPTOMS	− 6595.983	0.24/0.07	1.27 ***

(1) after adjustment on initial therapy (i.e. RT with or w/o single or bi-agent CT, combination CT, or RT + combination CT), treatment period (i.e. 1960-69, 1970-79 and 1980+), and staging laparotomy (performed or not performed)
(2) relative risk RR = exp (regression coefficient)
*(3) p value : ** < 0.01, *** < 0.001*

Table VIII-14. Stepwise proportional hazards model on survival for 2,592 CS IA patients *(1)*.

a) End point = death (all causes)

Step no	Variable	Log likelihood	Coeff./s.e.	RR[2]
0		- 2704.632		
1	AGE 60+ yrs	- 2608.961	2.24/0.13	9.41 ***[3]
2	AGE 50-59 yrs	- 2572.007	1.46/0.14	4.29 ***
3	AGE 40-49 yrs	- 2555.073	0.97/0.15	2.64 ***
4	FEMALE GENDER	- 2454.712	-0.45/0.10	0.64 ***
5	HISTOLOGY = LD	- 2537.488	1.45/0.29	4.27 ***
6	AGE 30-39 yrs	- 2534.086	0.40/0.15	1.48 **

(1) after adjustment on initial therapy (i.e. RT with or w/o single or bi-agent CT, combination CT, or RT + combination CT), treatment period (i.e. 1960-69, 1970-79 and 1980+), and staging laparotomy (performed or not performed)
(2) relative risk RR = exp (regression coefficient)
*(3) p value : ** < 0.01, *** < 0.001*

Table VIII-14. Stepwise proportional hazards model on survival for 2,592 CS IA patients (continued) [1].

b) End point = death from Hodgkin Disease

Step no	Variable	Log likelihood	Coeff./s.e.	RR[2]
0		− 1099.288		
1	AGE 60+ yrs	− 1081.508	1.45/0.19	4.26 ***[3]
2	HISTOLOGY = LD	− 1072.936	2.50/0.41	12.13 ***
3	HISTOLOGY = MC	− 1065.878	0.89/0.24	2.44 ***
4	FEMALE GENDER	− 1062.772	−0.44/0.17	0.65 **
5	AGE 40-49 yrs	− 1059.892	0.64/0.20	1.89 **
6	AGE 50-59 yrs	− 1055.834	0.66/0.21	1.94 **

c) End point = death from other causes than Hodgkin Disease

Step no	Variable	Log likelihood	Coeff./s.e.	RR[2]
0		− 1529.640		
1	AGE 60+ yrs	− 1446.079	3.15/0.21	23.44 ***[3]
2	AGE 50-59 yrs	− 1403.742	2.28/0.21	9.77 ***
3	AGE 40-49 yrs	− 1389.135	1.52/0.23	4.56 ***
4	AGE 30-39 yrs	− 1379.688	0.99/0.23	2.70 ***
5	FEMALE GENDER	− 1372.872	−0.50/0.14	0.61 ***

(1) after adjustment on initial therapy (i.e. RT with or w/o single or bi-agent CT, combination CT, or RT + combination CT), treatment period (i.e. 1960-69, 1970-79 and 1980+), and staging laparotomy (performed or not performed)
(2) relative risk RR = exp (regression coefficient)
*(3) p value : ** < 0.01, *** < 0.001*

Table VIII-15. Stepwise proportional hazards model on survival for 4,237 CS IIA patients (1).

a) End point = death (all causes)

Step no	Variable	Log likelihood	Coeff./s.e.	RR[(2)]
0		− 4841.197		
1	AGE 60+ yrs	− 4767.058	1.80/0.12	6.07 ***[(3)]
2	AGE 50-59 yrs	− 4727.764	1.16/0.11	3.19 ***
3	AGE 40-49 yrs	− 4709.753	0.63/0.10	1.88 ***
4	FEMALE GENDER	− 4701.195	−0.27/0.07	0.76 ***
5	HISTOLOGY = LD	− 4697.736	0.65/0.21	1.92 **

b) End point = death from Hodgkin Disease

Step no	Variable	Log likelihood	Coeff./s.e.	RR[(2)]
0		− 2659.238		
1	AGE 60+ yrs	− 2645.561	1.07/0.18	2.93 ***[(3)]
2	AGE 50-59 yrs	− 2633.006	0.84/0.16	2.31 ***
3	HISTOLOGY = LD	− 2629.804	0.82/0.26	2.26 **
4	HISTOLOGY = MC	− 2626.272	0.30/0.11	1.35 **

c) End point = death from other causes than Hodgkin Disease

Step no	Variable	Log likelihood	Coeff./s.e.	RR[(2)]
0		− 1955.280		
1	AGE 60+ yrs	− 1882.373	2.79/0.17	16.34 ***[(3)]
2	AGE 50-59 yrs	− 1856.054	1.72/0.18	5.57 ***
3	AGE 40-49 yrs	− 1830.034	1.29/0.16	3.64 **
4	FEMALE GENDER	− 1821.234	−0.45/0.11	0.64 **
5	AGE 30-39 yrs	− 2817.949	0.41/0.16	1.51 **

(1) after adjustment on initial therapy (i.e. RT with or w/o single or bi-agent CT, combination CT, or RT + combination CT), treatment period (i.e. 1960-69, 1970-79 and 1980+), and staging laparotomy (performed or not performed)
(2) relative risk RR = exp (regression coefficient)
*(3) p value : ** < 0.01, *** < 0.001*

Table VIII-16. Stepwise proportional hazards model on survival for 1,867 CS IB - IIB patients (1).

a) End point = death (all causes)

Step no	Variable	Log likelihood	Coeff./s.e.	RR[(2)]
0		- 2489.454		
1	AGE 60+ yrs	- 2444.677	1.34/0.13	3.83 ***[(3)]
2	FEMALE GENDER	- 2437.689	-0.34/0.09	0.71 ***
3	AGE 20-29 yrs	- 2432.269	-0.33/0.10	0.72 ***

b) End point = death from Hodgkin Disease

Step no	Variable	Log likelihood	Coeff./s.e.	RR[(2)]
0		- 1524.453		
1	AGE 60+ yrs	- 1516.490	0.90/0.20	2.46 ***[(3)]
2	HISTOLOGY = LD	- 1510.138	0.87/0.23	2.38 ***
3	FEMALE GENDER	- 1504.773	-0.39/0.12	0.68 ***
4	5+ LYMPH NODE AREAS INVOLVED	- 1500.934	0.50/0.19	1.65 **

c) End point = death from other causes than Hodgkin Disease

Step no	Variable	Log likelihood	Coeff./s.e.	RR[(2)]
0		- 802.875		
1	AGE 60+ yrs	- 754.076	2.94/0.23	18.97 ***[(3)]
2	AGE 50-59 yrs	- 741.996	1.76/0.26	5.83 ***
3	AGE 40-49 yrs	- 731.912	1.30/0.24	3.68 ***
4	AGE 30-39 yrs	- 728.247	0.66/0.24	1.94 **

(1) after adjustment on initial therapy (i.e. RT with or w/o single or bi-agent CT, combination CT, or RT + combination CT), treatment period (i.e. 1960-69, 1970-79 and 1980+), and staging laparotomy (performed or not performed)
(2) relative risk RR = exp (regression coefficient)
*(3) p value : ** < 0.01, *** < 0.001*

Table VIII-17. Stepwise proportional hazards model on survival for 1,486 CS IIIA patients (1).

a) End point = death (all causes)

Step no	Variable	Log likelihood	Coeff./s.e.	RR[2]
0		− 2114.044		
1	AGE 60+ yrs	− 2080.497	1.43/0.13	4.18 ***[3]
2	AGE 50-59 yrs	− 2062.136	1.04/0.14	2.84 ***
3	AGE 40-49 yrs	− 2052.931	0.57/0.13	1.77 ***
4	5+ LYMPH NODE AREAS INVOLVED	− 2048.627	0.32/0.10	1.38 **
5	FEMALE GENDER	− 2044.349	−0.31/0.11	0.73 **

b) End point = death from Hodgkin Disease

Step no	Variable	Log likelihood	Coeff./s.e.	RR[2]
0		− 1243.985		
1	AGE 60+ yrs	− 1230.402	0.91/0.16	2.48 ***[3]
2	5+ LYMPH NODE AREAS INVOLVED	− 1225.721	0.37/0.13	1.44 **
3	HISTOLOGY = MC	− 1221.762	0.42/0.13	1.52 ***
4	HISTOLOGY = LD	− 1218.015	0.87/0.29	2.39 **

c) End point = death from other causes than Hodgkin Disease

Step no	Variable	Log likelihood	Coeff./s.e.	RR[2]
0		− 672.692		
1	AGE 60+ yrs	− 645.180	2.19/0.22	8.91 ***[3]
2	AGE 50-59 yrs	− 622.059	1.84/0.23	6.27 ***
3	AGE 40-49 yrs	− 619.280	0.66/0.26	1.93 **

(1) after adjustment on initial therapy (i.e. RT with or w/o single or bi-agent CT, combination CT, or RT + combination CT), treatment period (i.e. 1960-69, 1970-79 and 1980+), and staging laparotomy (performed or not performed)
(2) relative risk RR = exp (regression coefficient)
(3) p value : ** < 0.01, *** < 0.001

Table VIII-18. Stepwise proportional hazards model on survival for 1,652 CS IIIB patients (1).

a) End point = death (all causes)

Step no	Variable	Log likelihood	Coeff./s.e.	RR[2]
0		- 3609.130		
1	AGE 60+ yrs	- 3558.019	1.39/0.11	4.00 ***[3]
2	AGE 50-59 yrs	- 3541.825	0.80/0.12	2.22 ***
3	AGE 40-49 yrs	- 3530.945	0.54/0.11	1.71 ***

b) End point = death from Hodgkin Disease

Step no	Variable	Log likelihood	Coeff./s.e.	RR[2]
0		- 2261.565		
1	AGE 60+ yrs	- 2235.056	1.09/0.13	2.99 ***[3]
2	AGE 50-59 yrs	- 2230.595	0.44/0.15	1.56 **
3	HISTOLOGY = LD	- 2227.469	0.47/0.18	1.61 **

c) End point = death from other causes than Hodgkin Disease

Step no	Variable	Log likelihood	Coeff./s.e.	RR[2]
0		- 880.011		
1	AGE 60+ yrs	- 854.246	2.17/0.22	8.75 ***[3]
2	AGE 50-59 yrs	- 834.749	1.66/0.21	5.25 ***
3	AGE 40-49 yrs	- 820.864	1.21/0.21	3.34 ***

(1) after adjustment on initial therapy (i.e. RT with or w/o single or bi-agent CT, combination CT, or RT + combination CT), treatment period (i.e. 1960-69, 1970-79 and 1980+), and staging laparotomy (performed or not performed)
(2) relative risk RR = exp (regression coefficient)
*(3) p value : ** < 0.01, *** < 0.001*

Table VIII-19. Stepwise proportional hazards model on survival for 1,601 CS IV patients [1].

a) End point = death (all causes)

Step no	Variable	Log likelihood	Coeff./s.e.	RR[2]
0		- 2877.616		
1	AGE 60+ yrs	- 2839.860	1.05/0.11	2.86 ***[3]
2	AGE 50-59 yrs	- 2829.165	0.64/0.13	1.90 ***
3	FEMALE GENDER	- 2820.331	-0.33/0.09	0.72 ***
4	HISTOLOGY = NS	- 2813.633	-0.31/0.09	0.73 ***
5	AGE 40-49 yrs	- 2810.437	0.32/0.12	1.37 **

b) End point = death from Hodgkin Disease

Step no	Variable	Log likelihood	Coeff./s.e.	RR[2]
0		- 1 669.005		
1	AGE 60+ yrs	- 1 655.195	0.74/0.14	2.10 ***[3]
2	HISTOLOGY = NS	- 1 648.908	-0.40/0.12	0.67 ***
3	EXTRA LOCALIZATION	- 1 643.113	-0.49/0.16	0.62 **
4	FEMALE GENDER	- 1 639.041	-0.34/0.12	0.71 **
5	AGE 50-59 yrs	- 1 635.303	0.47/0.16	1.60 **

c) End point = death from other causes than Hodgkin Disease

Step no	Variable	Log likelihood	Coeff./s.e.	RR[2]
0		- 486.149		
1	AGE 60+ yrs	- 448.466	2.65/0.27	14.15 ***[3]
2	AGE 50-59 yrs	- 441.287	1.28/0.35	3.60 ***
3	AGE 40-49 yrs	- 435.521	1.36/0.29	3.90 ***

(1) after adjustment on initial therapy (i.e. RT with or w/o single or bi-agent CT, combination CT, or RT + combination CT), treatment period (i.e. 1960-69, 1970-79 and 1980+), and staging laparotomy (performed or not performed)
(2) relative risk RR = exp (regression coefficient)
(3) p value : ** < 0.01, *** < 0.001

Table VIII-20. Deaths characteristics by type of initial therapy, treatment response, and clinical outcome

Treatment type	Patients at risk	All deaths	Hodgkin disease	Causes of death		
				Treatment related	Second cancer	Inter-current

NO COMPLETE REMISSION

Treatment type	Patients at risk	All deaths	Hodgkin disease	Treatment related	Second cancer	Intercurrent
All patients	1,868	1,380 (83.3)[a]	1,082 (7.0)[b]	69 (0.6)	28 (0.2)	85 (0.5)

INITIAL COMPLETE REMISSION, FURTHER RELAPSE

Treatment type	Patients at risk	All deaths	Hodgkin disease	Treatment related	Second cancer	Intercurrent
RT alone IF irradiation	291	139 (43.6)	104 (3.7)	4 (0.2)	15 (0.4)	14 (0.4)
Mantle or inverted Y RT	704	313 (39.6)	235 (3.3)	10 (0.1)	30 (0.3)	33 (0.4)
STNI or TNI	837	381 (43.3)	274 (3.6)	25 (0.3)	32 (0.3)	38 (0.4)
RT + single or bi-agent CT	110	76 (57.0)	65 (5.3)	1	7 (0.2)	3 (0.3)
Combination CT MOPP-like	616	336 (62.8)	235 (4.8)	8 (0.2)	18 (0.3)	11 (0.3)
Others	73	31 (50.0)[c]	28	0	3	0
RT + Combination CT IF irradiation + MOPP	238	131 (60.6)	87 (4.7)	2 (0.1)	4 (0.2)	4 (0.3)
+ Others	43	18 (33.0)[c]	17	0	1	0
Mantle or inverted Y RT + MOPP-like	156	93 (67.2)	78 (5.8)	4 (0.4)	8 (0.8)	3 (0.2)
+ Others	27	11 (40.0)	11	0	0	0
STNI or TNI + MOPP-like	229	156 (65.4)	141 (6.2)	1	5 (0.2)	6 (0.3)
+ Others	32	17 (24.0)[c]	13	0	1	2
All patients	3,422	1,738 (51.1)	1,315 (4.3)	55 (0.2)	126 (0.3)	121 (0.4)

Numbers with cause of death unspecified are not listed
a) *numbers and 10-year crude cumulative incidence rate (%)*; b) *numbers and mean annual probability calculated from the first 10 years of follow-up (%)*; c) *5-year survival rate*

Table VIII-20. Deaths characteristics by type of initial therapy, treatment response, and clinical outcome (continued)

Treatment type	Patients at risk	All deaths	Causes of death				
			Hodgkin disease	Treatment related	Second cancer	Inter-current
INITIAL COMPLETE REMISSION, NO FURTHER RELAPSE						
RT alone IF irradiation	445	68 (14.1)[a]	—	5 (0.1)[b]	17 (0.4)	38 (0.8)
Mantle or inverted Y RT	1,251	142 (11.3)	—	14 (0.1)	35 (0.2)	78 (0.6)
STNI or TNI	1,911	201 (9.3)	—	26 (0.1)	48 (0.2)	100 (0.5)
RT + single or bi-agent CT	206	36 (11.5)	—	3 (0.1)	9 (0.2)	15 (0.6)
Combination CT MOPP-like	1,278	202 (17.8)	—	15 (0.1)	38 (0.3)	54 (0.5)
Others	201	10 (6.8)[c]	—	5	1	4
RT + Combination CT						
IF irradiation + MOPP	830	80 (11.3)	—	6 (0.1)	19 (0.3)	14 (0.2)
+ Others	208	8 (6.2)	—	3	2	2
Mantle or inverted Y RT + MOPP-like	851	80 (12.6)	—	18 (0.3)	23 (0.3)	29 (0.5)
+ Others	302	3 (1.7)[c]	—	1	0	2
STNI or TNI + MOPP-like	1,062	135 (13.7)	—	17 (0.2)	52 (0.5)	53 (0.6)
+ Others	140	9 (8.7)[c]	—	0	1	8
All patients	8,821	990 (12.3)	—	111 (0.2)	247 (0.3)	409 (0.8)
OVERALL POPULATION	14,315	4,167 (32.1)*	2,404 (2.2)	237 (0.2)	404 (0.3)	589 (0.5)

* causes of death unspecified in 533 (12.8%) cases
a) numbers and 10-year crude cumulative incidence rate (%); b) numbers and mean annual probability calculated from the first 10 years of follow-up (%); c) 5-year survival rate

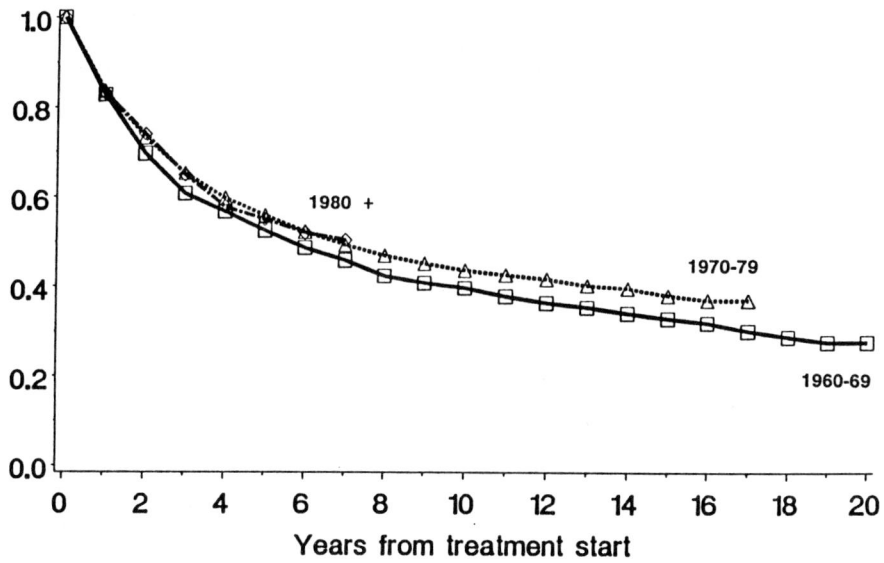

Figure VIII-16: *All stages. Survival after relapse by period. (1960-69 : 498 pts; 1970-79: 2,195 pts; 1980+ : 941 pts).*

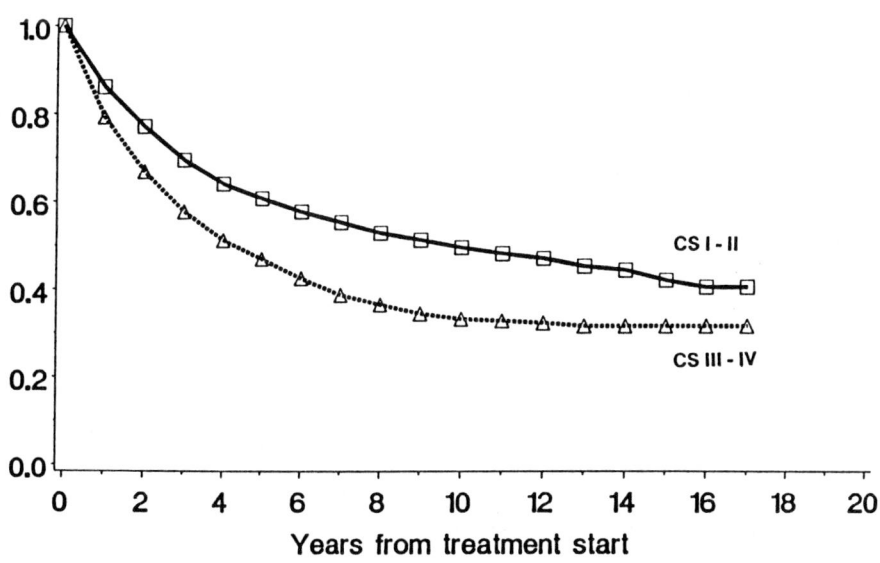

Figure VIII-17: *All stages. Survival after relapse in patients treated in year 1970 and after, by clinical stage. (I-II : 1,878 pts; III-IV : 1,257 pts).*

Table VIII-21. Survival after relapse by clinical stage

Clinical stage	IA	IIA	IB-IIB	IIIA	IIIB	IV
# of patients who relapsed (%)	564 (21.5)	1,134 (27.2)	460 (27.4)	422 (31.3)	439 (32.8)	403 (35.2)
Post relapse survival rates						
5-year (s.e)	.61 (.02)	.63 (.02)	.49 (.03)	.55 (.03)	.55 (.03)	.41 (.03)
10-year (s.e)	.48 (.03)	.50 (.02)	.41 (.03)	.42 (.03)	.42 (.03)	.23 (.03)
# of patients who died (%)	246 (44)	516 (46)	248 (54)	205 (49)	277 (63)	246 (61)
Causes of death						
progression	190	375	191	162	217	180
treatment related	7	24	10	3	6	5
second cancer	22	50	17	11	18	8
intercurrent	18	50	17	16	12	8
unspecified	9	17	13	13	24	45

Part IX - *Neuvième partie*

STUDY OF SECOND CANCER RISK

*RISQUE DE DEVELOPPEMENT D'UN DEUXIEME CANCER
ANALYSE PRONOSTIQUE*

Second cancer risk study

At time of data collection second cancer data were available for all series, that of the Southwest Oncology Group (SWOG) excepted. Therefore cases from the SWOG are excluded from the present study.

Overall data were available for 12,411 cases who had all survived at least one year post-treatment start and for whom initial type of therapy was specified (Table IX-1). In this cohort the total number of person-years at risk was 82,850.

Six-hundred eighty-eight second cancers were observed of which 177 were leukemias or pre-leukemias (AL), 112 were non-Hodgkin lymphomas (NHL), and 399 were solid tumors (ST). After second cancers occurring within one year post-treatment start were excluded, the series comprised 158 AL, 106 NHL, and 367 ST. Types of solid tumors observed are listed in Table IX-2. The most frequent ST were bronchus carcinomas (ICDO-162), basal cell carcinomas of the skin (ICDO-173) and digestive carcinomas (ICDO-150 to 159) in males; they were bronchus carcinomas, breast carcinomas (ICDO-174), basal cell carcinomas of the skin and in-situ cervix uteri carcinomas (ICDO-180) in females.

When compared to general population incidence rates matched for country, age, sex, and calendar-year, an increase in the relative risk (RR) for ST was observed in most of the sites potentially submitted to radiation therapy, both in males and females.

For AL and NHL the risk was similar to that reported by most of the authors in the literature, and similar in males and females.

RRs were calculated by calendar period since first primary for all ST (those from basal cell carcinomas of the skin and in-situ cervix uteri carcinomas being excluded), digestive, bronchus or breast carcinomas, NHL and AL, for males and females separately (Table IX-3).

For ST there was an increase in risk during the 5-9 year period and the 10-14 year period both in males and females overall. This increase was due to bronchus and digestive carcinomas in males. It was due to an excess of bronchus carcinomas in females. Moreover, female patients developed breast cancers more often in the 15-19 year period post initial therapy.

For NHL there was a continuously increased in risk with time in males, while in females a peak was observed during the 5-9 year period.

AL occurred more often within the first 10 years post diagnosis, after which the risk sharply decreased. The last case occurred 16 years after Hodgkin disease diagnosis in a relapsed patient. Again, RR were similar in magnitude when compared between males and females at each calendar period.

The mean numbers of second cancers observed by year are given by sex separately in Table IX-4. The incidence rates ranged between 3 cases per ten thousand person-years of observation (digestive carcinomas in females) to 2.1 cases per thousand person-years of observation (leukemias in males).

Overall the 10-year cumulative incidence rate of all second cancers was 6.4% (SD 0.1%) (Figure IX-1). After 15 years it was 11.2% (0.2%), and reached 18.6% (0.2%) after 20 years. For AL these rates were 1.8%, 2.2%, and 2.4%, respectively. For NHL they were 1.0%, 1.8% and 3.2%, while for ST they were 3.7%, 7.5%, and 13.6%.

The annual risks of second cancer are presented in Figure IX-2. While that risk was relatively constant with time, being null after 17 years, for AL and NHL, it continuously increased for ST.

Second cancer risk prognostic study

The search for prognostic factors to second cancer risk was performed on the entire cohort of patients for all second cancers, and for AL, NHL and ST, separately. Variables included in the model were those potentially linked to second cancer risk. They were: sex, age, bone marrow involvement, initial treatment type (including laparotomy) and clinical outcome. In addition histological subtypes (possibly linked to second NHL) were included in the model, as was the response to initial treatment since patients who did not reach initial complete remission had probably received heavier treatment, possibly more aggressive chemotherapy. Results are given in Tables IX-5 to IX-8.

The most important factors were:
- For *all types of second cancer*, age, treatment (combination chemotherapy including MOPP-like regimens or extended radiation therapy, these treatments having been given as first line treatment or when a relapse occurred) and sex (Table IX-5).

- For *leukemias*, they were age, combination chemotherapy with or without radiotherapy for a relapse or given as initial therapy (Table IX-6). In this series, laparotomy appeared to be associated whith a limited increased risk (RR = 1.33, p < 0.10).

- For *non-Hodgkin lymphoma*, associated factors were age, sex and relapse treatment (any type) (Table IX-7). Moreover, initial combined modality treatment with chemotherapy types other than MOPP-like regimes appeared associated with an increased risk, possibly because those treatments were more recently used than MOPP and patients were at low risk for relapse.

- For *solid tumors*, only age and, at lower level, extended radiation therapy significantly increased the risk (Table IX-8).

To analyze whether a specific type of therapy was associated with an increase in risk of second tumor, a second analysis limited to patients who achieved a complete remission was performed. For these patients time at risk began one year after initial treatment start and ended at date of second cancer occurrence, date of first relapse or date of last known vital status whichever came first. The series comprised 11,258 cases among whom 87 developed an AL, 68 a NHL, and 231 a ST. Incidence rates by sex and second cancer types are given in Table IX-9. Person-years and patient numbers at risk by treatment categories are listed in Table IX-10.

Compared to general population cancer incidence rates, ST were mostly associated with radiation therapy while NHL was associated with all types of initial therapy and AL mostly with combination chemotherapy with MOPP-like regimens or combinations of MOPP and radiotherapy (Table IX-10). Moreover some AL cases were observed after radiation therapy alone, either limited or extended field radiotherapy.

To quantify the risk associated with each of the variables studied, a stepwise regression analysis was performed which highlighted the strong association that exists between combined modality treatment with MOPP-like regimes and AL risk (Table IX-12). On the other hand MOPP-like treatments used alone only slightly increased the risk of AL, much less than age and stage. Again in this series limited to patients in first complete remission a small but significant relationship was observed between splenectomy and AL risk.

For NHL mostly age was associated with an increase in risk (Table IX-13) while for ST, besides age, extended radiotherapy was strongly associated with such a risk, as was combined modality treatments including MOPP-like regimes (Table IX-14).

In this series the 10-year cumulative incidence rate of AL was 1.3 % (Figure IX-3). After 15 years it was equal to 1.4 %. For NHL they were equal to 0.9 %, and 1.6 %, respectively, while for ST they were equal to 3.1 %, and to 6.2 %, respectively. Annual risks of second cancer are illustrated in Figure IX-4. While the risks of AL and NHL were moderate, that of ST was continuously increased.

A non negligible proportion of second cancers were observed after a relapse occurred. This was the case for 71 (45%) AL, 38 (36%) NHL, and 136 (37%) ST. No specific analysis was done for these cases. Nevertheless cumulative incidence rates and annual risks for AL, NHL, and ST are given in Figures IX-5 and IX-6, respectively. For patients who relapsed, the effect of various treatments on second cancer risk were about the same whether given initially or after relapse.

Table IX-1. Study population characteristics

		Patients at risk	Person-years at risk for developing a second cancer*
OVERALL POPULATION			
males		7,410	48,232
females		5,001	34,618
total		12,411	82,850
TIME SINCE HODGKIN DISEASE DIAGNOSIS			
1- 4 years	males	2,859	23,794
	females	1,781	16,472
5- 9 years	males	2,418	16,359
	females	1,645	11,746
10-14 years	males	1,491	6,591
	females	1,060	5,009
15-19 years	males	574	1,381
	females	450	1,273
20+ years	males	68	108
	females	65	119

* *time at risk beginning one year after initial treatment start*

Table IX-2. Observed (O) and expected (E) cases of second cancers occurring at least one year after initial treatment start (a)

Second cancer (ICDO-9)	MALES				FEMALES			
	O	E	O/E	95% CL (b)	O	E	O/E	95% CL
Lip (140)	1	0.974	1.03	0.03– 5.72	0	0.063	0	0 –58.55
Salivary gland (142)	3	0.386	7.77	1.60–22.71**	3	0.183	16.39	3.38–47.91**
Oral cavity (145)	0	2.607	0	0 – 1.41	1	0.360	2.78	0.07–15.48
Hypopharynx (148)	1	1.698	0.59	0.01– 3.28	0	0.118	0	0 –31.18
Esophagus (150)	3	3.529	0.85	0.18– 2.48	2	0.578	3.46	0.42–12.50
Stomach (151)	14	8.282	1.69	0.92– 2.84	2	2.570	0.78	0.09– 2.81
Small intestine (152)	3	0.313	9.58	1.98–28.01**	1	0.178	5.62	0.14–31.30
Colon (153)	18	9.726	1.85	1.10– 2.92*	5	5.694	0.88	0.29– 2.05
Rectum (154)	7	6.905	1.01	0.41– 2.09	3	2.868	1.05	0.22– 3.06
Liver (155)	2	1.511	1.32	0.16– 4.78	0	0.415	0	0 – 8.89
Pancreas (157)	6	3.525	1.70	0.62– 3.70	1	1.474	0.68	0.02– 3.78
Other digestive (159)	0				1			
Larynx (161)	3	3.805	0.79	0.16– 2.30	0	0.319	0	0 –11.56
Bronchus (162)	68	31.156	2.18	1.69– 2.77***	27	5.847	4.62	3.04– 6.72***
Pleura (163)	3	0.363	8.26	1.70–24.15**	2	0.065	30.77	3.73–111.2**
Thymus, heart (164)	1	0.220	4.55	0.12–25.33	0	0.039	0	0 –94.59
Other respiratory (165)	1				0			
Bone (170)	4	0.646	6.19	1.69–15.85**	2	0.310	6.45	0.78–23.31
Connective tissue (171)	3	1.081	2.78	0.57– 8.11	1	0.623	1.61	0.04– 2.94
Melanoma of skin (172)	7	3.784	1.85	0.74– 3.81	4	3.299	1.21	0.33– 3.10
Other skin (173)	31	8.518	3.64	2.47– 5.17***	14	4.038	3.47	1.90– 5.82***

a) in patients who survived one year or more
b) confidence limits of O/E assuming the Poisson distribution for O
* $p < 0.05$; ** $p < 0.01$; *** $p < 0.001$; two-sided test

Table IX-2. Observed (O) and expected (E) cases of second cancers occurring at least one year after initial treatment start (continued) (a)

Second cancer (ICDO-9)	MALES				FEMALES			
	O	E	O/E	95% CL [b]	O	E	O/E	95% CL
Female breast (174)	-				39	25.858	1.51	1.07- 2.06*
Uterus (179)	-				2	0.405	4.94	0.60-17.84
Cervix uteri (180)	-				9	6.600	1.36	0.62- 2.59
Corpus uteri (182)	-				2	4.891	0.41	0.05- 1.48
Ovary (183)	-				2	4.818	0.42	0.05- 1.50
Other female genital (184)	-				2	0.691	2.89	0.35-10.46
Prostate (185)	5	10.661	0.47	0.15- 1.09	-			
Testis (186)	5	3.847	1.30	0.42- 3.03	-			
Other male genital (187)	1	0.420	2.38	0.06-13.27				
Urinary bladder (188)	4	9.122	0.44	0.12- 1.12	3	1.627	1.84	0.38- 5.39
Kidney (189)	6	3.874	1.55	0.57- 3.37	1	1.225	0.82	0.02- 4.55
Eye (190)	1	0.292	3.42	0.09-19.08	0	0.131	0	0 -28.16
Brain (191)	4	4.028	0.99	0.27- 2.54	0	1.963	0	0 - 1.88
Thyroid (193)	5	0.978	5.11	1.66-11.93**	3	1.950	1.54	0.32- 4.50
Other endocrine gland (194)	1	0.131	7.63	0.19-42.53	0	0.086	0	0 -42.89
Others (195-199)	18				6			
Non-Hodgkin lymphoma (200)	79	2.222	35.55	28.15-44.31***	27	1.115	24.22	15.96-35.23***
Leukemia (204-208)	102	3.569	28.58	27.88-40.21***	56[c]	2.182	25.66	19.39-33.33***
All sites (140-208)	410	137.470	2.98	2.70- 3.29***	221	85.780	2.58	2.24- 2.93***

a) in patients who survived one year or more
b) confidence limits of O/E assuming the Poisson distribution for O
c) one patient simultaneously developed two second primaries: an acute leukemia and a breast cancer which were counted in both places
* $p < 0.05$; ** $p < 0.01$; *** $p < 0.001$; two-sided test

Table IX-3. Observed (O) and expected (E) cases of second cancers by calendar period since Hodgkin disease diagnosis

Second cancer (ICDO-9)		1-4 yrs	5-9 yrs	10-14 yrs	15-19 yrs	20+ yrs
MALES						
All sites (140-208)	O E O/E	145 58.93 2.46*** (2.0 - 2.80)[a]	154 47.15 3.27*** (2.69- 3.73)	79 23.60 3.35*** (2.65- 4.17)	30 7.31 4.10*** (2.77- 5.86)	2 0.88 2.27 (0.28- 8.21)
Solid tumors (173 excepted)	O E O/E	62 50.80 1.18 (0.94- 1.57)	76 40.95 1.86*** (1.46- 2.32)	48 20.61 2.33*** (1.72- 3.09)	11 6.35 1.73 (0.87- 3.10)	1 0.75 1.33 (0.03- 7.43)
Digestive (150-153, 157)	O E O/E	12 10.74 1.12 (0.58- 1.95)	20 8.73 2.29*** (1.40- 3.54)	12 4.40 2.73** (1.41- 4.76)	0 1.32 0 (0 - 2.80)	0 0.15 0 (0 -24.59)
Bronchus (162)	O E O/E	16 13.10 1.22 (0.70- 1.98)	25 10.67 2.34*** (1.52- 3.74)	22 5.46 4.03*** (2.53- 6.10)	4 1.68 2.38 (0.65- 6.10)	1 0.19 5.26 (0.13-29.32)
Non-Hodgkin lymphoma (200)	O E O/E	26 0.92 28.26*** (18.46-41.41)	23 0.72 31.94*** (20.25-47.93)	17 0.38 44.74*** (26.06-71.63)	12 0.10 120*** (62.01-210.0)	1 0.01 100* (2.53-557.0)
Leukemia (204-208)	O E O/E	49 1.59 30.82*** (22.80-40.74)	44 1.20 36.67*** (26.64-49.22)	7 0.54 12.96*** (5.21-26.71)	2 0.16 12.50* (1.51-45.15)	0 0.01 0 (0 -369.0)

a) confidence limits of O/E assuming the Poisson distribution for O
* $p < 0.05$; ** $p < 0.01$; *** $p < 0.001$; two-sided test

Table IX-3. Observed (O) and expected (E) cases of second cancers by calendar period since Hodgkin disease diagnosis (continued)

Second cancer (ICDO-9)		1-4 yrs	5-9 yrs	10-14 yrs	15-19 yrs	20+ yrs
FEMALES						
All sites (140-208)	O	64	90	45	18	4
	E	33.72	29.03	16.69	6.01	0.77
	O/E	1.90***	3.10***	2.70***	3.0***	5.20**
		(1.46- 2.42)[a]	(2.49- 3.81)	(1.97- 3.61)	(1.78- 4.73)	(1.42-13.30)
Solid tumors (173 excepted)	O	22	39	32	18	4
	E	31.22	19.59	13.73	5.0	0.64
	O/E	0.71	1.99***	2.33***	3.60***	6.25**
		(0.44- 1.07)	(1.42- 2.72)	(1.59- 3.29)	(2.13- 5.69)	(1.70-16.00)
Digestive (150-153, 157)	O	4	2	5	0	0
	E	4.27	3.51	1.99	0.68	0.06
	O/E	0.94	0.57	2.51	0	0
		(0.26- 2.40)	(0.07- 2.06)	(0.82- 5.86)	(0 - 5.43)	(0 -61.48)
Bronchus (162)	O	2	14	10	0	1
	E	2.26	1.94	1.15	0.41	0.03
	O/E	0.89	7.22***	8.70***	0	33.33
		(0.11- 3.20)	(3.95-12.11)	(4.17-15.99)	(0 - 9.00)	(0.84-186.0)
Breast (174)	O	5	12	9	13	0
	E	9.65	8.69	5.24	2.01	0.27
	O/E	0.52	1.38	1.72	6.47***	0
		(0.17- 1.21)	(0.71- 2.41)	(0.79- 3.26)	(3.44-11.06)	(0 -13.66)
Non-Hodgkin lymphoma (200)	O	9	15	3	0	0
	E	0.42	0.33	0.22	0.27	0.01
	O/E	21.43***	45.46***	13.64**	0	0
		(9.80-40.68)	(25.44-74.97)	(1.10-32.84)	(0 -92.22)	(0 -369.0)
Leukemia (204-208)	O	27	23	6	0	0
	E	0.86	0.71	0.41	0.13	0.01
	O/E	31.40***	32.39***	14.63***	0	0
		(20.69-45.68)	(20.54-48.61)	(5.37-31.85)	(0 -28.38)	(0 -369.0)

a) confidence limits of O/E assuming the Poisson distribution for O; * $p < 0.05$; ** $p < 0.01$; *** $p < 0.001$; two-sided test

Table IX-4. Second cancers occurring after Hodgkin disease: all cases who survived at least one year *(a)*

Second cancer (ICDO-9)	#	Patients at risk	PY[b] at risk	Rate[c]	95% CL[d]
MALES		7,410	48,232		
All sites (140-208)	410			85	77, 94
Solid tumors (173 excepted)	198			41	36, 47
Digestive (150-153, 157)	44			9	7, 12
Bronchus (162)	68			14	11, 18
Non-Hodgkin lymphoma (200)	79			16	13, 20
Leukemia (204-208)	102			21	17, 26
FEMALES		5,001	34,618		
All sites (140-208)	221			64	56, 73
Solid tumors (173 excepted)	115			33	27, 40
Digestive (150-153, 157)	11			3	2, 6
Bronchus (162)	27			8	5, 11
Breast (174)	39			11	8, 15
Non-Hodgkin lymphoma (200)	27			8	5, 11
Leukemia (204-208)	56			16	12, 21

a) *time at risk began one year after initial therapy start and ended at the date of second cancer, or the date of last known vital status whichever came first*
b) *person-years*
c) *numbers observed / 10,000 person-years at risk*
d) *confidence limits of O/PY assuming the Poisson distribution for O*

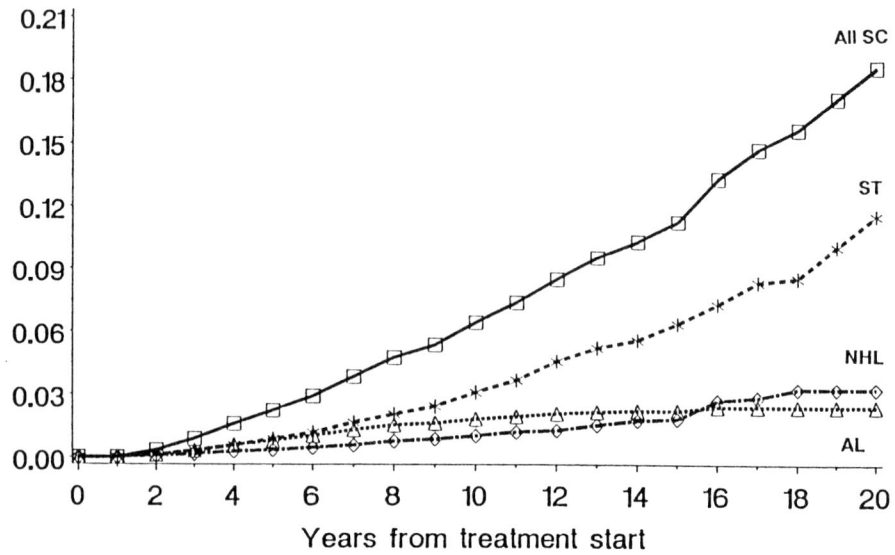

Figure IX-1 : *Cumulative incidence of second cancer (SC) in patients who survived at least one year post treatment initiation (N = 12,411). (All SC : 631 cases; Acute leukemia : 158 cases; Non-Hodgkin lymphoma : 106 cases; Solid tumors : 367 cases).*

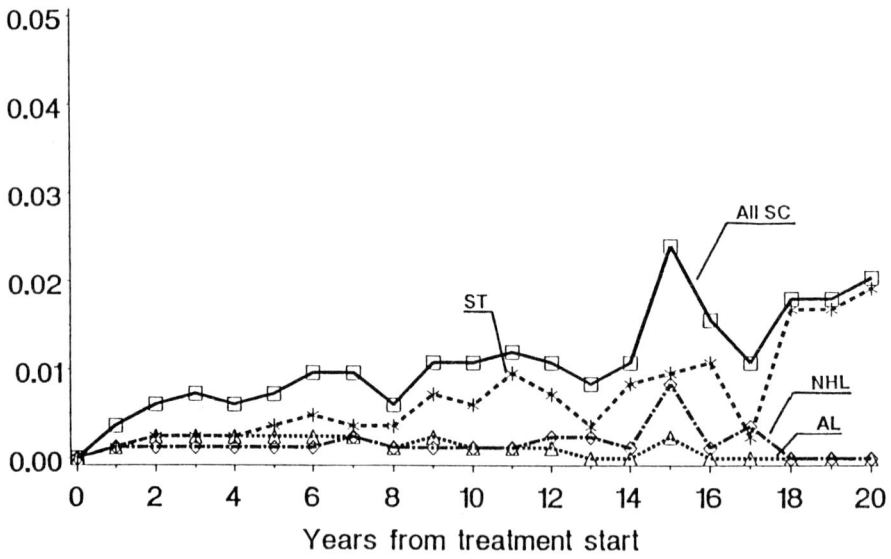

Figure IX-2 : *Annual second cancer (SC) risk in patients who survived at least one year post treatment initiation (N = 12,411). (All SC : 631 cases; Acute leukemia : 158 cases; Non-Hodgkin lymphoma : 106 cases; Solid tumors : 367 cases).*

Table IX-5. Proportional hazards model on second cancer risk (a) for 12,411 patients who survived at least one year after Hodgkin disease diagnosis.
Results for a model allowing all the variables simultaneously

Variables		Regression coefficient (s.e.)		RR(b)
SEX	Males	0		1.0(c)
	Females	− 0.23	(0.09)	0.79**
AGE	15-19 years	0		1.0
	20-29	0.06	(0.19)	1.06
	30-39	0.49	(0.19)	1.64**
	40-49	1.19	(0.19)	3.28***
	50-59	1.98	(0.19)	7.24***
	60+	2.32	(0.20)	10.18***
HISTOLOGY	LP	0		1.0
	NS	− 0.17	(0.14)	0.85
	MC	− 0.26	(0.15)	0.77+
	LD	− 0.39	(0.32)	0.68
	unclassified	0.30	(0.30)	1.35
BM INVOLVEMENT	no	0		1.0
	yes	− 0.12	(0.30)	0.88
RESPONSE TO INITIAL TREATMENT				
Complete remission		0		1.0
No complete remission		0.20	(0.21)	1.22
INITIAL TREATMENT TYPE				
Splenectomy	no	0		1.0
	yes	0.19	(0.09)	1.20*
IF irradiation alone		0		1.0
Mantle or inverted Y RT alone		0.08	(0.18)	1.08
STNI or TNI alone		0.37	(0.18)	1.44*
MOPP-like CT		0.51	(0.19)	1.67**
Other CT		0.56	(0.37)	1.75
Irradiation (any type) + MOPP-like		0.68	(0.17)	1.97***
+ other CT		0.53	(0.37)	1.70
CLINICAL OUTCOME (d)				
No relapse		0		1.0
First relapse treated with RT		0.47	(0.28)	1.60+
	CT	0.78	(0.14)	2.18***
	RT + CT	0.59	(0.12)	1.81***
Global chi-square		572.58		
p value (df)		< 0.0001	(22)	

a) ICDO-9 173, 180, and 195-199 excluded
b) relative risk RR = exp (regression coefficient)
c) reference category
d) time dependent covariates
p value : + < 0.10, * < 0.05, ** < 0.01, *** < 0.001; two-sided test

Table IX-6. Proportional hazards model on second leukemia risk (a) for 12,411 patients who survived at least one year after Hodgkin disease diagnosis.
Results for a model allowing all the variables simultaneously

Variables		Regression coefficient (s.e.)		RR[b]
SEX	Males	0		1.0[c]
	Females	− 0.09	(0.17)	0.91
AGE	15-19 years	0		1.0
	20-29	0.29	(0.32)	1.34
	30-39	0.35	(0.34)	1.42
	40-49	0.91	(0.35)	2.50**
	50-59	1.39	(0.36)	3.99***
	60+	1.50	(0.38)	4.49***
HISTOLOGY	LP	0		1.0
	NS	− 0.43	(0.26)	0.65
	MC	− 0.52	(0.29)	0.60+
	LD	− 0.89	(0.63)	0.41
	unclassified	− 0.52	(0.75)	0.59
BM INVOLVEMENT	no	0		1.0
	yes	0.34	(0.40)	1.41
RESPONSE TO INITIAL TREATMENT				
Complete remission		0		1.0
No complete remission		0.76	(0.30)	2.13**
INITIAL TREATMENT TYPE				
Splenectomy no		0		1.0
yes		0.29	(0.17)	1.33+
IF irradiation alone		0		1.0
Mantle or inverted Y RT alone		0.19	(0.48)	1.20
STNI or TNI alone		0.25	(0.47)	1.29
MOPP-like CT		1.25	(0.45)	3.50**
Other CT		1.45	(0.66)	4.28*
Irradiation (any type) + MOPP-like		1.67	(0.43)	5.32***
+ other CT		1.10	(0.72)	3.01
CLINICAL OUTCOME [d]				
No relapse		0		1.0
First relapse treated with RT		0.50	(0.72)	1.65
CT		1.67	(0.22)	5.29***
RT + CT		1.03	(0.22)	2.80***
Global chi-square		167.88		
p value (df)		< 0.0001	(22)	

a) ICDO-9 204-208
b) relative risk RR = exp (regression coefficient)
c) reference category
d) time dependent covariates
p value : + < 0.10, * < 0.05, ** < 0.01, *** < 0.001; two-sided test

Table IX-7. Proportional hazards model on second non-Hodgkin lymphoma risk (a) for 12,411 patients who survived at least one year after Hodgkin disease diagnosis.
Results for a model allowing all the variables simultaneously

Variables		Regression coefficient (s.e.)		RR[b]
SEX	Males	0		1.0[c]
	Females	− 0.64	(0.23)	0.53**
AGE	15-19 years	0		1.0
	20-29	0.37	(0.56)	1.44
	30-39	1.30	(0.54)	3.67**
	40-49	1.79	(0.55)	5.97***
	50-59	2.35	(0.56)	10.47***
	60+	3.07	(0.56)	21.64***
HISTOLOGY	LP	0		1.0
	NS	− 0.60	(0.28)	0.55*
	MC	− 0.58	(0.30)	0.56*
	LD	− 1.52	(1.03)	0.22
	unclassified	0.16	(0.63)	1.17
BM INVOLVEMENT	no	0		1.0
	yes	− 1.21	(1.02)	0.30
RESPONSE TO INITIAL TREATMENT				
Complete remission		0		1.0
No complete remission		− 0.17	(0.58)	0.85
INITIAL TREATMENT TYPE				
Splenectomy no		0		1.0
yes		0.37	(0.21)	1.44+
IF irradiation alone		0		1.0
Mantle or inverted Y RT alone		− 0.17	(0.39)	0.85
STNI or TNI alone		0.14	(0.39)	1.15
MOPP-like CT		0.68	(0.39)	1.97+
Other CT		0.86	(0.79)	2.36
Irradiation (any type) + MOPP-like		0.60	(0.37)	1.82
+ other CT		1.51	(0.61)	4.52**
CLINICAL OUTCOME [d]				
No relapse		0		1.0
First relapse treated with RT		1.32	(0.44)	3.73**
CT		0.82	(0.33)	2.27**
RT + CT		0.79	(0.27)	2.21**
Global chi-square		158.88		
p value (df)		< 0.0001	(22)	

a) ICDO-9 200
b) relative risk RR = exp (regression coefficient)
c) reference category
d) time dependent covariates
p value : + < 0.10, * < 0.05, ** < 0.01, *** < 0.001; two-sided test

Table IX-8. Proportional hazards model on second solid tumor risk (a) for 12,411 patients who survived at least one year after Hodgkin disease diagnosis.
Results for a model allowing all the variables simultaneously

Variables		Regression coefficient (s.e.)		RR[b]
SEX	Males	0		1.0[c]
	Females	− 0.15	(0.12)	0.86
AGE	15-19 years	0		1.0
	20-29	− 0.21	(0.25)	0.81
	30-39	0.29	(0.26)	1.34
	40-49	1.13	(0.25)	3.11***
	50-59	2.13	(0.24)	8.43***
	60+	2.48	(0.26)	11.95***
HISTOLOGY	LP	0		1.0
	NS	0.10	(0.20)	1.11
	MC	0.0	(0.21)	1.0
	LD	0.26	(0.40)	1.30
	unclassified	0.60	(0.39)	1.83
BM INVOLVEMENT	no	0		1.0
	yes	− 0.29	(0.52)	0.74
RESPONSE TO INITIAL TREATMENT				
Complete remission		0		1.0
No complete remission		− 0.06	(0.34)	0.96
INITIAL TREATMENT TYPE				
Splenectomy	no	0		1.0
	yes	0.01	(0.13)	1.01
IF irradiation alone		0		1.0
Mantle or inverted Y RT alone		0.15	(0.22)	1.16
STNI or TNI alone		0.52	(0.22)	1.69*
MOPP-like CT		0.15	(0.25)	1.16
Other CT		− 0.04	(0.62)	0.96
IF, mantle, or inverted Y RT + MOPP		− 0.24	(0.28)	0.78
STNI or TNI + MOPP-like		0.57	(0.25)	1.77*
Irradiation (any type) + other CT		− 0.41	(0.74)	0.66
CLINICAL OUTCOME [d]				
No relapse		0		1.0
First relapse treated with RT		0.09	(0.39)	1.10
	CT	0.16	(0.22)	1.17
	RT + CT	0.29	(0.17)	1.34+
Global chi-square		411.26		
p value (df)		< 0.0001	(23)	

a) ICDO-9 140-194 (173 and 180 excluded)
b) relative risk RR = exp (regression coefficient)
c) reference category
d) time dependent covariates
p value : + < 0.10, * < 0.05, ** < 0.01, *** < 0.001; two-sided test

Table IX-9. Second cancers occurring after Hodgkin disease: all cases in complete remission after initial therapy and who survived at least one year (a)

Second cancer (ICDO-9)	#	Patients at risk	PY[(b)] at risk	Rate[(c)]	95% CL[(d)]
MALES		6,674	36,586		
All sites (140-208)	267			73	64, 82
Solid tumors (173 excepted)	138			38	32, 45
Digestive (150-153, 157)	30			8	6, 12
Bronchus (162)	42			11	8, 16
Non-Hodgkin lymphoma (200)	50			14	10, 18
Leukemia (204-208)	57			16	12, 20
FEMALES		4,567	26,649		
All sites (140-208)	159			60	51, 70
Solid tumors (173+180 excepted)	93			35	28, 43
Digestive (150-153, 157)	8			3	1, 6
Bronchus (162)	21			8	5, 12
Breast (174)	36			14	9, 19
Non-Hodgkin lymphoma (200)	18			7	4, 11
Leukemia (204-208)	30			11	8, 16

a) time at risk began one year after initial therapy start and ended at the date of first relapse, the date of second cancer, or the date of last known vital status whichever came first
b) person-years
c) numbers observed / 10,000 person-years at risk
d) confidence limits of O/PY assuming the Poisson distribution for O

Table IX-10. Second cancers occurring after Hodgkin disease: all cases in complete remission after initial therapy and who survived at least one year (a)

Treatment category	#	Patients at risk	PY(b) at risk	Rate(c)	95% CL(d)
IF irradiation		748	6,108		
. solid tumor(e)	18			29	17, 47
. NHL	7			11	5, 24
. leukemia	1			2	0, 9
Mantle or inverted Y RT		2,063	18,178		
. solid tumor	42			23	17, 31
. NHL	8			4	2, 9
. leukemia	2			1	0, 4
STNI or TNI		2,681	21,520		
. solid tumor	77			36	28, 45
. NHL	17			8	5, 13
. leukemia	6			3	1, 6
MOPP-like alone		1,669	9,769		
. solid tumor	32			33	22, 46
. NHL	12			12	6, 21
. leukemia	19			19	12, 30
Other CT alone		344	1,268		
. solid tumor	2			16	2, 57
. NHL	1			8	0, 44
. leukemia	2			16	2, 57

a) time at risk began one year after initial therapy start and ended at the date of first relapse, the date of second cancer, or the date of last known vital status whichever came first
b) person-years
c) numbers observed / 10,000 person-years at risk
d) confidence limits of O/PY assuming the Poisson distribution for O
e) ICDO-9 173 and 180 excluded

Table IX-10. Second cancers occurring after Hodgkin disease: all cases in complete remission after initial therapy and who survived at least one year (continued) (a)

Treatment category	#	Patients at risk	PY[b] at risk	Rate[c]	95% CL[d]
IF irradiation + MOPP-like		835	5,028		
. solid tumor [e]	10			20	10, 37
. NHL	4			8	2, 20
. leukemia	11			22	11, 39
IF irradiation + other CT		243	696		
. solid tumor	0			0	0, 53
. NHL	0			0	0, 53
. leukemia	2			29	3, 104
Mantle or inverted Y RT + MOPP-like		975	5,877		
. solid tumor	11			19	9, 33
. NHL	6			10	4, 22
. leukemia	17			29	17, 46
Mantle or inverted Y RT + other CT		314	741		
. solid tumor	0			0	0, 50
. NHL	1			13	0, 75
. leukemia	0			0	0, 50
STNI or TNI + MOPP-like		1,335	9,843		
. solid tumor	36			37	26, 51
. NHL	11			11	6, 20
. leukemia	27			27	10, 40
STNI or TNI + other CT		51	262		
. solid tumor	1			38	1, 213
. NHL	0			0	0, 141
. leukemia	0			0	0, 141

a) time at risk began one year after initial therapy start and ended at the date of first relapse, the date of second cancer, or the date of last known vital status whichever came first
b) person-years
c) numbers observed / 10,000 person-years at risk
d) confidence limits of O/PY assuming the Poisson distribution for O
e) ICDO-9 173 and 180 excluded

Table IX-11. Stepwise proportional hazards model on second cancer risk (a) for 11,258 patients who achieved a complete remission after initial therapy and who survived at least one year after Hodgkin disease diagnosis (b)

Step no	Variable	Log likelihood	Coeff./s.e.	RR(c)
0		- 3411.880		
1	AGE 60+ yrs	- 3346.262	2.38/0.15	10.86 ***(d)
2	AGE 50-59 yrs	- 3293.084	1.89/0.15	6.61 ***
3	AGE 40-49 yrs	- 3277.590	1.06/0.16	2.87 ***
4	RT(e) + MOPP-like	- 3271.111	0.51/0.12	1.66 ***
5	STNI or TNI	- 3266.245	0.40/0.13	1.50 ***
6	AGE 30-39 yrs	- 3261.171	0.49/0.15	1.63 ***
7	CS III	- 3258.726	0.26/0.11	1.30 *

a) ICDO-9 173, 180, and 195-199 excluded
b) time at risk began one year after initial therapy start and ended at the date of first relapse, the date of second cancer, or the date of last known vital status whichever came first
c) relative risk RR = exp (regression coefficient)
d) p value : + < 0.10, * < 0.05, ** < 0.01, *** < 0.001; two-sided test
e) radiation therapy (any type)

Table IX-12. Stepwise proportional hazards model on second leukemia risk (a) for 11,258 patients who achieved a complete remission after initial therapy and who survived at least one year after Hodgkin disease diagnosis (b)

Step no	Variable	Log likelihood	Coeff./s.e.	RR(c)
0		- 758.012		
1	RT(d) + MOPP-like	- 731.927	1.96/0.31	17.11 ***(e)
2	AGE 50-59 yrs	- 722.047	1.57/0.28	4.81 ***
3	AGE 60+ yrs	- 715.176	1.52/0.34	4.56 ***
4	CS III	- 709.471	0.93/0.24	2.52 ***
5	CS IV	- 702.162	1.23/0.33	3.42 ***
6	SPLENECTOMY	- 700.334	0.50/0.23	1.65 *
7	AGE 40-49 yrs	- 698.369	0.66/0.32	1.93 *
8	MOPP-like alone	- 696.642	0.79/0.42	2.20 *

a) ICDO-9 204-208
b) time at risk began one year after initial therapy start and ended at the date of first relapse, the date of second cancer, or the date of last known vital status whichever came first
c) relative risk RR = exp (regression coefficient)
d) radiation therapy (any type)
e) p value : + < 0.10, * < 0.05, ** < 0.01, *** < 0.001; two-sided test

Table IX-13. Stepwise proportional hazards model on second non-Hodgkin lymphoma risk (a) for 11,258 patients who achieved a complete remission after initial therapy and who survived at least one year after Hodgkin disease diagnosis (b)

Step no	Variable	Log likelihood	Coeff./s.e.	RR(c)
0		- 557.265		
1	AGE 60+ yrs	- 541.535	3.02/0.41	20.40 ***(d)
2	AGE 50-59 yrs	- 530.913	2.18/0.43	8.81 ***
3	SEX Females	- 527.617	- 0.60/0.28	0.55 *
4	AGE 40-49 yrs	- 525.371	1.69/0.42	5.44 ***
5	AGE 30-39 yrs	- 520.774	1.30/0.40	3.67 ***
6	CS III	- 519.649	0.53/0.26	1.70 *

a) ICDO-9 200
b) time at risk began one year after initial therapy start and ended at the date of first relapse, the date of second cancer, or the date of last known vital status whichever came first
c) relative risk RR = exp (regression coefficient)
d) p value : + < 0.10, * < 0.05, ** < 0.01, *** < 0.001; two-sided test

Table IX-14. Stepwise proportional hazards model on second solid tumor risk (a) for 11,258 patients who achieved a complete remission after initial therapy and who survived at least one year after Hodgkin disease diagnosis (b)

Step no	Variable	Log likelihood	Coeff./s.e.	RR(c)
0		- 2081.420		
1	AGE 60+ yrs	- 2035.581	2.53/0.19	12.58 ***(d)
2	AGE 50-59 yrs	- 1999.625	1.92/0.18	6.80 ***
3	AGE 40-49 yrs	- 1990.132	1.03/0.20	2.81 ***
4	STNI or TNI	- 1983.752	0.61/0.14	1.84 ***
5	RT(e) + MOPP-like	- 1980.347	0.52/0.18	1.67 **
6	AGE 30-39 yrs	- 1978.445	0.39/0.20	1.48 *

a) ICDO-9 140-194 (173, 180, and 195-199 excluded)
b) time at risk began one year after initial therapy start and ended at the date of first relapse, the date of second cancer, or the date of last known vital status whichever came first
c) relative risk RR = exp (regression coefficient)
d) p value : + < 0.10, * < 0.05, ** < 0.01, *** < 0.001; two-sided test
e) radiation therapy (any type)

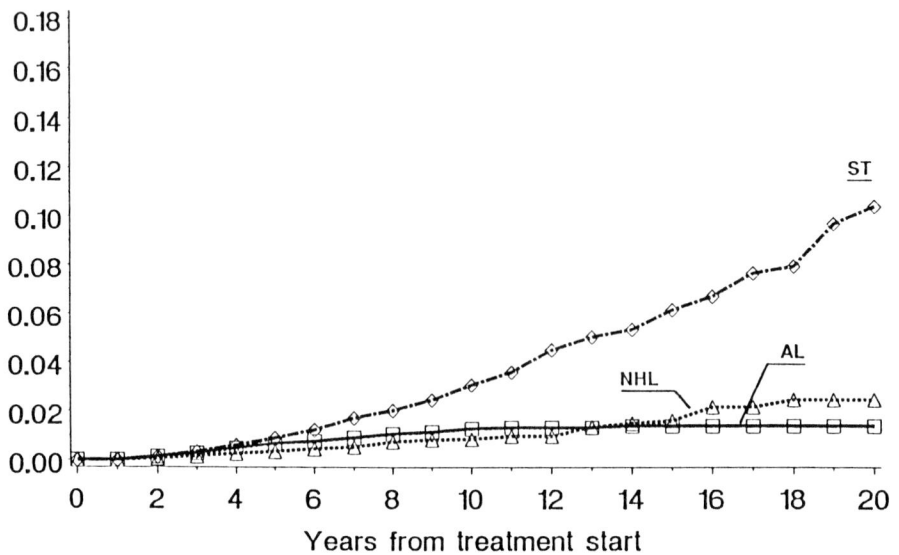

Figure IX-3 : *Cumulative incidence of second cancer in patients who achieved a complete remission and who survived at least one year post treatment initiation (N = 11,258). (Acute leukemia : 87 cases; Non-Hodgkin lymphoma : 68 cases; Solid tumors : 231 cases).*

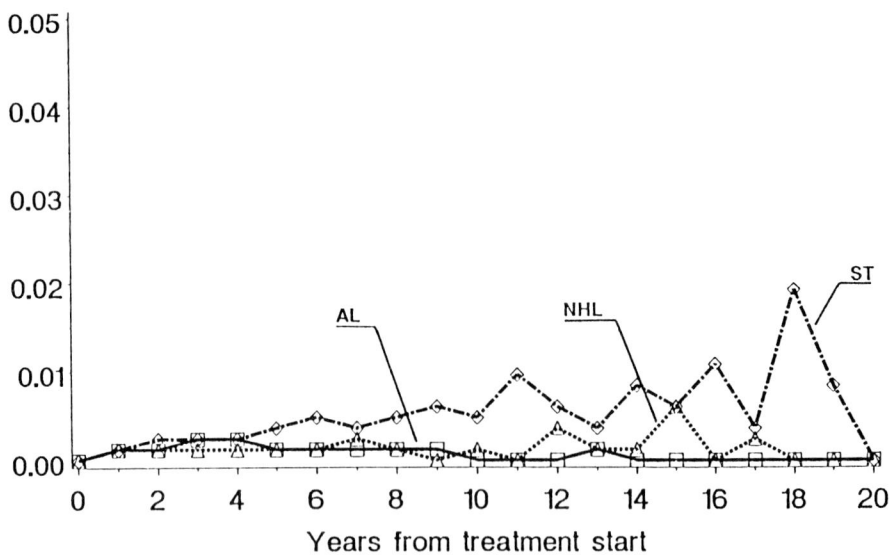

Figure IX-4 : *Annual second cancer risk in patients who achieved a complete remission and who survived at least one year post treatment initiation (N = 11,258). (Acute leukemia : 87 cases; Non-Hodgkin lymphoma : 68 cases; Solid tumors : 231 cases).*

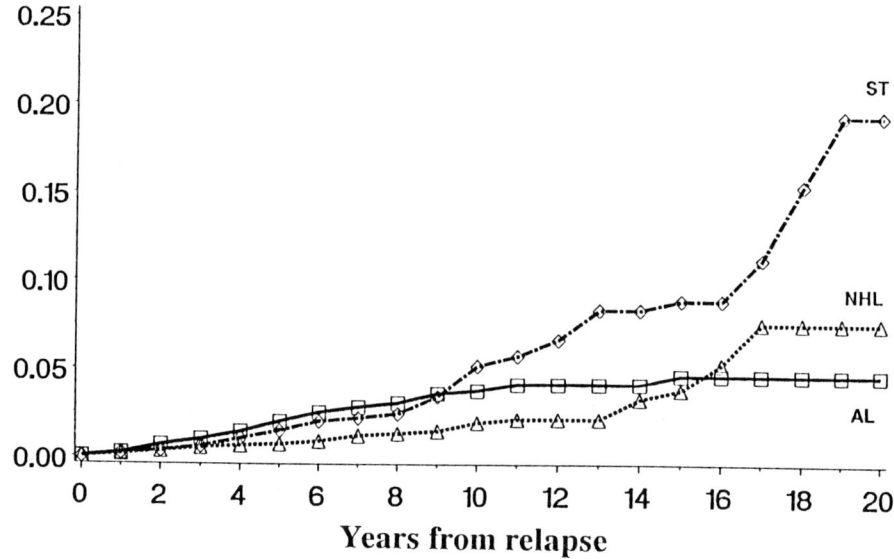

Figure IX-5 : *Cumulative incidence of second cancer in patients who relapsed. (N = 3,404). (Acute leukemia : 71 cases; Non-Hodgkin lymphoma : 38 cases; Solid tumors : 136 cases).*

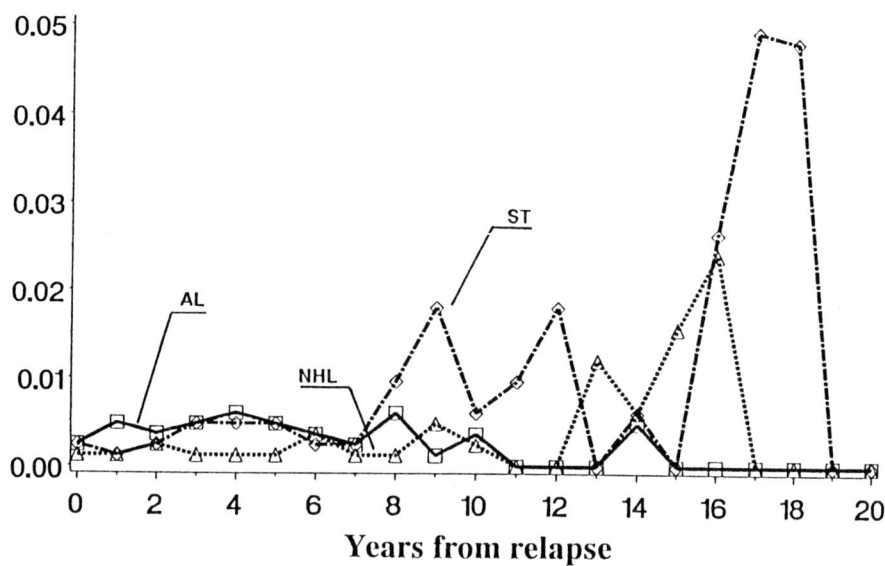

Figure IX-6 : *Annual second cancer risk in patients who relapsed (N = 3,404). (Acute leukemia : 71 cases; Non-Hodgkin lymphoma : 38 cases; Solid tumors : 136 cases).*

Part X - *Dixième partie*

LONG TERM SURVIVAL AND STUDY OF CAUSES OF DEATH

SURVIE A LONG TERME ET ANALYSE DES CAUSES DE DECES

Long term survival and analysis of causes of death

The population study is composed of the 14,225 (99.4%) cases for whom age, sex, initial clinical stage and survival data were available. In this cohort the total number of person-years at risk was 103,717 (Table X-1).

Overall, 4,139 patients died. In 2,777 (67%) patients the death followed Hodgkin disease progression; 233 (6%) patients died from treatment-related adverse effect without evidence of active disease; 413 (10%) patients developed a second cancer (147 leukemias, 61 non-Hodgkin lymphomas, and 205 solid tumors including 82 bronchus carcinomas, 45 tumors of the digestive tract and 12 breast carcinomas) that caused death; 577 (14%) patients died from another intercurrent disease. In the remaining 139 (3%) patients the cause of death was unspecified.

Life table figures for all causes of death adjusted for age, sex and country show 539.14 expected (E) deaths compared with 4,139 observed (O), giving a relative risk (O/E) of 7.68 ($p<0.001$) (Table X-2). The corresponding plots are given Figure X-1.

Most of the disease-related or treatment-related deaths occurred within the first 10-year interval posttreatment start. Therefore, the proportion of deaths due to other causes than disease progression or treatment complication increased with time. It was 18% of all deaths that occurred during the first 4-year interval, 38% during the 5-9 year interval, 56% during the 10-14 year interval, 69% during the 15-19 year interval, and 93% (13 out of 14) thereafter (Table X-2). Consequently, a decrease of the O/E ratio was observed from year 2 to year 10 posttreatment initiation, whereas its value remained quite unchanged in the following years (Table X-2 and Figure X-2). This observation is better shown in Figures X-3 and X-4 where it can be seen that after year 10 the annual rate of death unrelated to Hodgkin disease or its treatment became preponderant.

When these deaths unrelated to Hodgkin disease are detailed, it can be shown that the most important are intercurrent disease and second cancer deaths. By contrast, treatment-related deaths never exceeded 3% in cumulative rate (Figures X-5 and X-6).

The same analysis was performed *i)* by sex, *ii)* by age, and *iii)* by clinical stage :

In both sexes, the distribution of deaths by cause was similar except for intercurrent deaths which were more frequent in males than in females (Table X-3). Overall, the O/E ratio was higher in males than in females highlighting the general knowledge of worse survival in males compared to females. The same observation was made when only deaths not related to Hodgkin disease were considered (Tables X-4a and X-4b, Figure X-7).

According to age, proportions of deaths unrelated to Hodgkin disease were 17% in patients aged 15-19 years at Hodgkin disease diagnosis, 18% in those aged 20-29 years, 24% in those aged 30-39 years, 30% in those aged 40-49 years, 36% in those aged 50-59 years, and 38% in those aged 60 years or more. Among these deaths, second cancers represented 39%, 38%, 39%, 39%, 44%, and 27% in the six age categories, respectively (Tables X-6a to X-6f). The O/E ratio for death unrelated to Hodgkin disease decreased from 4.13 ($p<0.001$) in the youngest patients to 1.42 ($p<0.001$) in the oldest but remained statistically significant. This observation was also made when analyzed by time interval. Expected and observed survival by age are shown in Figures X-8 and X-9, and the corresponding O/E ratios as a function of time in Figure X-10. Whatever the category considered, there was a decrease of the O/E ratio until year 10, while its value remained constant thereafter, except in the younger category where a peak was observed between years 9 and 11. Figures X-11 and X-12 show the cumulative incidence of death by age. While deaths related to Hodgkin disease tend to reach a plateau level whatever the age (Figure X-11), that from other causes regularly increased with time, especially in patients aged 50 years or more (Figure X-12).

In clinical stage I-II patients the proportion of deaths unrelated to Hodgkin disease was 37% while it was only 19% in patients with clinical stage III-IV. On the other hand, O/E ratios were similar in early and advanced stage patients, 2.07 ($p < 0.001$) and 2.13 ($p < 0.001$), respectively (Tables X-8a and X-8b). Again, the O/E ratio showed a decrease with time until year 10 in both groups, and remained constant thereafter (Figure X-13). While cumulative incidence of death showed similar impact on survival for Hodgkin disease-related-deaths and deaths not disease related in early stages (Figure X-14), Hodgkin disease was the main cause of death in advanced stages (Figure X-15).

The influence of time period of initial treatment on survival was also analyzed (Tables X-10a to X-10c). Deaths unrelated to Hodgkin disease represented 36% of the overall deaths observed in patients treated during the sixties. They represented 27% and 23% of the total number of deaths for patients initially treated during the seventies and the eighties, respectively. Despite this slight decrease, corresponding O/E ratios were similar. On the other hand treatment-related deaths were 1%, 6%, and 8% in proportion, respectively.

In order to assess the possible impact of initial treatment on the causes of death, the following analysis was restricted to patients who achieved an initial complete remission. For patients who further relapsed, time at risk was then censored at the time the patient relapsed. Initial treatments were grouped into three categories: radiotherapy alone followed or not by adjuvant single or bi-agent chemotherapy, chemotherapy alone, and combined modality treatment.

Cumulative incidence and annual death rate were analyzed by age. Figure X-16 shows the dramatic increase of death (all causes) rates in patients older than 50 with an increase of the annual death rate with time, whereas the force of mortality (ie annual death rate) remained constant in the younger patients (Figure X-17).

Cumulative incidence of second cancer death and other intercurrent deaths increased with time while that of treatment-related death did not (Figure X-18). The annual death rate wasnot negligible in these patients, approximately 1% yearly for all causes, mainly due to deaths other than treatment-related (Figure X-19).

When deaths other than treatment-related were analyzed separately by age, there was evidence that patients older than 50 years at diagnosis were at high risk for death from second cancer or intercurrent disease (Figures X-20 and X-21).

Overall, no difference in survival was observed whether patients initially achieved a complete remission after one or the other treatment (Figure X-22). The annual death rates were similar in the three groups showing a slight increase with time after year 10 (Figure X-23). While no difference was observed in treatment-related death rates (Figure X-24), second cancer deaths occurred more often and earlier in patients initially treated by chemotherapy alone or combined modality treatments (Figure X-25), a figure which can be related to second leukemia risk associated with these treatment types (see part IX of the present report). On the other hand, there was no obvious difference in cumulative incidence of intercurrent death by treatment category (Figure X-26).

Table X-1. Study population characteristics by sex

		Patients at risk *	Person-years at risk
OVERALL POPULATION			
males		8,614	60,963
females		5,611	42,754
total		14,225	103,717
TIME SINCE HODGKIN DISEASE DIAGNOSIS			
0- 4 years	males	3,598	33,444
	females	2,127	22,597
5- 9 years	males	2,481	18,301
	females	1,693	12,962
10-14 years	males	1,696	7,539
	females	1,221	5,658
15-19 years	males	665	1,561
	females	494	1,394
20+ years	males	74	118
	females	76	143

* *patients for whom the following information are available: age, sex, clinical stage and last known vital status*

Table X-2. Observed (O) and expected (E) deaths overall and by follow-up time

Causes of death	O	E	Excess of deaths[a]	O/E	95% CL[b]
OVERALL POPULATION					
All causes	4,139	539.14		7.68***	7.44- 7.91
Hodgkin disease	2,777				
Treatment related	233				
Second cancer	413				
Intercurrent	577				
Unspecified	139				
Not related to HD[c]	1,129		0.57	2.09***	1.97- 2.22
TIME SINCE HODGKIN DISEASE DIAGNOSIS					
0- 4 yrs All causes	2,735	279.96		9.77***	9.41-10.14
Not related to HD	500		0.39	1.79***	1.63- 1.95
5- 9 yrs All causes	963	161.71		5.96***	5.58- 6.34
Not related to HD	368		0.66	2.28***	2.05- 2.52
10-14 yrs All causes	344	77.60		4.43***	3.98- 4.93
Not related to HD	191		0.86	2.46***	2.12- 2.84
15-19 yrs All causes	83	18.52		4.48***	3.57- 5.56
Not related to HD	57		1.30	3.08***	2.33- 3.99
20+ yrs All causes	14	1.34		10.45***	5.70-17.53
Not related to HD	13		4.47	9.70***	5.71-17.53

a) excess of deaths = (O - E) x 100 / numbers of person-years at risk
b) confidence limits of O/E assuming the Poisson distribution for O
c) all deaths except those from Hodgkin disease progression or relapse, or treatment related (see text)
* $p < 0.05$; ** $p < 0.01$; *** $p < 0.001$; two-sided test

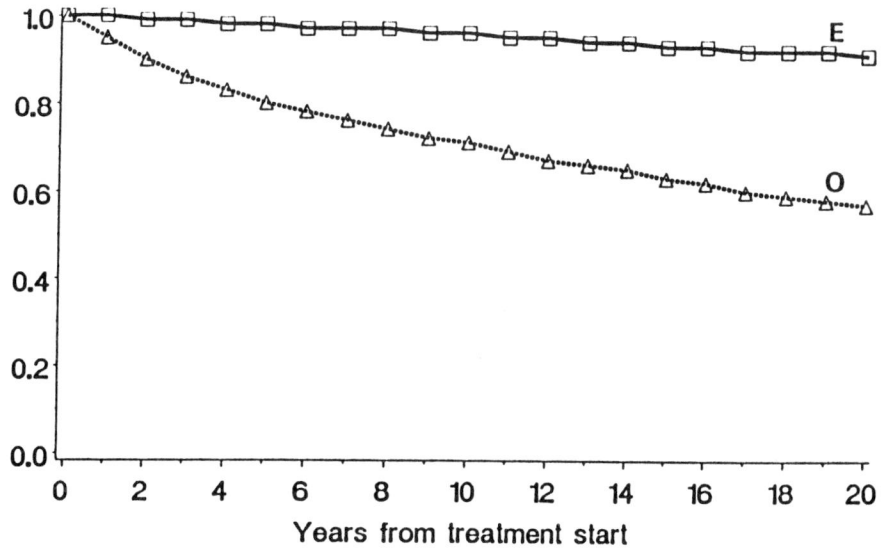

Figure X-1: *All stages. Expected (E) and observed (O) survival (N = 14,225).*

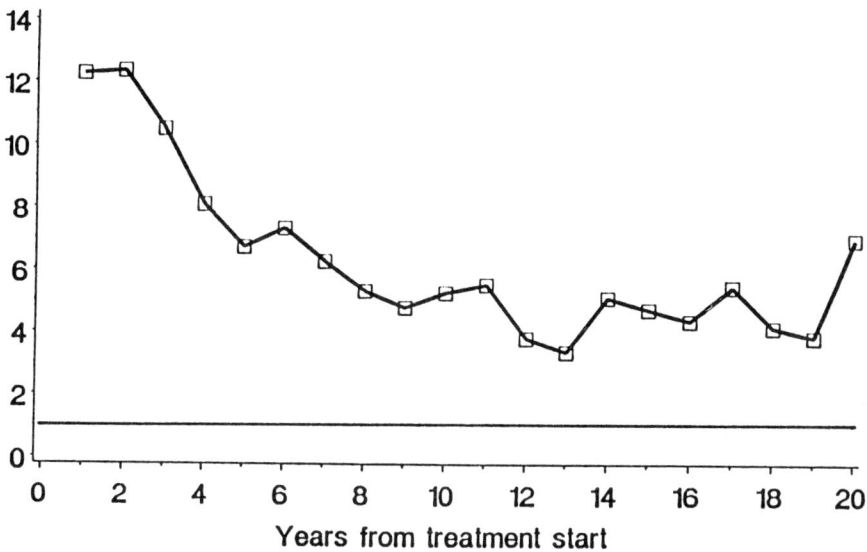

Figure X-2: *All stages. Standardized Mortality Ratio (SMR) as a function of time (All causes of death)*

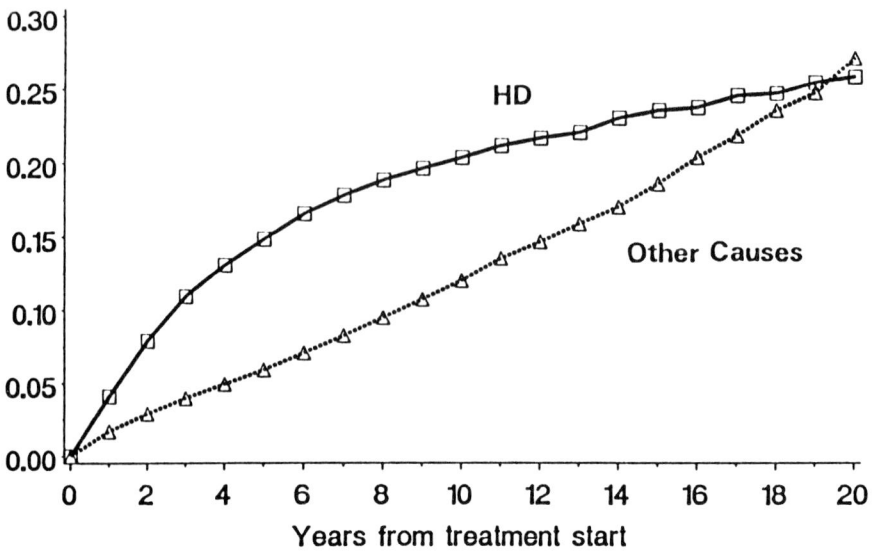

Figure X-3: *All stages. Cumulative incidence of death among the overall population study (N = 14,225). (HD : Hodgkin disease related death, 3,010 cases; Other causes : 1,129 cases).*

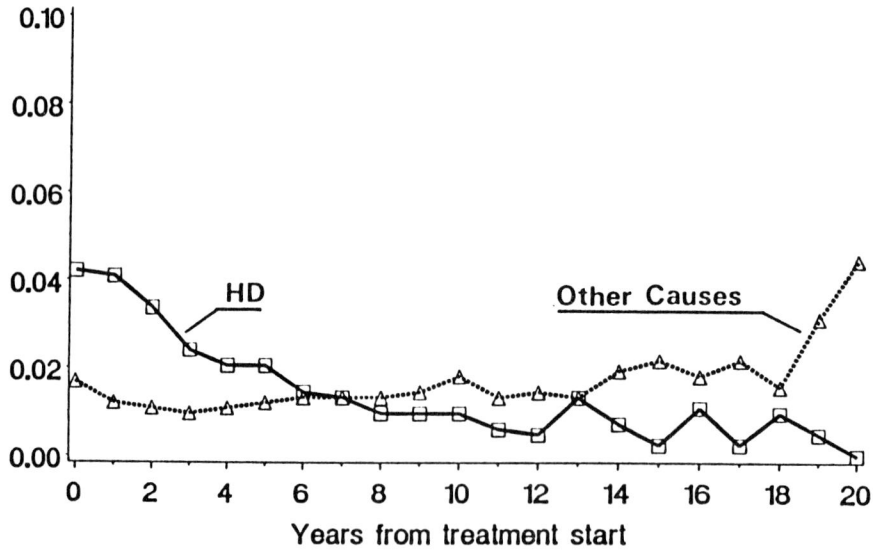

Figure X-4: *All stages. Annual risk of death among the overall population study (N = 14,225). (HD : Hodgkin disease related death, 3,010 cases; Other causes : 1,129 cases).*

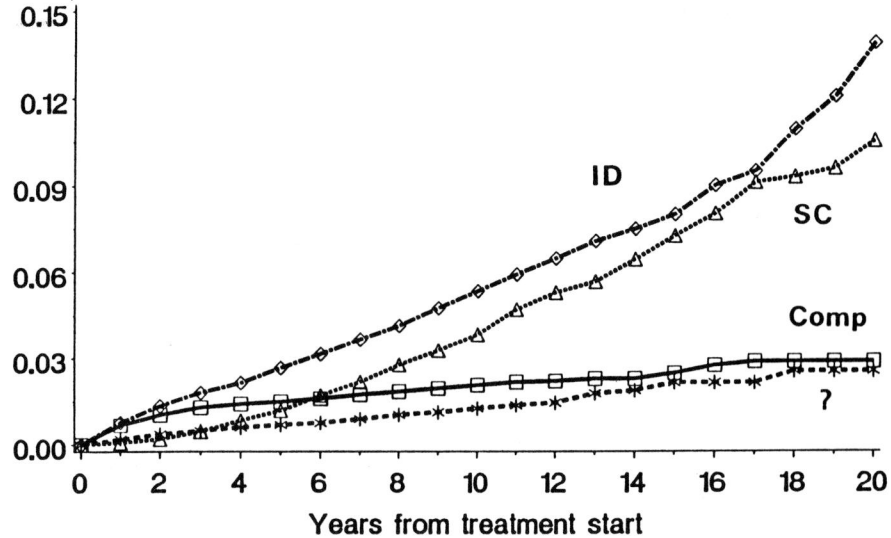

Figure X-5 : *All stages. Cumulative incidence of death among the overall population study (N = 14,225). (ID : intercurrent disease, 577 cases; SC: second cancer, 413 cases; Comp : treatment-related death, 233 cases; ? : cause unspecified, 139 cases).*

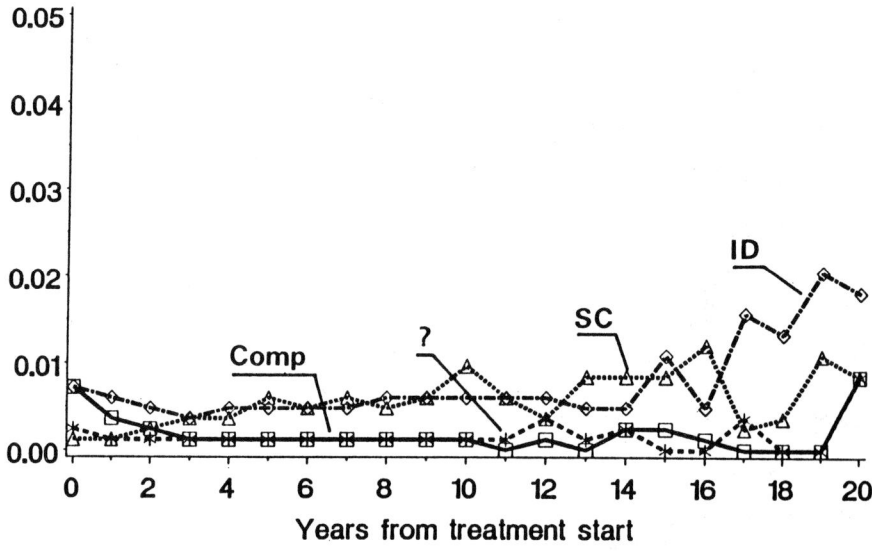

Figure X-6 : *All stages. Annual risk of death among the overall population study (N = 14,225). (ID : intercurrent disease, 577 cases; SC: second cancer, 413 cases; Comp : treatment-related death, 233 cases; ? : cause unspecified, 139 cases).*

Table X-3. Deaths characteristics by sex

Causes of death	Males				Females			
OVERALL POPULATION								
All causes			2,763				1,376	
Hodgkin dis.			1,839	(67%)			938	(68%)
Treatment rel.			139	(5%)			94	(7%)
2nd cancer			280	(10%)			133	(10%)
	95	47	138	(58, 35)[a]	52	14	67	(24, 10, 12)[b]
Intercurrent			420	(15%)			157	(11%)
Unspecified			85	(3%)			54	(4%)
TIME SINCE HODGKIN DISEASE DIAGNOSIS								
0- 4 yrs All causes			1,820				915	
Hodgkin dis.			1,374	(75%)			680	(74%)
Treatment rel.			110	(6%)			71	(8%)
2nd cancer			81	(5%)			42	(5%)
	40	10	31	(7, 10)[a]	25	4	13	(3, 5, 3)[b]
Intercurrent			208	(11%)			90	(10%)
Unspecified			47	(3%)			32	(3%)
5- 9 yrs All causes			653				310	
Hodgkin dis.			360	(55%)			198	(64%)
Treatment rel.			22	(3%)			15	(5%)
2nd cancer			122	(19%)			46	(15%)
	48	18	56	(27, 12)[a]	22	3	21	(9, 1, 4)[b]
Intercurrent			128	(20%)			37	(12%)
Unspecified			21	(3%)			14	(4%)
10-14 yrs All causes			224				120	
Hodgkin dis.			96	(43%)			48	(40%)
Treatment rel.			4	(2%)			5	(4%)
2nd cancer			58	(26%)			37	(31%)
	7	10	41	(19, 13)[a]	5	7	25	(11, 4, 4)[b]
Intercurrent			53	(24%)			22	(18%)
Unspecified			13	(5%)			8	(7%)
15-19 yrs All causes			57				26	
Hodgkin dis.			9	(16%)			12	(46%)
Treatment rel.			3	(4%)			2	(8%)
2nd cancer			18	(32%)			5	(19%)
	0	9	9	(4, 0)[a]	0	0	5	(0, 0, 1)[b]
Intercurrent			25	(44%)			7	(27%)
Unspecified			2	(4%)			0	
20+ yrs All causes			9				5	
Hodgkin dis.			0				0	
Treatment rel.			0				1	
2nd cancer			1				3	
	0	0	1	(1, 0)[a]	0	0	3	(1, 0, 0)[b]
Intercurrent			6				1	
Unspecified			2				0	

a) # of leukemias, non-Hodgkin lymphomas, and solid tumors, respectively; in ( ) # of lung and digestive cancers
b) # of leukemias, non-Hodgkin lymphomas, and solid tumors, respectively; in ( ) # of lung, digestive, and breast cancers

Table X-4a. Observed (O) and expected (E) deaths in male patients, overall and by follow-up time

Causes of death		O	E	Excess of deaths[a]	O/E	95% CL[b]
OVERALL POPULATION						
All causes		2,763	389.75		7.09***	6.83- 7.36
Hodgkin disease		1,839				
Treatment related		139				
Second cancer		280				
Intercurrent		420				
Unspecified		85				
Not related to HD[c]		785		0.65	2.01***	1.88- 2.16
TIME SINCE HODGKIN DISEASE DIAGNOSIS						
0- 4 yrs	All causes	1,820	204.97		8.88***	8.48- 9.30
	Not related to HD	336		0.39	1.64***	1.47- 1.82
5- 9 yrs	All causes	653	116.84		5.59***	5.17- 6.03
	Not related to HD	271		0.84	2.32***	2.25- 2.61
10-14 yrs	All causes	224	54.69		4.10***	3.58- 4.67
	Not related to HD	124		0.92	2.27***	1.89- 2.70
15-19 yrs	All causes	57	12.32		4.63***	3.50- 5.99
	Not related to HD	45		2.09	3.65***	2.66- 4.88
20+ yrs	All causes	9	0.91		9.89***	4.52-18.77
	Not related to HD	9		6.86	9.89***	4.52-18.77

a) excess of deaths = (O - E) x 100 / numbers of person-years at risk
b) confidence limits of O/E assuming the Poisson distribution for O
c) all deaths except those from Hodgkin disease progression or relapse, or treatment related (see text)
* $p < 0.05$; ** $p < 0.01$; *** $p < 0.001$; two-sided test

Table X-4b. Observed (O) and expected (E) deaths in female patients, overall and by follow-up time

Causes of death	O	E	Excess of deaths[a]	O/E	95% CL[b]
OVERALL POPULATION					
All causes	1,376	149.41		9.21***	8.73- 9.71
Hodgkin disease	938				
Treatment related	94				
Second cancer	133				
Intercurrent	157				
Unspecified	54				
Not related to HD[c]	344		0.46	2.30***	2.07- 2.56
TIME SINCE HODGKIN DISEASE DIAGNOSIS					
0- 4 yrs All causes	915	75.03		12.20***	11.42-13.01
Not related to HD	164		0.39	2.19***	1.86- 2.55
5- 9 yrs All causes	310	44.86		6.91***	6.16- 7.72
Not related to HD	97		0.40	2.16***	1.75- 2.64
10-14 yrs All causes	120	23.92		5.02***	4.16- 6.00
Not related to HD	67		0.76	2.80***	2.17- 3.56
15-19 yrs All causes	26	6.22		4.18***	2.73- 6.13
Not related to HD	12		0.41	1.93*	1.00- 3.37
20+ yrs All causes	5	0.42		11.90***	3.87-27.78
Not related to HD	4		2.50	9.52**	2.59-24.38

a) excess of deaths = (O - E) x 100 / numbers of person-years at risk
b) confidence limits of O/E assuming the Poisson distribution for O
c) all deaths except those from Hodgkin disease progression or relapse, or treatment related (see text)
* $p < 0.05$; ** $p < 0.01$; *** $p < 0.001$; two-sided test

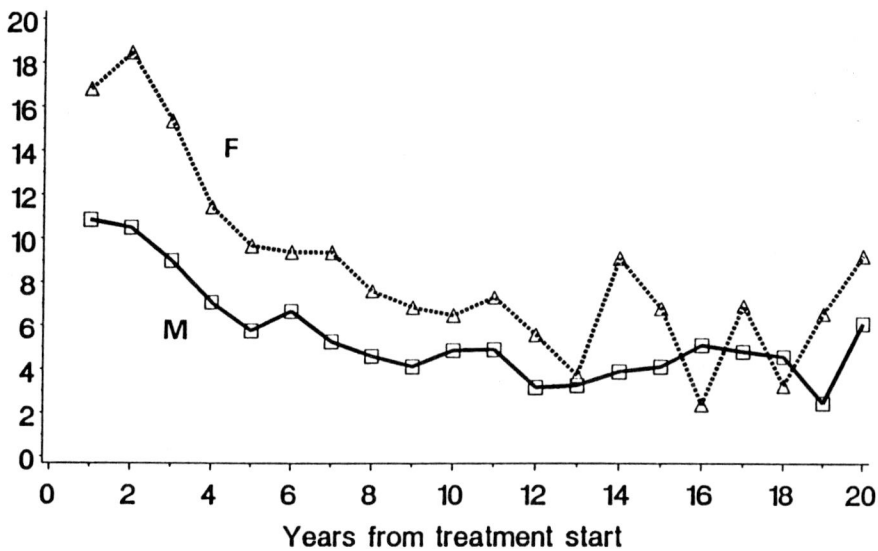

Figure X-7 : *All stages. Standardized Mortality Ratio (SMR) as a function of time in males (N = 8,614) and in females (N = 5,611) (All causes of death).*

Table X-5. Study population characteristics by age

		Patients at risk *	Person-years at risk
OVERALL POPULATION			
Age 15-19 years		1,675	13,907
20-29 years		5,013	40,621
30-39 years		3,246	24,096
40-49 years		1,826	12,492
50-59 years		1,282	7,560
60+ years		1,183	5,041
total		14,225	103,717
TIME SINCE HODGKIN DISEASE DIAGNOSIS			
0- 4 years	15-19 yrs	559	7,039
	20-29 yrs	1,690	20,876
	30-39 yrs	1,220	13,176
	40-49 yrs	816	6,933
	50-59 yrs	663	4,520
	60+ yrs	777	3,497
5- 9 years	15-19 yrs	517	4,272
	20-29 yrs	1,558	12,538
	30-39 yrs	1,064	7,357
	40-49 yrs	499	3,718
	50-59 yrs	346	2,174
	60+ yrs	290	1,206
10-14 years	15-19 yrs	380	2,009
	20-29 yrs	1,171	5,762
	30-39 yrs	690	2,859
	40-49 yrs	367	1,526
	50-59 yrs	212	731
	60+ yrs	97	310
15-19 years	15-19 yrs	181	527
	20-29 yrs	528	1,316
	30-39 yrs	239	646
	40-49 yrs	135	305
	50-59 yrs	57	133
	60+ yrs	19	28
20+ years	15-19 yrs	38	61
	20-29 yrs	66	129
	30-39 yrs	33	58
	40-49 yrs	9	11
	50-59 yrs	4	2
	60+ yrs	0	0

* *patients for whom the following information are available: age, sex, clinical stage and last known vital status*

Table X-6a. Observed (O) and expected (E) deaths in patients aged 15 to 19 years at diagnosis, overall and by follow-up time

Causes of death	O	E	Excess of deaths[a]	O/E	95% CL[b]
OVERALL POPULATION					
All causes	326	13.57		24.02***	21.49-26.78
Hodgkin disease	251				
Treatment related	19				
Second cancer	22				
Intercurrent	28				
Unspecified	6				
Not related to HD[c]	56	0.31		4.13***	3.12- 5.36
TIME SINCE HODGKIN DISEASE DIAGNOSIS					
0- 4 yrs All causes	196	6.62		29.61***	25.61-34.05
Not related to HD	22	0.22		3.32***	2.08- 5.03
5- 9 yrs All causes	87	4.23		20.57***	16.47-25.37
Not related to HD	13	0.21		3.07***	1.64- 5.26
10-14 yrs All causes	31	2.03		15.27***	10.37-21.67
Not related to HD	14	0.60		6.90***	3.77-11.57
15-19 yrs All causes	9	0.72		12.50***	5.72-23.72
Not related to HD	5	0.81		6.94**	2.25-16.21
20+ yrs All causes	3	0.10		30.00**	6.19-87.67
Not related to HD	2	3.11		20.00**	2.42-72.25

a) excess of deaths = (O - E) x 100 / numbers of person-years at risk
b) confidence limits of O/E assuming the Poisson distribution for O
c) all deaths except those from Hodgkin disease progression or relapse, or treatment related (see text)
* $p < 0.05$; ** $p < 0.01$; *** $p < 0.001$; two-sided test

Table X-6b. Observed (O) and expected (E) deaths in patients aged 20 to 29 years at diagnosis, overall and by follow-up time

Causes of death	O	E	Excess of deaths[a]	O/E	95% CL[b]
OVERALL POPULATION					
All causes	1,016	52.58		19.32***	18.15-20.55
Hodgkin disease	787				
Treatment related	50				
Second cancer	68				
Intercurrent	91				
Unspecified	20				
Not related to HD[c]	179	0.31		3.40***	2.92- 3.94
TIME SINCE HODGKIN DISEASE DIAGNOSIS					
0- 4 yrs All causes	639	23.61		27.06***	25.01-29.25
Not related to HD	76	0.25		3.22***	2.54- 4.03
5- 9 yrs All causes	253	16.05		15.76***	13.88-17.83
Not related to HD	49	0.26		3.05***	2.26- 4.04
10-14 yrs All causes	98	9.57		10.24***	8.31-12.48
Not related to HD	40	0.53		4.18***	2.99- 5.69
15-19 yrs All causes	22	2.95		7.46***	4.67-11.29
Not related to HD	10	0.54		3.39**	1.63- 6.23
20+ yrs All causes	4	0.50		8.00**	2.18-20.48
Not related to HD	4	2.71		8.00**	2.18-20.48

a) excess of deaths = (O - E) x 100 / numbers of person-years at risk
b) confidence limits of O/E assuming the Poisson distribution for O
c) all deaths except those from Hodgkin disease progression or relapse, or treatment related (see text)
* p < 0.05; ** p < 0.01; *** p < 0.001; two-sided test

Table X-6c. Observed (O) and expected (E) deaths in patients aged 30 to 39 years at diagnosis, overall and by follow-up time

Causes of death		O	E	Excess of deaths[a]	O/E	95% CL[b]
OVERALL POPULATION						
All causes		757	59.37		12.75***	11.86-13.69
Hodgkin disease		541				
Treatment related		37				
Second cancer		69				
Intercurrent		89				
Unspecified		21				
Not related to HD[c]		179		0.50	3.01***	2.59- 3.49
TIME SINCE HODGKIN DISEASE DIAGNOSIS						
0- 4 yrs	All causes	466	24.81		18.78***	17.12-20.57
	Not related to HD	56		0.24	2.26***	1.71- 2.93
5- 9 yrs	All causes	204	19.71		10.35***	8.98-11.87
	Not related to HD	70		0.68	3.55***	2.77- 4.49
10-14 yrs	All causes	57	10.84		5.26***	3.98- 6.81
	Not related to HD	26		0.53	2.40***	1.57- 3.51
15-19 yrs	All causes	24	3.78		6.35***	4.07- 9.45
	Not related to HD	21		2.67	5.56***	3.44- 8.49
20+ yrs	All causes	6	0.50		12.00***	4.40-26.12
	Not related to HD	6		9.48	12.00***	4.40-20.48

a) excess of deaths = (O - E) x 100 / numbers of person-years at risk
b) confidence limits of O/E assuming the Poisson distribution for O
c) all deaths except those from Hodgkin disease progression or relapse, or treatment related (see text)
* $p < 0.05$; ** $p < 0.01$; *** $p < 0.001$; two-sided test

Table X-6d. Observed (O) and expected (E) deaths in patients aged 40 to 49 years at diagnosis, overall and by follow-up time

Causes of death	O	E	Excess of deaths[a]	O/E	95% CL[b]
OVERALL POPULATION					
All causes	642	82.63		7.77***	7.18- 8.39
Hodgkin disease	405				
Treatment related	39				
Second cancer	78				
Intercurrent	103				
Unspecified	17				
Not related to HD[c]	198		0.92	2.40***	2.07- 2.75
TIME SINCE HODGKIN DISEASE DIAGNOSIS					
0- 4 yrs All causes	421	34.87		12.07***	10.95-13.28
Not related to HD	81		0.67	2.32***	1.84- 2.89
5- 9 yrs All causes	141	27.34		5.16***	4.34- 6.08
Not related to HD	67		1.07	2.45***	1.90- 3.11
10-14 yrs All causes	66	15.91		4.15***	3.21- 5.28
Not related to HD	41		1.64	2.58***	1.85- 3.50
15-19 yrs All causes	14	4.25		3.29***	1.80- 5.53
Not related to HD	9		1.56	2.12	0.96- 4.02
20+ yrs All causes	0	0.16		0	0 -23.06
Not related to HD	0		0	0	0 -23.06

a) excess of deaths = (O - E) x 100 / numbers of person-years at risk
b) confidence limits of O/E assuming the Poisson distribution for O
c) all deaths except those from Hodgkin disease progression or relapse, or treatment related (see text)
* $p < 0.05$; ** $p < 0.01$; *** $p < 0.001$; two-sided test

Table X-6e. Observed (O) and expected (E) deaths in patients aged 50 to 59 years at diagnosis, overall and by follow-up time

Causes of death	O	E	Excess of deaths[a]	O/E	95% CL[b]
OVERALL POPULATION					
All causes	600	119.47		5.02***	4.63- 5.44
Hodgkin disease	351				
Treatment related	32				
Second cancer	95				
Intercurrent	106				
Unspecified	16				
Not related to HD[c]	217		1.29	1.82***	1.58- 2.07
TIME SINCE HODGKIN DISEASE DIAGNOSIS					
0- 4 yrs All causes	400	58.30		6.86***	6.21- 7.57
Not related to HD	92		0.75	1.58***	1.27- 1.94
5- 9 yrs All causes	132	39.13		3.37***	2.82- 4.00
Not related to HD	74		1.60	1.89***	1.48- 2.37
10-14 yrs All causes	55	18.31		3.00***	2.26- 3.91
Not related to HD	40		2.97	2.18***	1.56- 2.97
15-19 yrs All causes	12	4.45		2.70**	1.39- 4.71
Not related to HD	10		4.17	2.25*	1.08- 4.13
20+ yrs All causes	1	0.23		4.35	0.11-24.22
Not related to HD	1		-	4.35	0.11-24.22

a) excess of deaths = (O - E) x 100 / numbers of person-years at risk
b) confidence limits of O/E assuming the Poisson distribution for O
c) all deaths except those from Hodgkin disease progression or relapse, or treatment related (see text)
* $p < 0.05$; ** $p < 0.01$; *** $p < 0.001$; two-sided test

Table X-6f. Observed (O) and expected (E) deaths in patients aged 60 years or more at diagnosis, overall and by follow-up time

Causes of death	O	E	Excess of deaths[a]	O/E	95% CL[b]
OVERALL POPULATION					
All causes	798	211.41		3.77***	3.52- 4.05
Hodgkin disease	442				
Treatment related	56				
Second cancer	81				
Intercurrent	160				
Unspecified	59				
Not related to HD[c]	300		1.76	1.42***	1.26- 1.59
TIME SINCE HODGKIN DISEASE DIAGNOSIS					
0- 4 yrs All causes	613	132.81		4.62***	4.26- 5.00
Not related to HD	173		1.15	1.30***	1.12- 1.51
5- 9 yrs All causes	146	57.00		2.56***	2.16- 3.01
Not related to HD	95		3.15	1.67***	1.35- 2.04
10-14 yrs All causes	37	20.42		1.81**	1.28- 2.50
Not related to HD	30		3.09	1.47	0.99- 2.10
15-19 yrs All causes	2	2.22		0.90	0.11- 3.25
Not related to HD	2		-	0.90	0.11- 3.25
20+ yrs All causes	-				
Not related to HD	-				

a) excess of deaths = (O - E) x 100 / numbers of person-years at risk
b) confidence limits of O/E assuming the Poisson distribution for O
c) all deaths except those from Hodgkin disease progression or relapse, or treatment related (see text)
* $p < 0.05$; ** $p < 0.01$; *** $p < 0.001$; two-sided test

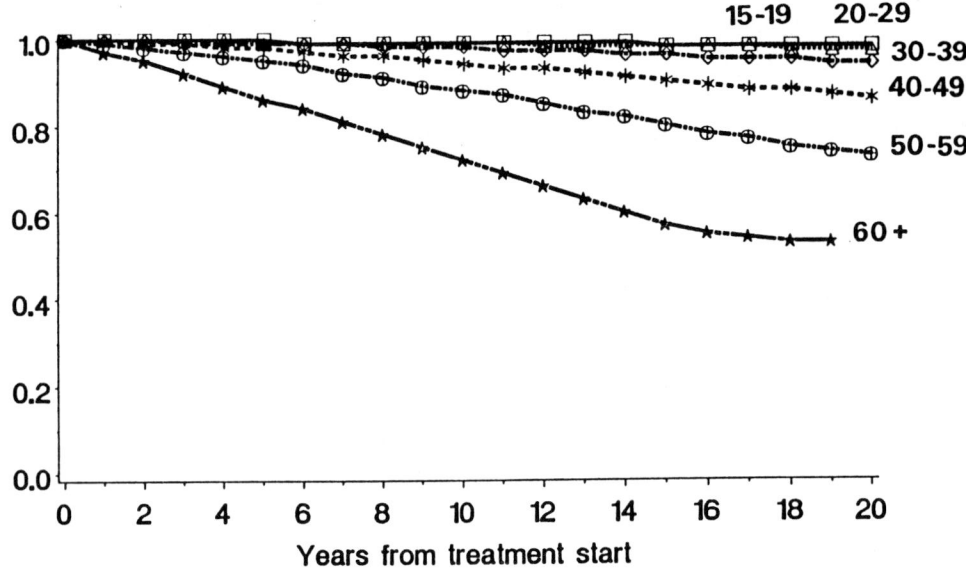

Figure X-8 : *All stages. Expected survival by age at Hodgkin disease diagnosis.*

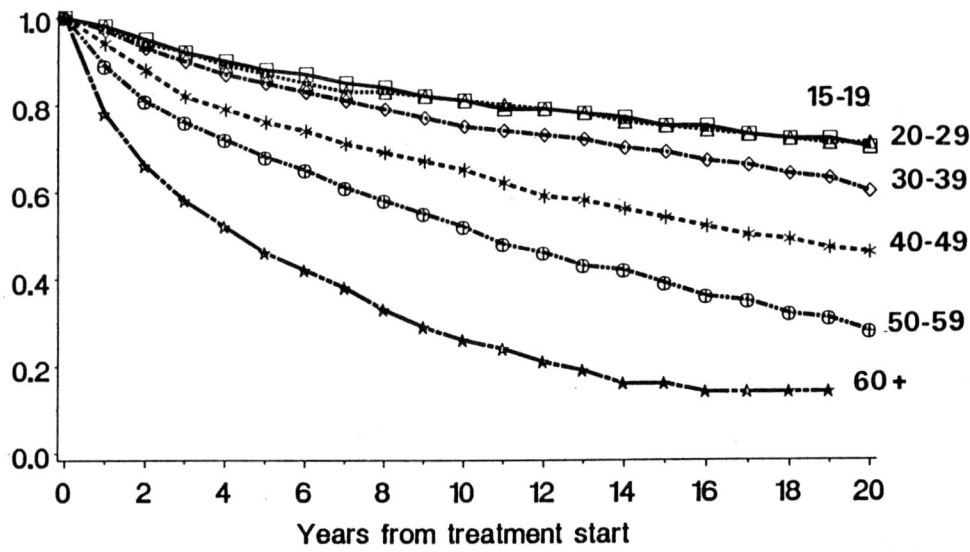

Figure X-9 : *All stages. Observed survival by age at Hodgkin disease diagnosis (15-19 yrs : 1,675 pts; 20-29 yrs : 5,013 pts; 30-39 yrs : 3,246 pts; 40-49 yrs : 1,826 pts; 50-59 yrs : 1,282 pts; 60+ yrs : 1,183 pts).*

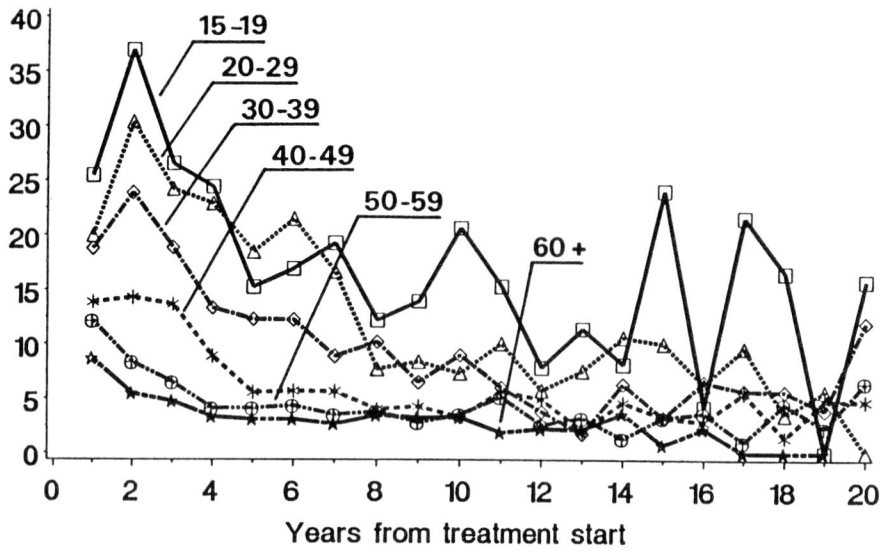

Figure X-10: *All stages. Standardized Mortality Ratio (SMR) as a function of time by age at Hodhkin disease diagnosis (All causes of death).*

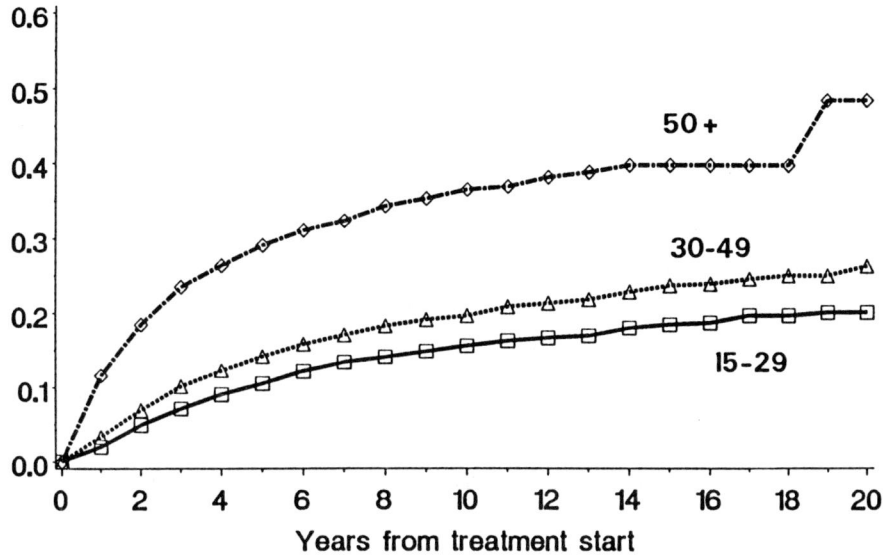

Figure X-11: *All stages. Cumulative incidence of disease-related death by age at diagnosis (15-29 yrs : 6,688 pts; 30-49 yrs : 5,072 pts; 50+ yrs : 2,465 pts).*

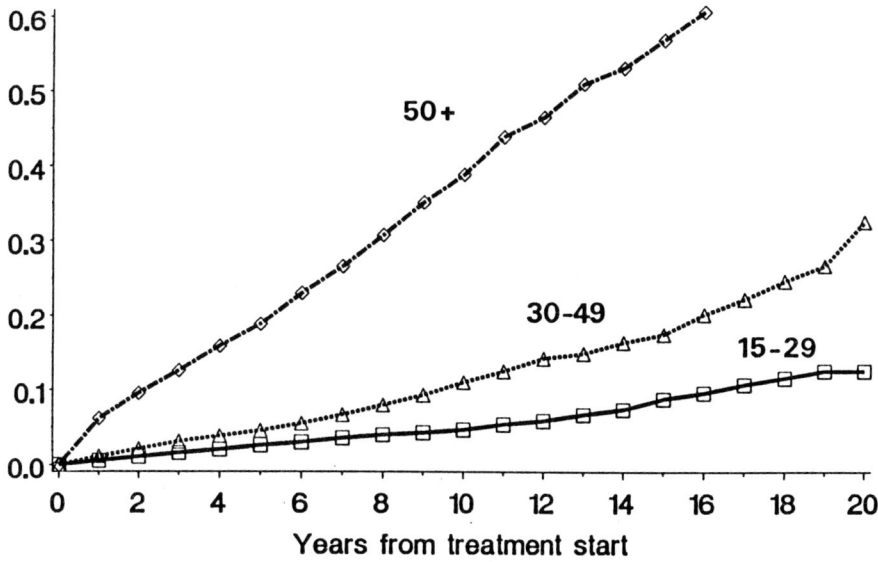

Figure X-12: *All stages. Cumulative incidence of intercurrent death by age at diagnosis (15-29 yrs : 6,688 pts; 30-49 yrs : 5,072 pts; 50+ yrs : 2,465 pts).*

Table X-7. Study population characteristics by clinical stage

		Patients at risk *	Person-years at risk
OVERALL POPULATION			
CS I-II		9,041	71,743
CS III-IV		5,184	31,974
total		14,225	103,717
TIME SINCE HODGKIN DISEASE DIAGNOSIS			
0- 4 years	CS I-II	3,079	37,662
	CS III-IV	2,646	18,378
5- 9 years	CS I-II	2,985	22,134
	CS III-IV	1,289	9,129
10-14 years	CS I-II	2,029	9,474
	CS III-IV	888	3,724
15-19 years	CS I-II	821	2,247
	CS III-IV	338	708
20+ years	CS I-II	127	226
	CS III-IV	23	35

* *patients for whom the following information are available: age, sex, clinical stage and last known vital status*

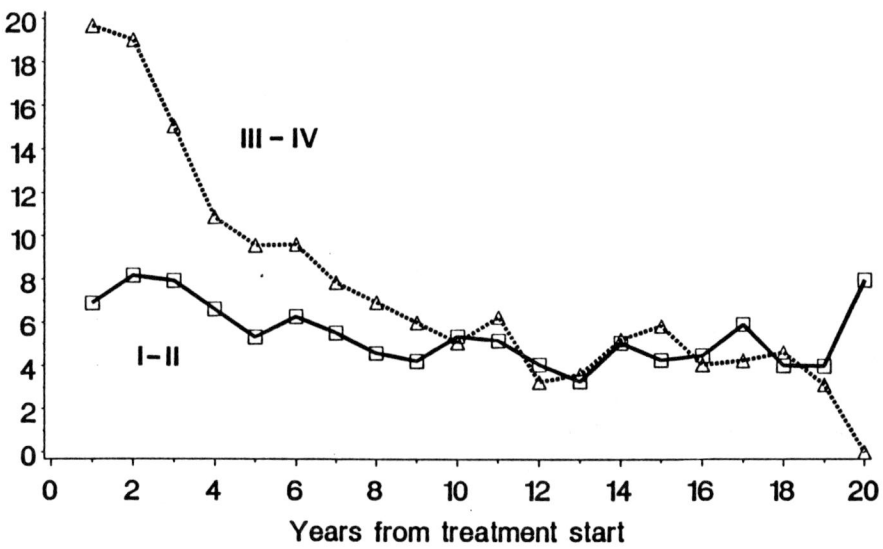

Figure X-13 : *All stages. Standardized Mortality Ratio (SMR) as a function of time by clinical stage (CS I-II : 9,041 pts; CS III-IV : 5,184 pts) (All causes of death)*

Table X-8a. Observed (O) and expected (E) deaths in CS I-II patients, overall and by follow-up time

Causes of death		O	E	Excess of deaths[a]	O/E	95% CL[b]
OVERALL POPULATION						
All causes		1,957	344.72		5.68***	5.43- 5.93
Hodgkin disease		1,117				
Treatment related		125				
Second cancer		246				
Intercurrent		383				
Unspecified		86				
Not related to HD[c]		715		0.52	2.07***	1.92- 2.23
TIME SINCE HODGKIN DISEASE DIAGNOSIS						
0- 4 yrs	All causes	1,119	170.14		6.58***	6.20- 6.97
	Not related to HD	282		0.30	1.66***	1.47- 1.86
5- 9 yrs	All causes	546	107.13		5.10***	4.58- 5.54
	Not related to HD	248		0.64	2.31***	2.04- 2.68
10-14 yrs	All causes	217	51.97		4.18***	3.64- 4.77
	Not related to HD	134		0.87	2.58***	2.16- 3.05
15-19 yrs	All causes	64	14.08		4.55***	3.50- 5.80
	Not related to HD	42		1.24	2.98***	2.15- 4.03
20+ yrs	All causes	11	1.14		9.65***	4.82-17.26
	Not related to HD	11		4.36	9.65***	4.82-17.26

a) excess of deaths = (O - E) x 100 / numbers of person-years at risk
b) confidence limits of O/E assuming the Poisson distribution for O
c) all deaths except those from Hodgkin disease progression or relapse, or treatment related (see text)
* $p < 0.05$; ** $p < 0.01$; *** $p < 0.001$; two-sided test

Table X-8b. Observed (O) and expected (E) deaths in CS III-IV patients, overall and by follow-up time

Causes of death		O	E	Excess of deaths[a]	O/E	95% CL[b]
OVERALL POPULATION						
All causes		2,182	194.42		11.22***	10.76-11.70
Hodgkin disease		1,660				
Treatment related		108				
Second cancer		167				
Intercurrent		194				
Unspecified		53				
Not related to HD[c]		414		0.69	2.13***	1.93- 2.34
TIME SINCE HODGKIN DISEASE DIAGNOSIS						
0- 4 yrs	All causes	1,616	109.65		14.74***	14.03-15.47
	Not related to HD	220		0.60	2.01***	1.75- 2.29
5- 9 yrs	All causes	417	54.65		7.63***	6.92- 8.40
	Not related to HD	120		0.72	2.20***	1.82- 2.63
10-14 yrs	All causes	127	25.52		4.98***	4.15- 5.92
	Not related to HD	57		0.85	2.23***	1.69- 2.89
15-19 yrs	All causes	19	4.42		4.30***	2.59- 6.71
	Not related to HD	15		1.49	3.39***	1.90- 5.60
20+ yrs	All causes	3	0.19		15.79**	3.26-46.14
	Not related to HD	2		5.17	10.53*	1.27-38.02

a) excess of deaths = (O - E) x 100 / numbers of person-years at risk
b) confidence limits of O/E assuming the Poisson distribution for O
c) all deaths except those from Hodgkin disease progression or relapse, or treatment related (see text)
* $p < 0.05$; ** $p < 0.01$; *** $p < 0.001$; two-sided test

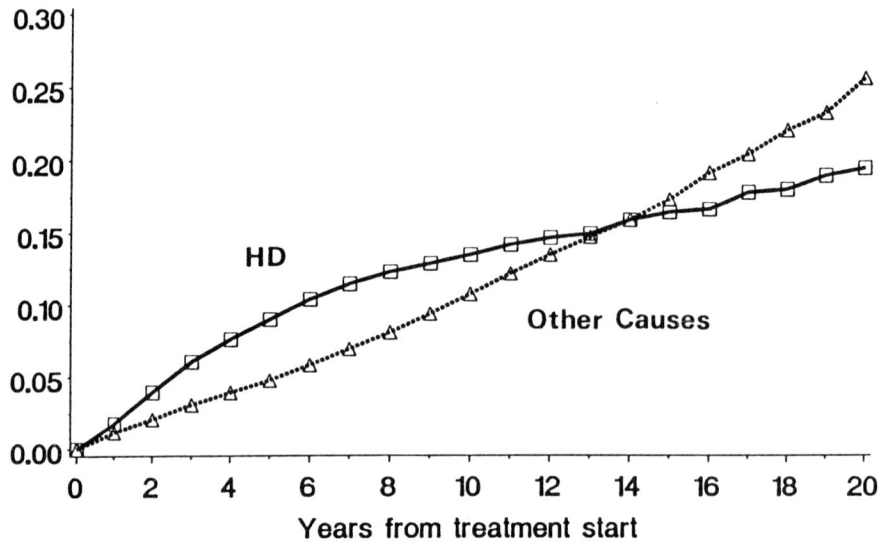

Figure X-14: *Early stages. Cumulative incidence of death (N = 9,041). (HD : Hodgkin disease related death, 1,242 cases; Other causes : 715 cases).*

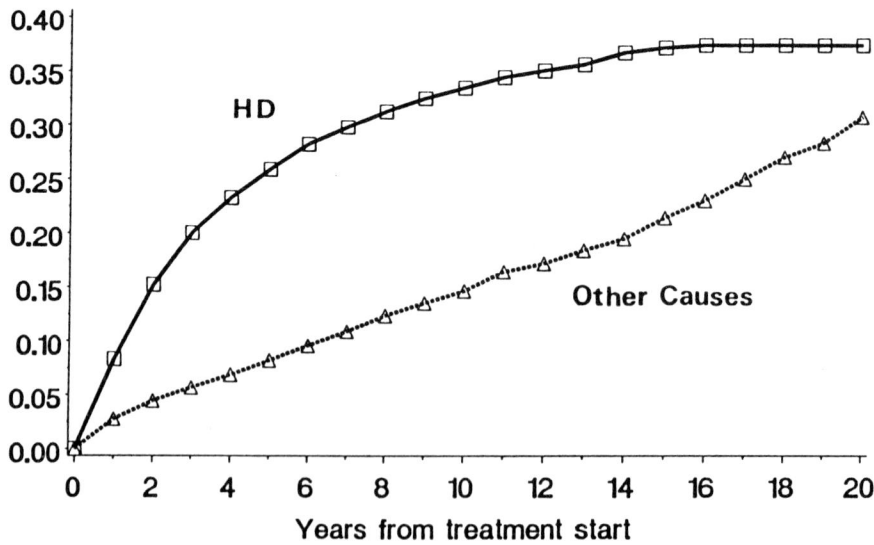

Figure X-15: *Advanced stages. Cumulative incidence of death (N = 5,184). (HD : Hodgkin disease related death, 1,768 cases; Other causes : 414 cases).*

Table X-9. Study population characteristics according to treatment period

		Patients at risk *	Person-years at risk
OVERALL POPULATION			
1960 - 1969		1,095	13,180
1970 - 1979		8,057	70,457
1980 +		5,073	20,080
total		14,225	103,717
TIME SINCE HODGKIN DISEASE DIAGNOSIS			
0- 4 years	1960-1969	300	4,509
	1970-1979	2,038	34,048
	1980 +	3,387	17,485
5- 9 years	1960-1969	141	3,602
	1970-1979	2,447	25,065
	1980 +	1,686	2,596
10-14 years	1960-1969	130	2,941
	1970-1979	2,787	10,257
	1980 +	0	0
15-19 years	1960-1969	374	1,867
	1970-1979	785	1,088
	1980 +	0	0
20+ years	1960-1969	150	260
	1970-1979	0	0
	1980 +	0	0

* *patients for whom the following information are available: age, sex, clinical stage and last known vital status*

Table X-10a. Observed (O) and expected (E) deaths in patients treated during the 1960-69 period, overall and by follow-up time

Causes of death		O	E	Excess of deaths[a]	O/E	95% CL[b]
OVERALL POPULATION						
All causes		556	91.17		6.10***	5.60- 6.63
Hodgkin disease		348				
Treatment related		7				
Second cancer		68				
Intercurrent		112				
Unspecified		21				
Not related to HD[c]		201		0.83	2.20***	1.91- 2.53
TIME SINCE HODGKIN DISEASE DIAGNOSIS						
0- 4 yrs	All causes	290	29.59		9.80***	8.70-11.00
	Not related to HD	53		0.52	1.79***	1.34- 2.34
5- 9 yrs	All causes	120	24.12		4.98***	4.12- 5.95
	Not related to HD	41		0.47	1.70***	1.22- 2.31
10-14 yrs	All causes	81	21.08		3.84***	3.05- 4.78
	Not related to HD	53		1.09	2.51***	1.88- 3.29
15-19 yrs	All causes	51	14.72		3.46***	2.58- 4.56
	Not related to HD	41		1.41	2.78***	2.00- 3.78
20+ yrs	All causes	14	1.78		7.87***	4.30-13.20
	Not related to HD	13		4.32	7.30***	3.89-12.49

a) excess of deaths = (O - E) x 100 / numbers of person-years at risk
b) confidence limits of O/E assuming the Poisson distribution for O
c) all deaths except those from Hodgkin disease progression or relapse, or treatment related (see text)
* $p < 0.05$; ** $p < 0.01$; *** $p < 0.001$; two-sided test

Table X-10b. Observed (O) and expected (E) deaths in patients treated during the 1970-79 period, overall and by follow-up time

Causes of death	O	E	Excess of deaths[a]	O/E	95% CL[b]
OVERALL POPULATION					
All causes	2,760	369.07		7.48***	7.20- 7.76
Hodgkin disease	1,860				
Treatment related	163				
Second cancer	283				
Intercurrent	362				
Unspecified	92				
Not related to HD[c]	737		0.52	2.00***	1.86- 2.15
TIME SINCE HODGKIN DISEASE DIAGNOSIS					
0- 4 yrs All causes	1,689	172.39		9.80***	9.34-10.28
Not related to HD	279		0.31	1.62***	1.43- 1.82
5- 9 yrs All causes	776	130.17		5.96***	5.55- 6.40
Not related to HD	304		0.69	2.34***	2.08- 2.61
10-14 yrs All causes	263	59.77		4.40***	3.88- 4.97
Not related to HD	138		0.76	2.31***	1.94- 2.73
15-19 yrs All causes	32	6.74		4.75***	3.25- 6.70
Not related to HD	16		0.85	2.37**	1.36- 3.85
20+ yrs All causes	-				
Not related to HD	-				

a) excess of deaths = $(O - E) \times 100$ / numbers of person-years at risk
b) confidence limits of O/E assuming the Poisson distribution for O
c) all deaths except those from Hodgkin disease progression or relapse, or treatment related (see text)
* $p < 0.05$; ** $p < 0.01$; *** $p < 0.001$; two-sided test

Table X-10c. Observed (O) and expected (E) deaths in patients treated during the 1980+ period, overall and by follow-up time

Causes of death	O	E	Excess of deaths[a]	O/E	95% CL[b]
OVERALL POPULATION					
All causes	823	98.43		8.36***	7.80- 8.95
Hodgkin disease	569				
Treatment related	63				
Second cancer	62				
Intercurrent	103				
Unspecified	26				
Not related to HD[c]	191		0.46	1.95***	1.68- 2.24
TIME SINCE HODGKIN DISEASE DIAGNOSIS					
0- 4 yrs All causes	756	84.87		8.91***	8.28- 9.57
Not related to HD	168		0.48	1.98***	1.69- 2.30
5- 9 yrs All causes	67	12.55		5.34***	4.14- 6.78
Not related to HD	23		0.40	1.83**	1.16- 2.75
10-14 yrs All causes	-				
Not related to HD	-				
15-19 yrs All causes	-				
Not related to HD	-				
20+ yrs All causes	-				
Not related to HD	-				

a) excess of deaths = $(O - E) \times 100$ / numbers of person-years at risk
b) confidence limits of O/E assuming the Poisson distribution for O
c) all deaths except those from Hodgkin disease progression or relapse, or treatment related (see text)
* $p < 0.05$; ** $p < 0.01$; *** $p < 0.001$; two-sided test

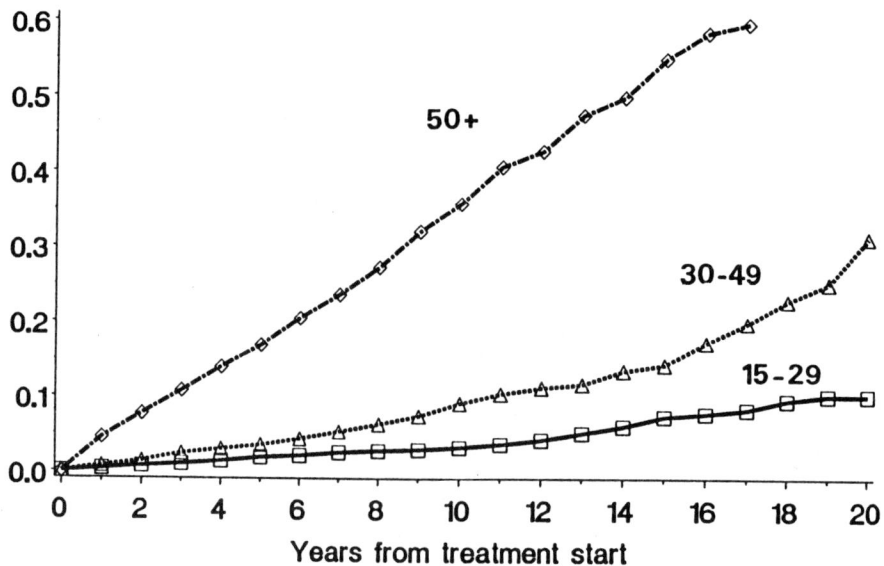

Figure X-16 : *All stages. Cumulative incidence of death (all causes) by age at Hodgkin disease diagnosis in patients who achieved a complete remission (N = 12,301). (15-29 yrs : 5,952 pts; 30-49 yrs : 4,459 pts; 50+ yrs : 1,890 pts).*

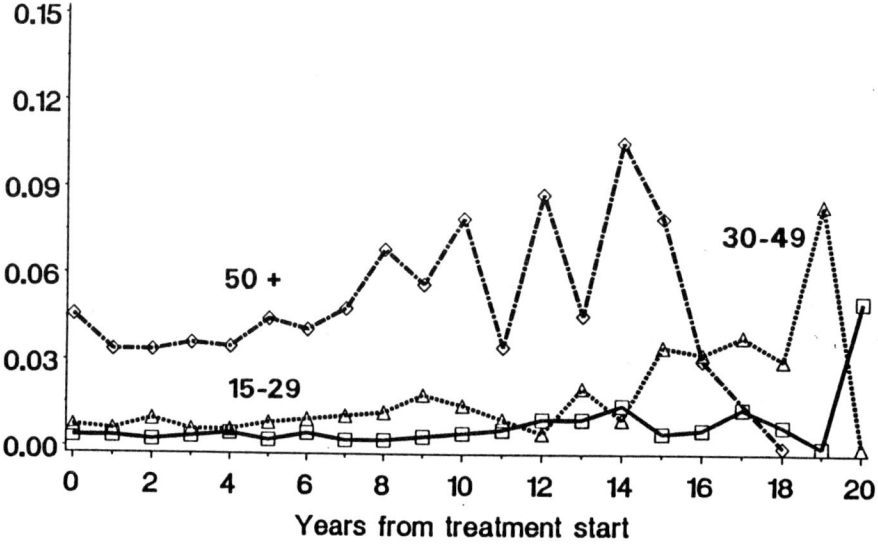

Figure X-17 : *All stages. Annual risk of death (all causes) by age at Hodgkin disease diagnosis in patients who achieved a complete remission (N = 12,301). (15-29 yrs : 5,952 pts; 30-49 yrs : 4,459 pts; 50+ yrs : 1,890 pts).*

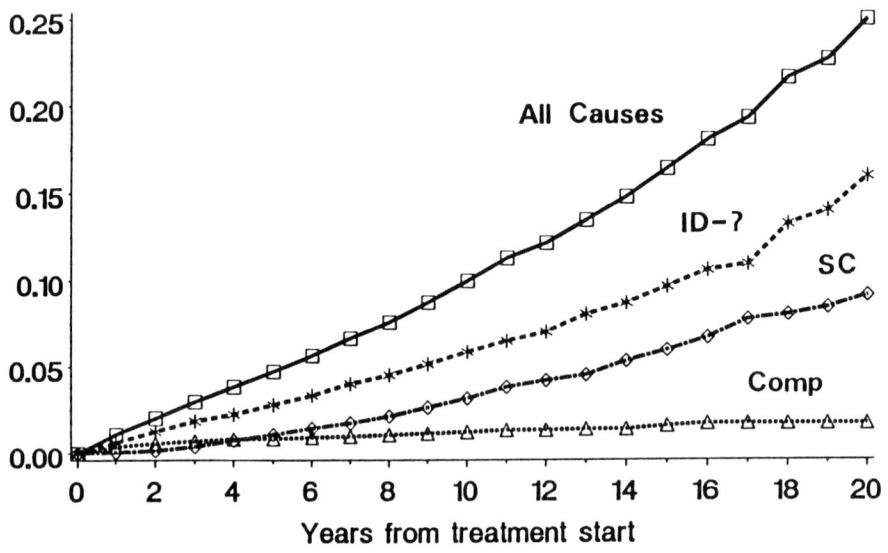

Figure X-18: *All stages. Cumulative incidence of death in patients who achieved a complete remission (N = 12,301). (All causes: 2,738 cases; ID-? : intercurrent disease and cause unspecified, 638 cases; SC: second cancer, 383 cases; Comp : treatment-related death, 168 cases).*

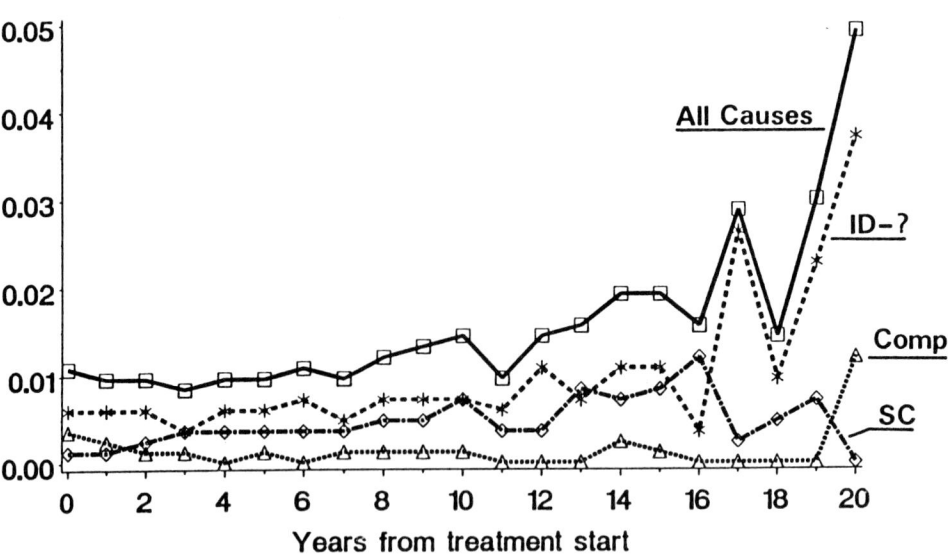

Figure X-19: *All stages. Annual risk of death in patients who achieved a complete remission (N = 12,301). (All causes: 2,738 cases; ID-? : intercurrent disease and cause unspecified, 638 cases; SC: second cancer, 383 cases; Comp : treatment-related death, 168 cases).*

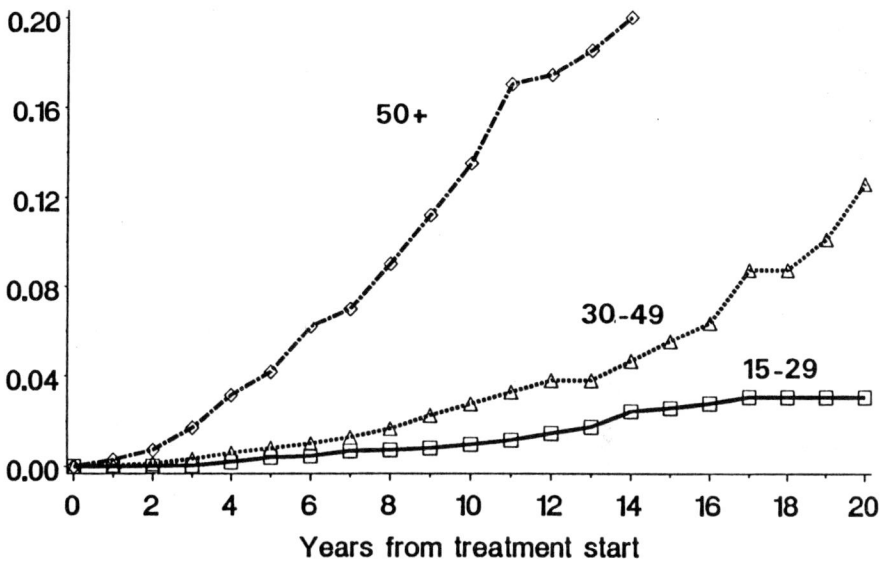

Figure X-20: *All stages. Cumulative incidence of death from second cancer, by age, in patients who achieved a complete remission (N = 12,301). (Second cancer deaths: 383 cases).*

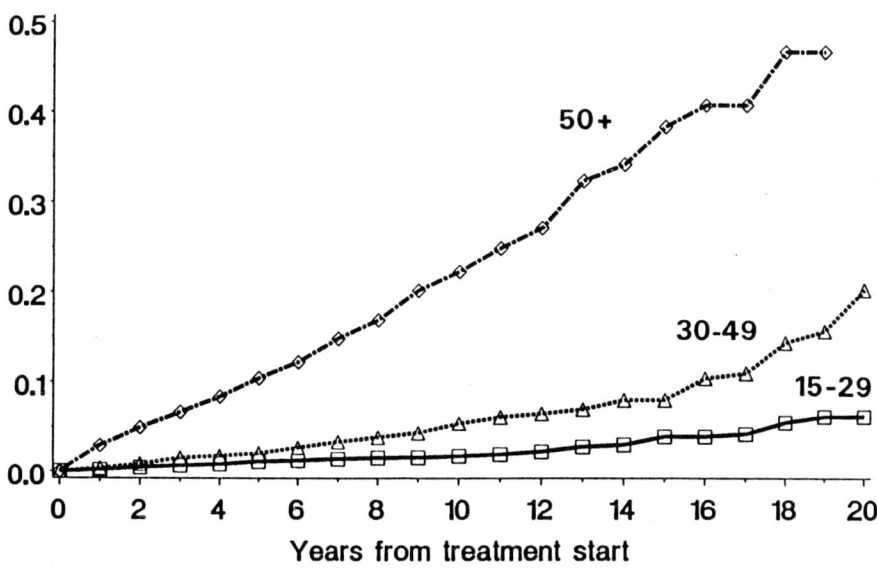

Figure X-21: *All stages. Cumulative incidence of death from intercurrent disease and cause unspecified, by age, in patients who achieved a complete remission (N = 12,301). (Death observed in 638 cases).*

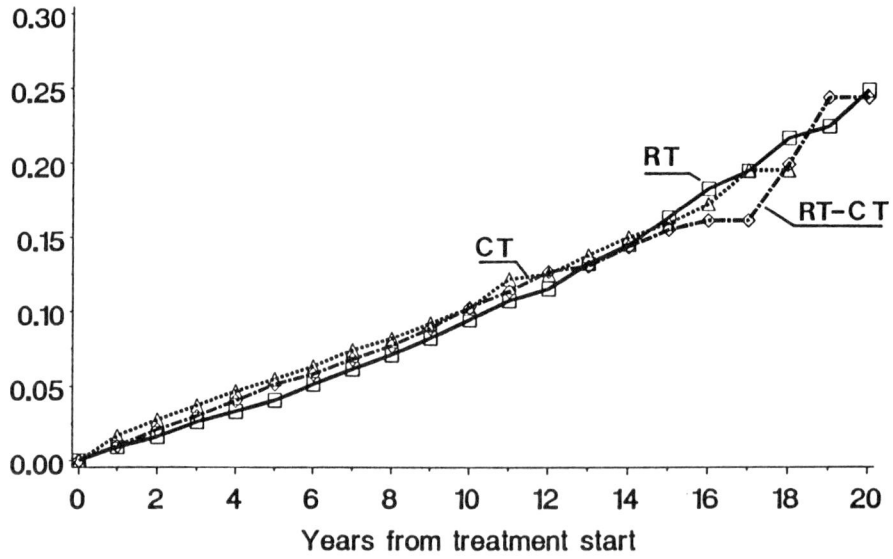

Figure X-22 : *All stages. Cumulative incidence of death (all causes) by initial treatment type in patients who achieved a complete remission (N = 12,283). (RT : radiation therapy alone, 5,799 pts; CT : chemotherapy alone, 2,201 pts; RT-CT : combined modalities, 4,283 pts).*

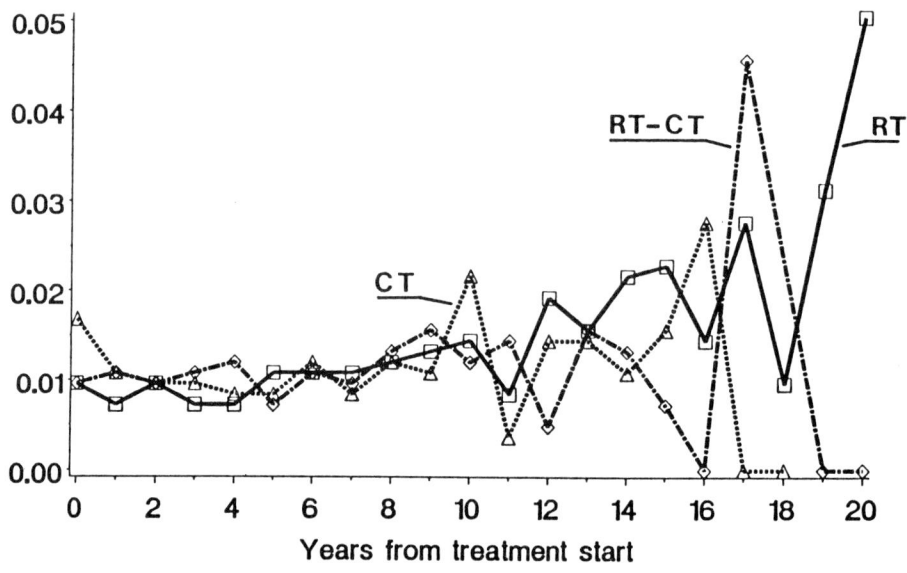

Figure X-23 : *All stages. Annual risk of death (all causes) by initial treatment type in patients who achieved a complete remission (N = 12,283). (RT : radiation therapy alone, 5,799 pts; CT : chemotherapy alone, 2,201 pts; RT-CT : combined modalities, 4,283 pts).*

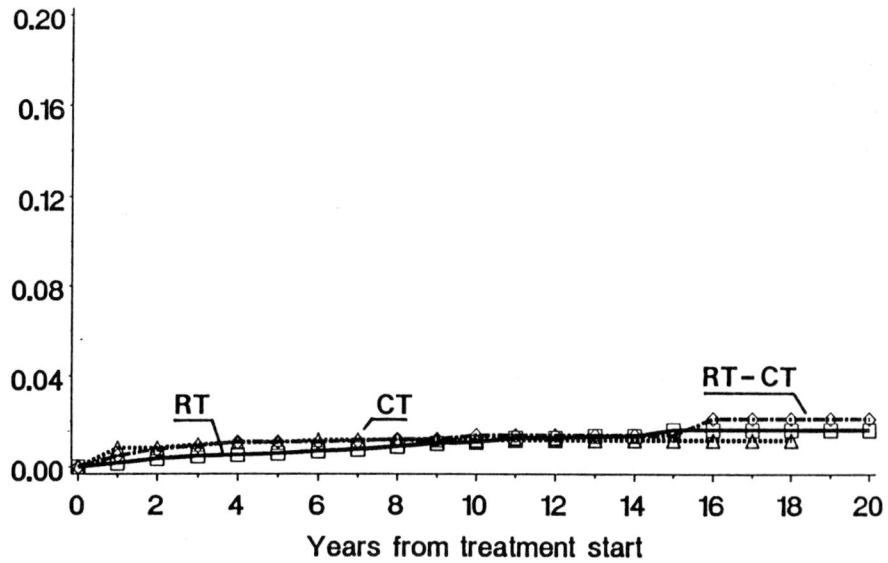

Figure X-24 : *All stages. Cumulative incidence of treatment-related death by initial treatment type in patients who achieved a complete remission. (RT : radiation therapy alone, 5,799 pts; CT : chemotherapy alone, 2,201 pts; RT-CT : combined modalities, 4,283 pts).*

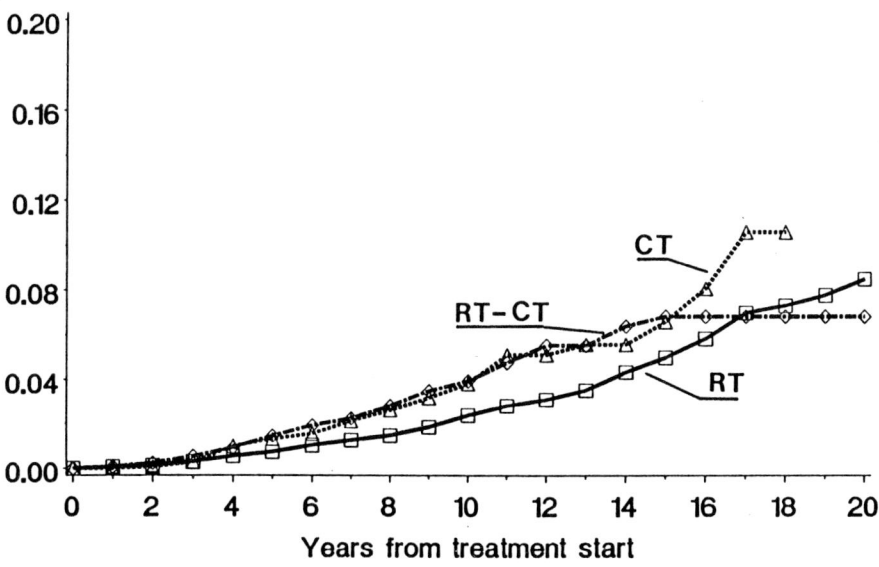

Figure X-25 : *All stages. Cumulative incidence of second cancer related death by initial treatment type in patients who achieved a complete remission. (RT : radiation therapy alone, 5,799 pts; CT : chemotherapy alone, 2,201 pts; RT-CT : combined modalities, 4,283 pts).*

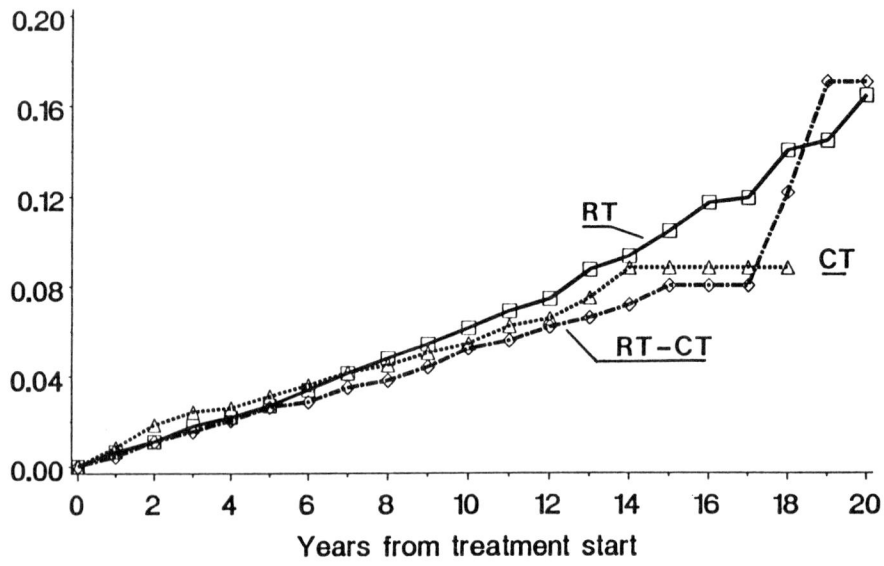

Figure X-26: *All stages. Cumulative incidence of death from intercurrent cause or cause unspecified, by initial treatment type, in patients who achieved a complete remission. (RT: radiation therapy alone, 5,799 pts; CT: chemotherapy alone, 2,201 pts; RT-CT: combined modalities, 4,283 pts).*

REFERENCES

BIBLIOGRAPHIE

References

Carde, P., et al. (1988): Clinical stages I and II Hodgkin's disease : A specifically tailored therapy according to prognostic factors. *J. Clin. Oncol.* 6, 239-252.

Carde, P., et al. (1990): H6 EORTC controlled trials in clinical stage I-II Hodgkin's disease. First report on the results of a randomized staging laparotomy in favorable cases and of a randomized MOPP versus ABVD combined radiotherapy modality in unfavorable cases. *Proc. Am. Soc. Clin. Oncol.* (in press).

Christensen, E. (1987): Multivariate survival analysis using Cox's regression model. *Hepatology* 6, 1346-1358.

Cooper, M.R., et al. (1980): A new effective four-drug combination of CCNU (1-(2-chloroethyl)-3-cyclohexyl-1-nitrosourea) (NSC-79038), vinblastine, prednisone, and procarbazine for the treatment of advanced Hodgkin's disease. *Cancer* 46, 654-662.

Cox, D.R. (1972): Regression models and life tables (with discussion). *J. R. Statist. Soc.* B 34, 187-220.

Dixon, W.J., et al. (1987a): *BMDP Statistical Software*. Berkeley, Los Angeles, London: University of California Press.

Dixon, D.O., et al. (1987b): Reporting outcomes in Hodgkin's disease and lymphoma. *J. Clin. Oncol.* 5, 1670-1672.

Fuller, L.M., et al. (1982): Collaborative clinical trial for stage I and II Hodgkin's disease: Significance of mediastinal and non-mediastinal disease in laparotomy- and non-laparotomy-stages patients. *Cancer Treat. Rep.* 66, 775-787.

Fuller, L.M., et al. (1988): The adjuvant role of two cycles of MOPP oand low-dose lung irradiation in stage IA through IIB Hodgkin's disease: Preliminary results. *Int. J. Radiat. Oncol. Biol. Phys.* 14, 683-692.

Gobbi, P.G., et al. (1986): Prognostic significance of serum albumin in Hodgkin's disease. *Haematologica (Pavia)* 71, 95-102.

Gobbi, P.G., el al. (1988): Hodgkin's disease: A directly predictive equation. *Lancet* i, 675-679.

Hagemeister, F.B., et al. (1982): Stages I and II Hodgkin's disease: Involved field versus extended field versus involved field followed by 6 MOPP. *Cancer Treat. Rep.* 66, 789-798.

Hancock, B.W. (1986): Randomised study of MOPP against LOPP in advanced Hodgkin's disease (British National Lymphoma Investigation). *Radiot. Oncol.* 7, 215-221.

Hayat, M. (1972): A randomized study of irradiation and vinblastine in clinical stages I and II of Hodgkin's disease. Preliminary results. *Eur. J. Cancer* 8, 353-362.

Haybittle, J.L., et al. (1985): Review of British National Lymphoma Investigation studies of Hodgkin's disease and development of prognostic index. *Lancet* i, 967-972.

Hoerni, B., et al. (1980): Hodgkin's disease clinical stages I and II: Results of radical irradiation with or without chemotherapy. *Acta Radiol. Oncol.* 19, 183-191.

Hoppe, R.T. et al. (1985): The concept, evolution and preliminary results of the current Stanford trials for Hodgkin's disease. *Cancer Surveys* 4, 459-475.

Hoppe, R.T., et al. (1989): Current Stanford clinical trials for Hodgkin's disease. In *New aspects in the diagnosis and treatment of Hodgkin's disease*, V. Diehl, M. Pfreundschuh & M. Löffler, pp. 182-190. Recent Results in Cancer Research 117. Berlin, Heidelberg: Springer Verlag.

Kleinbaum, D., et al. (1982): *Epidemiologic research: Principles and quantitative methods*. Belmont, CA: Lifetime Learning.

Krikorian, J.G., et al. (1986): Hodgkin's disease presenting below the diaphragm: A review. *J. Clin. Oncol.* 4, 1551-1562.

Lagarde, P., et al. (1988): Brief chemotherapy associated with extended field radiotherapy in Hodgkin's disease. Long-term results in a series of 1092 patients with clinical stages I-IIIA. *Eur. J. Cancer Clin. Oncol.* 24, 1191-1198.

Lee, C.K.K., et al. (1978): Hodgkin's disease: A reassessment of prognostic factors following modification of radiotherapy. *Int. J. Radiat. Oncol. biol. Phys.* 13, 983-991.

Löffler, M., et al. (1989): Risk factor adapted treatment of Hodgkin's ltmphoma: Strategies and perspectives. In *New aspects in the diagnosis and treatment of Hodgkin's disease*, V. Diehl, M. Pfreundschuh & M. Löffler, pp. 142-162. Recent Results in Cancer Research 117. Berlin, Heidelberg: Springer Verlag.

Mauch, P., et al. (1985): Stage III Hodgkin's disease: Improved survival with combined modality therapy as compared with radiation therapy alone. *J. Clin. Oncol.* 3, 1166-1173.

Mauch, P., et al. (1988): Stage IA and IIA supradiaphragmatic Hodgkin's disease: Prognostic factors in surgically staged patients treated with mantle and paraaortic irradiation. *J. Clin. Oncol.* 6, 1576-1583.

Morgenfield, M., et al. (1979): Combined chemotherapy cyclophosphamide, vinblastine, procarbazine and prednisone (CVPP) vs CVPP plus CCNU (CCVP) in Hodgkin's disease. *Cancer* 43, 1579-1586.

Nissen, N.I., et al. (1979): A comparative study of BCNU containing 4-drug program versus MOPP versus 3-drug combinations in advanced Hodgkin's disease. A cooperative study of the cancer and Leukemia Group B. *Cancer* 43, 31-40.

Pavlovsky, S., et al. (1988): Radomized trial of chemotherapy versus chemotherapy plus radiotherapy for stage I-II Hodgkin's disease. *J. Nat. Cancer Inst.* 80, 1466-1473.

Specht, L., et al. (1988): Tumor burden as the most important prognostic factor in early stage Hodgkin's disease. Relation to other prognostic factors and implication for choice of treatment. *Cancer* 61, 1719-1727.

Tubiana, M., et al. (1981): Five-year results of the EORTC randomized study of splenectomy and spleen irradiation in clinical stages I and II of Hodgkin's disease. *Eur. J. Cancer* 17, 355-363.

Tubiana, M., et al. (1989): Toward comprehensive management tailored to prognostic factors of patients with clinical stages I and II in Hodgkin's disease. The EORTC Lymphoma Group controlled clinical trials : 1964-1987. *Blood* 73, 47-56.

Wartelle, M., et al. (1983): Pigas: An interactive statistical database management system. In *Proceedings on the Second International Workshop on Statistical Database Management*, ed. R. Hammond & J.L. McCarthy, pp. 124-132. Los Altos, CA, Sept. 27-29, 1983.

Waterhouse, J., et al. (1982): *Cancer Incidence in Five Continents Vol. IV*. IARC Scientific Publication n° 42. Lyon: International Agency for Research on Cancer.

World Health Statistics Annual (1965 to 1988). Ed. World Health Organization. Geneva: World Health Organization.

World Health Organization (1976): *International classification of diseases for Oncology*. Geneva: World Health Organization.

Zittoun, R., et al. (1985): Extended versus involved fields irradiation combined MOPP chemotherapy in early clinical stages of Hodgkin's disease. *J. Clin. Oncol.* 3, 207-214.

GLOSSARY OF THE CHEMOTHERAPY REGIMENS USED

GLOSSAIRE : DESCRIPTION DES CHIMIOTHERAPIES UTILISEES

Glossary of the chemotherapy regimens used

MOPP-like regimens :

MOPP : mustard, vincristine, procarbazine, prednisone
C-MOPP : cyclophosphamide, mustard, vincristine, procarbazine, prednisone
Bleo-MOPP : bleomycin, mustard, vincristine, procarbazine, prednisone
PAVe : procarbazine, melphalan, vinblastine
LOPP : chlorambucil, vincristine, procarbazine, prednisone
BOPP : bleomycin, vincristine, procarbazine, prednisone
COPP : cyclophosphamide, vincristine, procarbazine, prednisone
MVPP : mustine, vinblastine, procarbazine, prednisone
CVPP : cyclophosphamide, vinblastine, procarbazine, prednisone
LVPP : chlorambucil, vinblastine, procarbazine, prednisone

Adriamycin containing regimens :

ABVD : doxorubicin, bleomycin, vinblastine, dacarbazine
ABV : doxorubicin, bleomycin, vinblastine
EBVD : epirubicin, bleomycin, vinblastine, dacarbazine
BAP : bleomycin, doxorubicin, prednisone
BCAVe : bleomycin, cyclophosphamide, doxorubicin, vinblastine
MCAVe-CEC : methotrexate, cyclophosphamide, doxorubicin, vinblastine, lomustine, etoposide, chlorambucil
BEVA : bleomycin, etoposide, vinblastine, doxorubicin
ABDIC : doxorubicin, bleomicin, dacarbazine, lomustine, prednisone

Colloques **INSERM**
ISSN 0768-3154

Other *Colloques* published as co-editions by John Libbey Eurotext and INSERM

153 Hormones and Cell Regulation (11th European Symposium). *Hormones et Régulation Cellulaire (11ᵉ Symposium Européen).*
Edited by J. Nunez and J.E. Dumont.
ISBN : John Libbey Eurotext 0 86196 104 8
INSERM 2 85598 324 X

158 Biochemistry and Physiopathology of Platelet Membrane. *Biochimie et Physiopathologie de la Membrane Plaquettaire.*
Edited by G. Marguerie and R.F.A. Zwaal.
ISBN : John Libbey Eurotext 0 86196 114 5
INSERM 2 85598 345 2

162 The Inhibitors of Hematopoiesis. *Les Inhibiteurs de l'Hématopoïèse.*
Edited by A. Najman, M. Guignon, N.C. Gorin and J.Y. Mary.
ISBN : John Libbey Eurotext 0 86196 125 0
INSERM 2 85598 340 1

164 Liver Cells and Drugs. *Cellules Hépatiques et Médicaments.*
Edited by A. Guillouzo.
ISBN : John Libbey Eurotext 0 86196 128 5
INSERM 2 85598 341 X

165 Hormones and Cell Regulation (12th European Symposium). *Hormones et Régulation Cellulaire (12ᵉ Symposium Européen).*
Edited by J. Nunez, J.E. Dumont and E. Carafoli.
ISBN : John Libbey Eurotext 0 86196 133 1
INSERM 2 85598 347 9

167 Sleep Disorders and Respiration. *Les Evénements Respiratoires du Sommeil.*
Edited by P. Lévi-Valensi and D. Duron.
ISBN : John Libbey Eurotext 0 86196 127 7
INSERM 2 85598 344 4

169 Neo-Adjuvant Chemotherapy. *Chimiothérapie Néo-Adjuvante.*
Edited by C. Jacquillat, M. Weil, D. Khayat.
ISBN : John Libbey Eurotext 0 86196 150 1
INSERM 2 85598 349 5

171 Structure and Functions of the Cytoskeleton. *La Structure et les Fonctions du Cytosquelette.*
Edited by B.A.F. Rousset.
ISBN : John Libbey Eurotext 0 86196 149 8
INSERM 2 85598 351 7

Colloques INSERM
ISSN 0768-3154

172 The Langerhans Cell. *La Cellule de Langerhans.*
Edited by J. Thivolet, D. Schmitt.
ISBN : John Libbey Eurotext 0 86196 181 1
INSERM 2 85598 352 5

173 Cellular and Molecular Aspects of Glucuronidation. *Aspects Cellulaires et Moléculaires de la Glucuronoconjugaison.*
Edited by G. Siest, J. Magdalou, B. Burchell
ISBN : John Libbey Eurotext 0 86196 182 X
INSERM 2 85598 353 3

174 Second Forum on Peptides. *Deuxième Forum Peptides.*
Edited by A. Aubry, M. Marraud, B. Vitoux
ISBN : John Libbey Eurotext 0 86196 151 X
INSERM 2 85598 354 1

176 Hormones and Cell Regulation (13th European Symposium). *Hormones et Régulation Cellulaire (13ᵉ Symposium Européen).*
Edited by J. Nunez, J.E. Dumont, R. Denton
ISBN : John Libbey Eurotext 0 86196 183 8
INSERM 2 85598 356 8

179 Lymphokine Receptors Interactions. *Interactions Lymphokines-récepteurs.*
Edited by D. Fradelizi, J. Bertoglio
ISBN : John Libbey Eurotext 0 86196 148 X
INSERM 2 85598 359 2

191 Anticancer Drugs (1st International Interface of Clinical and Laboratory responses to anticancer drugs). *Médicaments anticancéreux (1ʳᵉ Confrontation internationale des réponses cliniques et expérimentales aux médicaments anticancéreux).*
Edited by H. Tapiero, J. Robert, T.J. Lampidis
ISBN : John Libbey Eurotext 0 86196 223 0
INSERM 2 85598 393 2

193 Living in the Cold (2nd International Symposium). *La Vie au Froid (2ᵉ Symposium International).*
Edited by A. Malan, B. Canguilhem
ISBN : John Libbey Eurotext 0 86196 234 9
INSERM 2 85598 395 9

Colloques INSERM
ISSN 0768-3154

194 Progress in Hepatitis B Immunization. *La vaccination contre l'hépatite B.*
Edited by P. Coursaget, M.J. Tong
ISBN : John Libbey Eurotext 0 86196 249 4
INSERM 2 85598 396 7

196 Treatment strategy in Hodgkin's disease. Stratégie dans la maladie de Hodgkin.
Edited by P. Sommers, M. Henry-Amar, J.H. Meezwaldt, P. Carde
ISBN : John Libbey Eurotext 0 86196 226 5
INSERM 2 85598 398 3

198 Hormones and Cell Regulation (14th European Symposium). *Hormones et Régulation Cellulaire (14ᵉ Symposium Européen).*
Edited by J. Nunez, J.E. Dumont
ISBN : John Libbey Eurotext 0 86196 229 X
INSERM 2 85598 400 9

199 Placental Communications : Biochemical, Morphological and Cellular Aspects. Communications placentaires : aspects biochimique, morphologique et cellulaire.
Edited by L. Cedard, E. Alsat, J.-C. Challier, G. Chaouat, A. Malassiné

Reproduction photomécanique
IMPRIMERIE LOUIS-JEAN
BP 87 — 05003 GAP Cedex
Tél. : 92.51.35.23
Dépôt légal : 536 — Juillet 1990
Imprimé en France